The Complete Book of
mother
& babycare

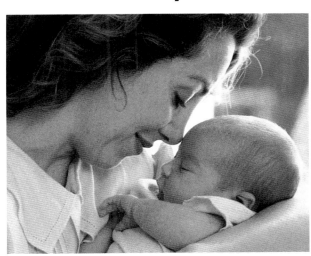

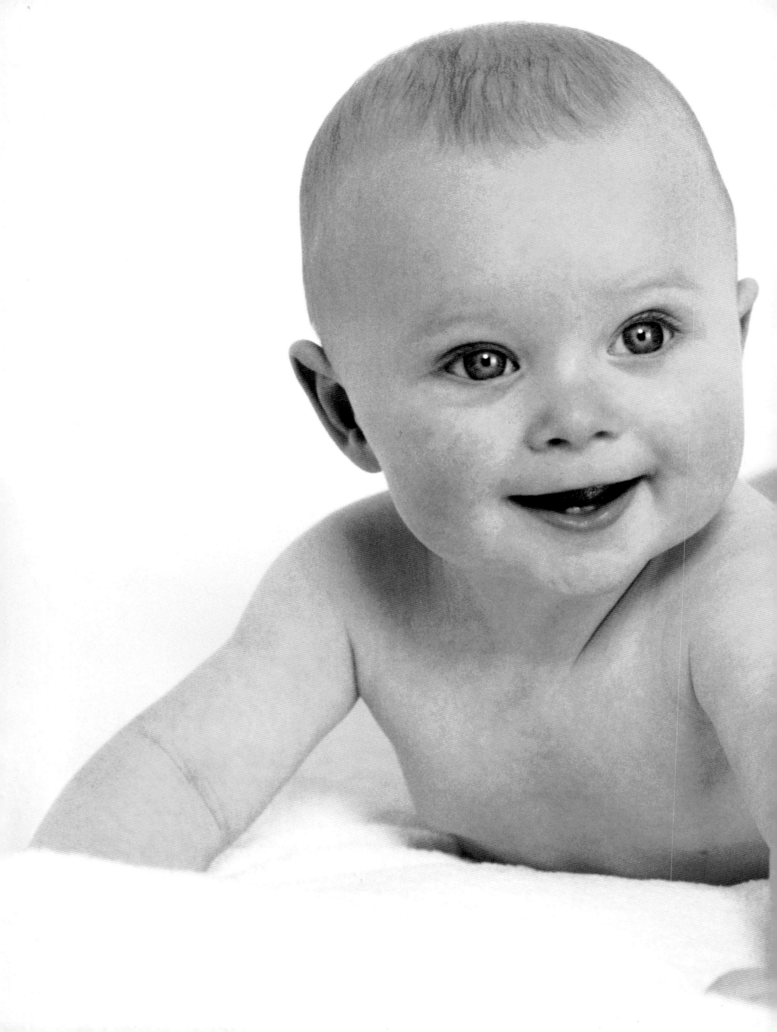

Elizabeth Fenwick

The Complete Book of
mother
& babycare

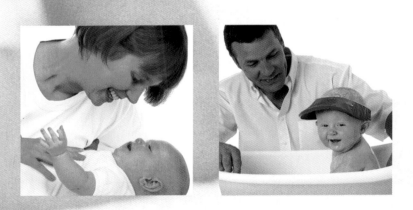

NEW FULLY UPDATED EDITION

LONDON, NEW YORK, MUNICH, MELBOURNE, DELHI

THIS REVISED EDITION

DK London
Senior Art Editor Sarah Ponder
Project Editor Suhel Ahmed
Publishing Manager Anna Davidson
Managing Editor Penny Warren
Managing Art Editor Glenda Fisher
Medical Consultants Ann Peters RN HV,
Elizabeth Owen MD FRCOG MHPEd, Dr Su Laurent FRCPCH
Senior Production Editor Jennifer Murray
Senior Production Controller Alice Sykes
DTP Miriam Dangerfield
Category Publisher Peggy Vance

DK India
Editorial Manager Suchismita Banerjee
Senior Editors Saloni Talwar, Neha Gupta
Design Managers Arunesh Talapatra, Ashita Murgai
Senior Designer Navidita Thapa
Designers Neerja Rawat, Akanksha Gupta, Pallavi Narain,
Anchal Kaushal, Rajnish Kashyap
DTP Co-ordinator Balwant Singh, Pankaj Sharma
DTP Designers Tarun Sharma, Jaipal Singh Chauhan,
Nand Kishore, Mohd. Usman, Chetan Singh

ORIGINAL EDITION CONSULTANTS
Professor R.W. Taylor, MD, FRCOG, Head of
Department of Gynaecology, The United Medical Schools
of Guy's and St Thomas's Hospital, London
Professor Jon Scopes, MB, PhD, FRCP, Department
of Paediatrics, St Thomas's Hospital, London
Christine Williams, RGN, HV, FWT, Health Visitor
and Family Planning Nurse
Janice Leighton, RGN, RM, Community Midwife
Alan McLaughlin, RGN, Department of Clinical
Neurology, St Thomas's Hospital, London

ISBN 978-1-40534-850-8

Printed and bound in Toppan, China

See our complete catalogue at
www.dk.com

Introduction

Every pregnancy, and every baby, is special. Even though it's an experience that has happened countless times to countless couples, it will still be momentous for you. Having a baby opens up a new and exciting world – but it can seem a dauntingly unfamiliar world, too. This book guides you through your pregnancy stage-by-stage, showing you how to make it a happy and healthy time for yourself, and give your baby the best possible start in life.

Most of us know very little about pregnancy and babycare at first and we may assume that there is a "right" or "wrong" way of doing things. There seldom is. But there's often an easy way. So what we have tried to do in this book is to show you what parents have found works best, and what makes life easiest, by offering practical solutions to common problems.

Since the first edition of this book was published I have become a grandmother and been reminded all over again of what parenthood actually means, of the highs and lows, the hard work, the anxieties, the exhaustion, as well as the moments of sheer joy and wonder. Over the last decade our ideas about how a family works have been changing too. More women are trying to find ways of combining work and family responsibilities. More are having to cope alone with bringing up a family. And more fathers are involved in their child's care, sometimes indeed as the child's primary carer. But parental anxieties do not change much over the years. What all parents want is their children's health and happiness.

I hope you will quickly discover that parenthood, for all its responsibilities, can be fun. You don't have to aim to be perfect parents, just the parents who are right for your baby. A baby is a personality in his or her own right almost from the moment of birth. Perhaps one of the harder tasks of parenthood is to accept each child as an individual in his or her own right, and to tolerate and encourage your children's differences from you and from each other. If you feel you need a philosophy to see you through the next few years, you cannot do better than to remember the words of psychologist Anthony Storr: "Children develop most satisfactorily if they are loved for what they are, not for what anyone thinks they ought to be."

Elizabeth Fenwick

Contents

Your child's health   **178–253**

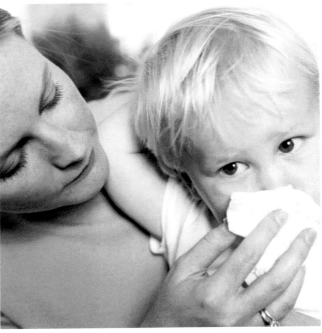

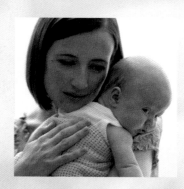

pregnancy and **birth**

An illustrated guide to a healthy and happy pregnancy, incorporating practical self-help advice for labour and birth.

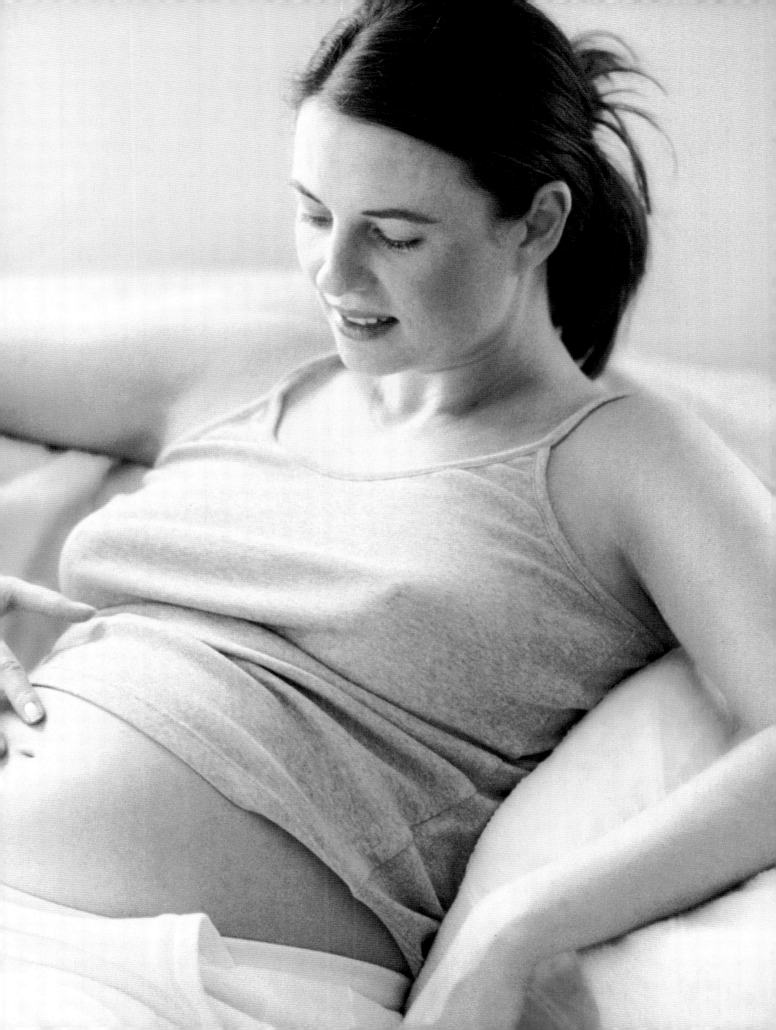

Thinking about pregnancy

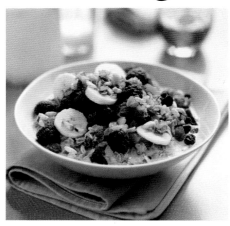

There are a number of steps you can take to increase your chances of conceiving and giving birth to a normal, healthy baby. Ideally, you and your partner should plan for pregnancy at least three months before you conceive as it is in the first few weeks, when you may not even know you are pregnant, that a baby's development can be most easily affected. Planning for pregnancy gives you the time you need to consider any risks, and, if necessary, to do something positive about them.

Checklist for pregnancy

Use these questions as a checklist if you want to have a baby or you find that you are pregnant. A few may not apply to you, but it's important to ask yourself all of them. Talk to your partner, too, as some of the questions relate directly to him. If you feel worried by any of the points, see your doctor.

Are you immune to rubella?
Rubella, or German measles, can cause serious defects in the baby if you develop it in pregnancy, especially during early pregnancy. At least three months before you start trying to become pregnant, ask your doctor for a blood test to make sure that you are immune. If you are not, he can give you a vaccination.

Have you or your partner a family history of inherited disease?
If either you or your partner has a close relative with an inherited disease there is a chance that it might be passed on to your baby. See your doctor before trying to become pregnant, and if necessary he can refer you to a genetic counsellor who can assess the level of risk that you will be taking. It's reassuring to know that, in many cases, only if both partners carry the gene that causes the disease does the child run a real risk of inheriting it.

Do you have a long-standing medical condition?
If you have a medical disorder, such as diabetes or epilepsy, you should talk to your doctor before trying to become pregnant. Your doctor may want to change your drug treatment, either because the drugs you are on might

affect the baby, or because they might make it more difficult for you to conceive.

If you are on the pill, when should you stop taking it?
It is best to stop taking the pill well before trying to conceive to allow your body time to return to its normal cycle. Wait until you have had three menstrual periods before trying to become pregnant

Q&A

"At what age are you in the best physical condition to have a baby?"
This is probably in your twenties, although more women are deciding to start a family at a later date, when they feel emotionally and financially ready for a baby. Risks of a difficult pregnancy do increase if you are over 35 years old, but this reduces if you lead a healthy lifestyle. The risk of having a Down's syndrome baby increases if you are over 35. Women under 18 run a greater risk of having a stillbirth or low-birthweight baby, but regular visits to the antenatal clinic and keeping healthy minimize this.

as conceiving during this stage will make it more difficult to predict your baby's due date (you can use a condom or cap during this time).

Might you be at risk from sexually transmitted infections (STIs)?
Although you will be routinely screened for some sexually transmitted infections once pregnant, such as HIV (see page 36), the most common STI in young women is chlamydia, which at present is not routinely screened for. Although it can be easily treated with antibiotics, unfortunately in about 75 per cent of people there are no symptoms. If undetected, it can be transmitted to your baby and lead to possible pregnancy complications, so make sure you ask for a screening test if you think you might be at risk. If you are under 25 and sexually active, you have a one in 10 chance of having chlamydia. If you have had two partners within a year, or recently changed partners, your risk is also increased.

Does your work bring you into contact with any risks?
Your employer has a responsibility to make sure that you are not exposed to any risks in your work that might affect your chances of conception or put your

baby at risk. Your employer should carry out a specific risk assessment once you notify them in writing that you are pregnant. This must take into account any advice provided by your health professional. One rare infection, *Chlamydia psittaci*, which can cause miscarriage, may be caught from sheep at lambing time. Therefore, if you work on a farm, you should not help with lambing during your pregnancy, or come into contact with newborn lambs or milk ewes that have recently given birth.

How much do you weigh?

Ideally, your weight should be normal for your height for at least six months before conceiving, so if you are seriously overweight or underweight see your doctor for advice on attaining the right weight. Unless you have a serious weight problem, never diet in pregnancy.

Are you eating healthily?

Your chances of conceiving, and of having a healthy baby, increase if you eat a healthy balanced diet.

Do you smoke or drink?

You and your partner should both stop smoking and drinking as soon as you want to become pregnant – tobacco and alcohol affect fertility and can harm the growing baby before and after birth.

Folic acid

From the time you stop using contraception until the 12th week of pregnancy you should take a folic acid supplement. Folic acid, also called folate or folacin, is one of the B vitamins. It is one of the few nutrients that is known to prevent neural tube defects (NTDs) such as spina bifida or anencephaly. The neural tube, which goes on to form the baby's spine, develops very soon after conception, probably even before you realize that you are pregnant. Without sufficient folic acid, the neural tube may fail to fuse completely along its length, exposing the spinal cord and resulting in the condition known as spina bifida. Infants with anencephaly die shortly after birth because a large part of the brain is absent.

Sources of folic acid

Research has shown that an increased intake of folic acid can prevent up to 70 per cent of cases of spina bifida.

Good natural food sources of folic acid include dark green leafy vegetables (spinach and broccoli), citrus fruits, legumes (kidney beans, chick peas), wheatgerm, yeast, and egg yolk. Try to eat vegetables lightly steamed or raw. Some foods have also been fortified with folic acid. These include grain products such as bread, rice, pasta, and breakfast cereals.

However, you should not depend on food sources alone. To be on the safe side you should start to take a folic acid supplement as soon as you decide to stop using contraception. Multivitamin tablets often contain some folic acid, but not enough to protect your baby. To reduce the risk of spina bifida, you need to take one 400 microgram folic acid tablet every day until week 12 of pregnancy. Tablets can be bought over the counter without a prescription, from any pharmacy or health food shop and most supermarkets. If you have had one child with a neural tube defect, you have a higher risk of having a second child with the same defect. In this instance, your doctor will advise you to take a higher dose (5 milligrams) of folic acid each day.

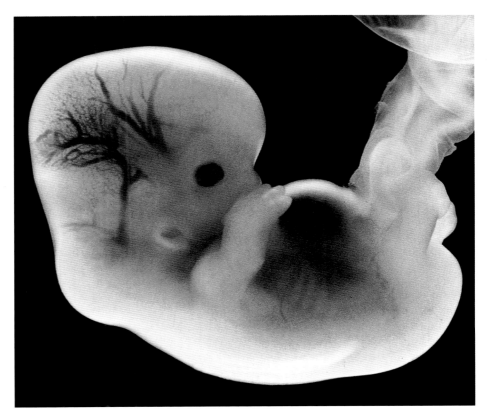

The developing embryo
Your unborn baby will stand a better chance of developing normally if you take a folic acid supplement. This should be taken before conception and during the first 12 weeks of pregnancy.

A pregnancy calendar

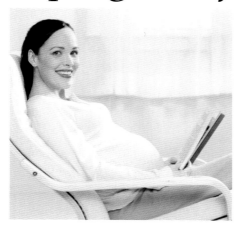

This month-by-month calendar charts the progress of one woman's pregnancy. There is advice on what to do at each stage, as well as reassuring answers to questions and worries you might have. Every pregnancy varies, so don't be surprised if some of the changes described don't happen to you at exactly the same time. The calendar counts day one of pregnancy as the first day of your last menstrual period. So two weeks after conception, you are four weeks pregnant.

Becoming pregnant

If you are thinking of becoming pregnant, check that your lifestyle involves nothing that might harm the baby. All the major organs of his body are formed during the first three months of pregnancy and it is now that his health can be harmed most easily. Once you have conceived you will experience a number of changes, such as heavy breasts or feeling sick. Most of these changes are set off by the increase in hormone levels during the early weeks as your body prepares to nurture and accommodate your baby.

Early signs of pregnancy

One or more of the changes listed below can signify that you are pregnant. You may not notice any of them at first, but still instinctively know you are pregnant because you "feel" different.

● A missed period (amenorrhoea). This is usually one of the first signs of pregnancy, but if your periods are irregular, or you are anxious, busy, or ill, or are underweight, this may not be a reliable guide. It is also possible to have slight bleeding around the time you would normally expect your period, after you have conceived.

● Breasts are enlarged and tender, and perhaps tingle a little. The veins over the surface of the breasts may become more prominent.

● A feeling of deep tiredness, not just in the evening, but also during the day.

● Feeling faint, and perhaps dizzy.

● An increase in normal vaginal discharge.

● Nausea and perhaps vomiting; this can happen at any time of day. Certain odours may make you feel nauseous, particularly cooking smells.

● Some foods taste different from normal, and you may develop a strong dislike of some things, such as alcohol, coffee, and cigarette smoke, and a craving for others.

● Feeling unusually emotional. This is due primarily to the changes in your hormones.

● A frequent need to pass water, although this may be only in very small quantities.

● A strange metallic taste in the mouth.

Confirming the pregnancy

Two weeks after conception a pregnancy hormone, HCG (human chorionic gonadotrophin), appears in your urine. At this stage, a test of the urine will confirm whether or not you are pregnant. Your GP or community contraception clinic will give you a free test. Pregnancy tests are also available at NHS walk-in centres and many pharmacies and pregnancy advisory services will also do a test for a fee.

Home pregnancy testing kits

If you would rather do the pregnancy test yourself, buy a testing kit from a chemist. The kit comes in the form of a stick that you urinate directly onto. The first urine that you pass in the morning is best, as it contains the most HCG hormone. It is important to catch a mid-stream sample. Modern digital testing kits are very accurate but since a large proportion of pregnancies at this stage fail to carry on, it is advisable to wait for at least a week after a missed period to know for certain whether or not you are still pregnant.

Calculating your delivery date

Pregnancy lasts about 266 days from conception to birth. The most likely time of conception is when you ovulate. In a normal 28-day cycle this happens about 14 days before the next period is due, so to calculate your approximate delivery date count 280 days (266 plus

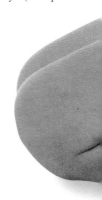

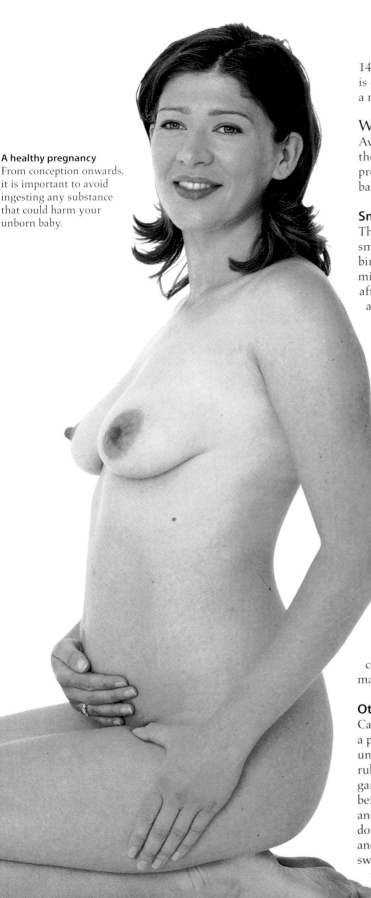

A healthy pregnancy
From conception onwards, it is important to avoid ingesting any substance that could harm your unborn baby.

14) from the first day of your last period. Remember, this is only a guide. Although the average pregnancy is 40 weeks, a normal pregnancy can last for up to 42 weeks.

What to avoid
Avoid smoking, alcohol, and any form of medication (unless the medication is confirmed as safe by your doctor) throughout pregnancy, but especially in the first three months when the baby's organs are forming.

Smoking
This deprives the baby of oxygen. Babies of mothers who smoke are more likely to be premature and have a low birthweight. Smoking also increases the chances of having a miscarriage, a stillbirth, a malformed baby, or a baby that dies after birth, so stop smoking completely. Even a few cigarettes a day can harm your baby, so simply cutting down is not enough. Passive smoking poses similar risks to your baby's health and could be a factor in causing cot death, so avoid smoky atmospheres when pregnant. If your partner smokes, encourage him to give up.

Alcohol
A glass of wine once or twice a week is unlikely to do you or your baby any harm, but it is better to give up altogether as no one is sure of the safe limit. Regular excessive alcohol consumption can cause serious harm and "binge drinking" is particularly dangerous.

Medication
Many drugs can have harmful or unknown effects on your unborn baby, so avoid taking medication in pregnancy unless it is prescribed by a doctor who knows that you are pregnant. This includes many of the remedies you would normally take for minor complaints, such as aspirin. Herbal remedies are sometimes perceived as being safer than pharmaceutical drugs, but many contain powerful active ingredients and all should be avoided without the advice of a qualified medical herbalist. If you need medication to control an existing condition such as diabetes, your doctor may have to alter your dose.

Other risks
Cat and dog faeces, and raw or undercooked meat, may contain a parasite called toxoplasma, which can seriously harm the unborn baby. Avoid emptying pet litter trays (if you must, wear rubber gloves and then wash your hands). Wear gloves for all gardening jobs and thoroughly wash all fruit and vegetables before eating to remove any soil. To avoid the risk of listeriosis and salmonella, wash your hands after handling raw meat, and don't eat undercooked meat or fish, raw/lightly cooked egg, soft and blue-veined cheeses, or pâté. Avoid eating shellfish, shark, swordfish, and marlin, which may carry the risk of food poisoning. Refer to page 53 for more on foods to avoid.

The start of life

During the first eight weeks of pregnancy the baby develops from a single cell at conception to a fetus approximately 2.5cm (1in) long, and begins to look human.

Conception to week four

1 Ovulation
Around day 14 of your menstrual cycle, a ripe egg is released from one of your ovaries, and fertilization becomes possible. The egg is caught by the fingers at the end of the Fallopian tube, and drawn into it. The egg can survive for up to 24 hours as it waits to be fertilized. If it isn't fertilized, it passes out of the vagina with the lining of the womb in your next monthly period.

3 The cell divides
The cell starts to divide and carries on dividing into more cells as it travels down the Fallopian tube.

4 Reaching the womb
On about the fourth day after fertilization, the cells reach the womb. They form a ball of about 100 cells with a fluid-filled centre, which produces HCG hormone, and floats about in the cavity for the next few days.

The swim of the sperm
During orgasm, a man may ejaculate between 200 and 400 million sperm into a woman's vagina. Most will perish, but some swim through the mucus secreted by the cervix (the neck of the womb), and cross the womb into the Fallopian tube. If an egg hasn't been released, the sperm can survive in the tube for up to 48 hours.

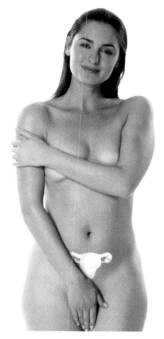

Position of the womb

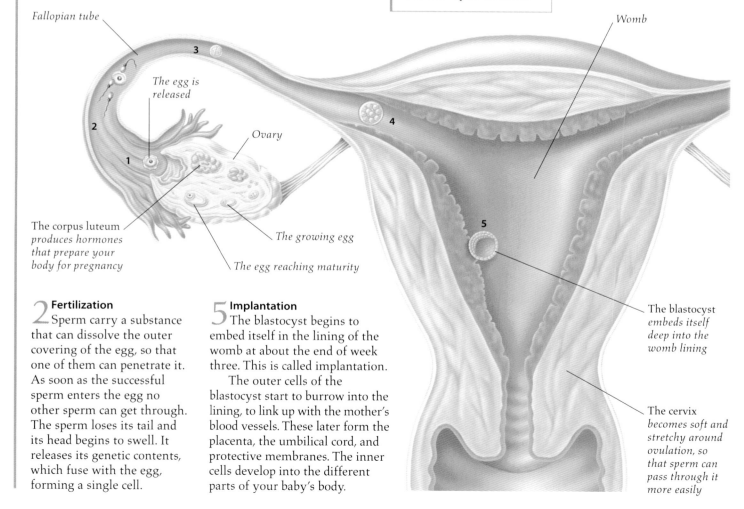

Fallopian tube

3

The egg is released

2

Ovary

1

The corpus luteum *produces hormones that prepare your body for pregnancy*

The growing egg

The egg reaching maturity

4

Womb

5

The blastocyst *embeds itself deep into the womb lining*

The cervix *becomes soft and stretchy around ovulation, so that sperm can pass through it more easily*

2 Fertilization
Sperm carry a substance that can dissolve the outer covering of the egg, so that one of them can penetrate it. As soon as the successful sperm enters the egg no other sperm can get through. The sperm loses its tail and its head begins to swell. It releases its genetic contents, which fuse with the egg, forming a single cell.

5 Implantation
The blastocyst begins to embed itself in the lining of the womb at about the end of week three. This is called implantation.
The outer cells of the blastocyst start to burrow into the lining, to link up with the mother's blood vessels. These later form the placenta, the umbilical cord, and protective membranes. The inner cells develop into the different parts of your baby's body.

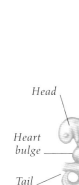
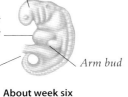

Head

Heart bulge

Tail

Arm bud

About week six

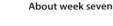
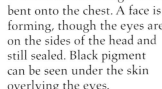

Eye

Umbilical cord

Arm bud

Leg bud

About week seven

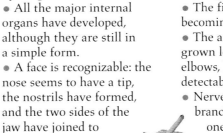

Eye

Mouth

Hand

Umbilical cord

Brain

Ear

Arm

Elbow

Leg

About week eight

Weeks five to six

● The embryo is floating in a fluid-filled sac.
● It has a simple brain, spine, and central nervous system.
● Four shallow pits have appeared on the head, which will later become the baby's eyes and ears.
● The embryo has the beginnings of a digestive system, a mouth, and a jaw.
● The stomach and chest are developing. The heart can be seen as a large bulge at the front of the chest; by the end of the week it will start beating.
● A system of blood vessels is forming.
● Protruding buds mark the beginning of the baby's arms and legs.

Week seven

● The head looks large and is bent onto the chest. A face is forming, though the eyes are on the sides of the head and still sealed. Black pigment can be seen under the skin overlying the eyes.
● The arms and legs are clearly visible, with clefts at the end, which become fingers and toes.
● The heart starts to circulate blood around the embryo's body.
● The outline of the baby's nervous system is already nearly complete.
● Bone cells are beginning to develop.
● The embryo has lungs, an intestine, a liver, kidneys, and internal sex organs, but none are yet fully formed.

Week eight

● The embryo can now be called a fetus, which means "young one".
● All the major internal organs have developed, although they are still in a simple form.
● A face is recognizable: the nose seems to have a tip, the nostrils have formed, and the two sides of the jaw have joined to make a mouth. There is already a tongue.

● The inner parts of the ears, responsible for balance and hearing, are forming.
● The fingers and toes are becoming more distinct.
● The arms and legs have grown longer, and shoulders, elbows, hips, and knees are detectable.
● Nerve cells in the brain are branching to connect with one another to form a primitive neural pathway.
● The baby moves around quite a lot, though you can't feel him yet.

Length: The embryo is now 6mm (¼in), about the size of an apple seed.

Length: The embryo is now 1.3cm (½in), about the size of a small grape.

Length: The fetus is now 2.5cm (1in), about the size of an average strawberry.

Twins

Currently, about one in 32 pregnancies results in twins. This figure has increased dramatically since 1980, and it's mainly due to fertility treatments. However, it is steadily coming down again as fertility treatments become more refined.
Fraternal twins occur when two separate eggs are fertilized by two separate sperm. The twins each have their own placenta, may or may not be the same sex, and are no more alike than any other brothers or sisters.
Identical twins are produced when the egg is fertilized and divides into two separate halves, each of which develops into an identical baby. The twins usually share a placenta, are always of the same sex, and have the same physical characteristics and genetic makeup.

"Can I do anything to influence the baby's sex?"

Q&A

The baby's sex is determined by the man's sperm, which can be either male or female. Research suggests that male sperm do not survive as long as female sperm, so you may increase your chances of having a boy if you make love when you are most fertile (about 14 days before your period is due); and of having a girl if you have intercourse up to three days before you expect to be fertile. It might, therefore, be a good idea to keep a chart of your cycle before you try to get pregnant. None of these techniques have been proven, however.

week 12

The baby looks much more human although his head is still large in proportion to his body, and his limbs, although fully formed, are small. You should find that the discomforts of early pregnancy are beginning to wear off. Make sure you have your first visit to the antenatal clinic and your first ultrasound scan around now.

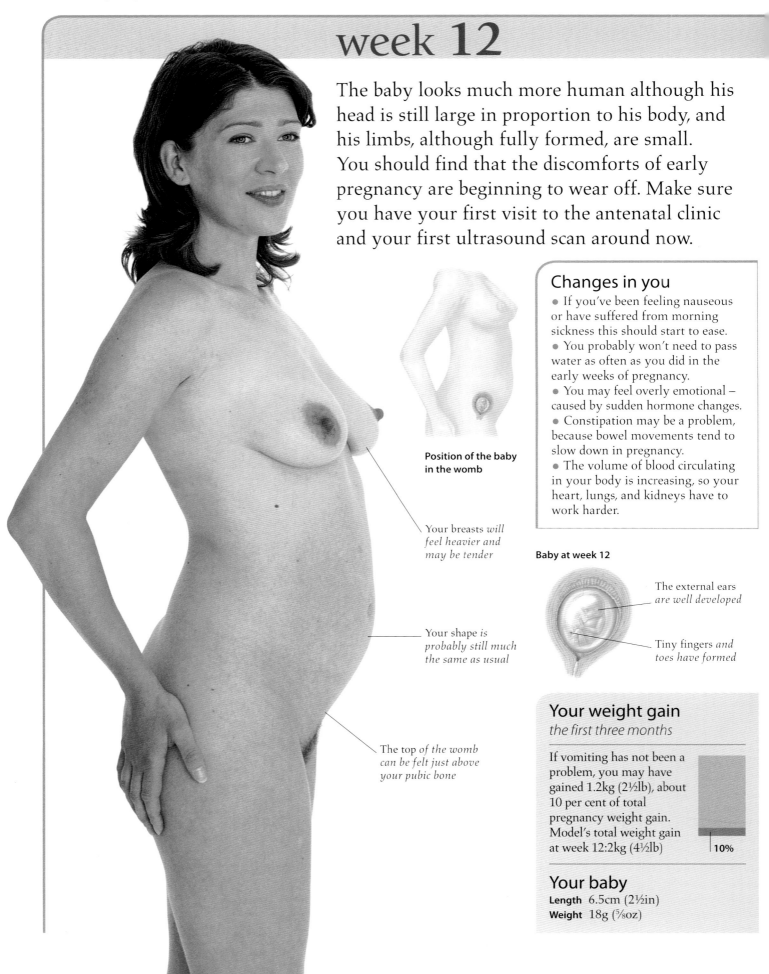

Position of the baby in the womb

Your breasts *will feel heavier and may be tender*

Your shape *is probably still much the same as usual*

The top *of the womb can be felt just above your pubic bone*

Changes in you

● If you've been feeling nauseous or have suffered from morning sickness this should start to ease.
● You probably won't need to pass water as often as you did in the early weeks of pregnancy.
● You may feel overly emotional – caused by sudden hormone changes.
● Constipation may be a problem, because bowel movements tend to slow down in pregnancy.
● The volume of blood circulating in your body is increasing, so your heart, lungs, and kidneys have to work harder.

Baby at week 12

The external ears *are well developed*

Tiny fingers *and toes have formed*

Your weight gain
the first three months

If vomiting has not been a problem, you may have gained 1.2kg (2½lb), about 10 per cent of total pregnancy weight gain. Model's total weight gain at week 12:2kg (4½lb)

10%

Your baby
Length 6.5cm (2½in)
Weight 18g (⅝oz)

What to do
- Buy a bra that will support your breasts well.
- Check that you are eating a varied diet of fresh foods.
- Guard against constipation by drinking a lot of water and including high-fibre foods in your diet.
- Tell your employer that you are pregnant, so that you can take paid time off work to go to the antenatal clinic and antenatal classes.
- Make sure you have your first appointment with your midwife and your first ultrasound scan now.
- Ask at the clinic how to claim for free dental treatment and prescriptions during pregnancy.
- Make an appointment with your dentist for a check-up.
- Find out about antenatal classes in your area.
- Practise antenatal exercises regularly. Go swimming.

Your growing baby
- All of the internal organs are formed, and most are working, so the baby is less likely to be harmed by infections or drugs.
- The eyelids have developed, and are closed over the eyes.
- The baby has earlobes.
- The limbs are formed. Miniature fingernails and toenails are growing.
- Muscles are developing, so the baby moves much more. He can curl and fan his toes. He can make a fist with his tiny fingers.
- He can move the muscles of his mouth to frown, purse his lips, and open and close his mouth.
- He can suck. He swallows the fluid that surrounds him. He passes urine.

See also:
Antenatal clinic *pages 34–5*
Antenatal exercises *pages 45–7*
Eating healthily *pages 50–3*
Frequent urination *page 41*
Morning sickness *page 41*
Pregnancy bra *page 23*
Protecting your back *page 44*

Antenatal classes

Start thinking about the type of class that will best suit you and your partner. Often you can go to introductory classes now – on ways to keep healthy in pregnancy, for example – and then start antenatal classes eight to 10 weeks before the baby is due. Antenatal exercise classes may continue throughout your pregnancy.

Choosing a class
Different classes emphasize different subjects, so select a class that is going to cover in most detail the topics that concern you. There are three main types of classes, and you may want to go to more than one. All of these classes cover labour and birth.

Hospital classes
These free classes are an invaluable source of information on the procedures and routines followed in the hospital where you are having your baby, and you will probably go on a tour of the delivery room and maternity wards. The only

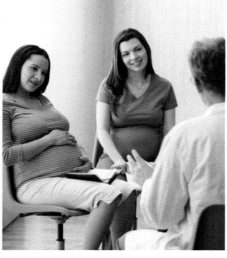

Antenatal class
You will meet trained teachers and other prospective mothers in these classes.

drawback is that the classes can be large, and may take the form of lectures with films, so it can be hard to ask questions.

Local classes
Ask your midwife where these classes are held. They are run by teachers trained by the organization offering the class, who may or may not be health professionals. They are also free, usually smaller, and with a friendlier atmosphere than hospital classes. You will also get to meet other prospective mothers.

These classes emphasize how to care for your new baby; labour and birth will be covered, too. If you are having a hospital birth, you may be able to go on a tour of the hospital where you are having your baby. Your partner will be invited to some classes.

Other classes
These are run by organizations such as the National Childbirth Trust (NCT), and a fee is usually charged. The classes concentrate on antenatal exercises, as well as techniques such as relaxation, to help you cope with labour and birth, and are a good place to meet other mothers-to-be in your area. Your partner will be encouraged to attend, too.

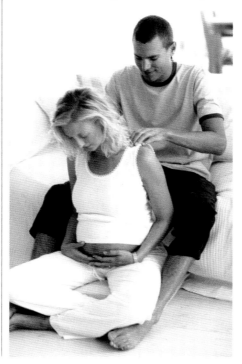

Tips for labour
Massage is one of the techniques you and your partner may be taught at an antenatal class to help you cope with labour.

week 16

You are now into the second three months of pregnancy and you will definitely begin to look pregnant and start feeling energized. Your baby is fully formed, and has been nourished by the placenta since week 14. Over the remaining weeks he grows and matures so that he is capable of independent life.

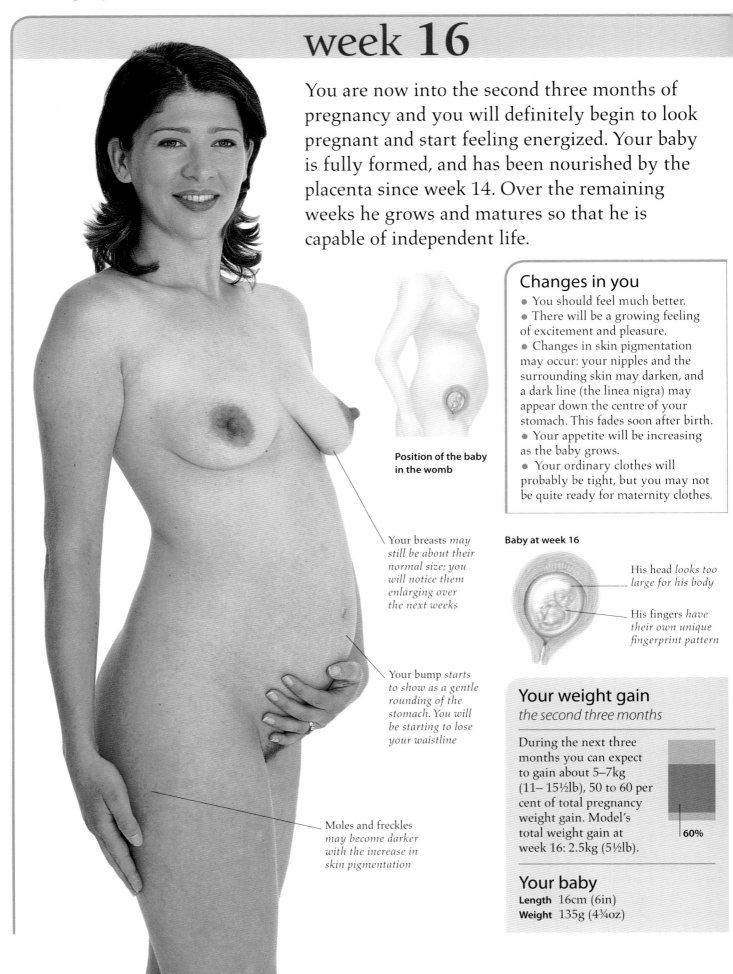

Position of the baby in the womb

Changes in you
- You should feel much better.
- There will be a growing feeling of excitement and pleasure.
- Changes in skin pigmentation may occur: your nipples and the surrounding skin may darken, and a dark line (the linea nigra) may appear down the centre of your stomach. This fades soon after birth.
- Your appetite will be increasing as the baby grows.
- Your ordinary clothes will probably be tight, but you may not be quite ready for maternity clothes.

Your breasts *may still be about their normal size; you will notice them enlarging over the next weeks*

Baby at week 16

His head *looks too large for his body*

His fingers *have their own unique fingerprint pattern*

Your bump *starts to show as a gentle rounding of the stomach. You will be starting to lose your waistline*

Moles and freckles *may become darker with the increase in skin pigmentation*

Your weight gain
the second three months

During the next three months you can expect to gain about 5–7kg (11– 15½lb), 50 to 60 per cent of total pregnancy weight gain. Model's total weight gain at week 16: 2.5kg (5½lb).

60%

Your baby
Length 16cm (6in)
Weight 135g (4¾oz)

What to do

- Give up smoking if you have not already done so and encourage your partner to do the same. Make the living area a smoke-free zone.
- Don't indulge in overeating; eat healthy and watch your weight gain.
- Start to take iron supplements, if prescribed by your doctor.
- After the first trimester you can stop taking folic acid.
- Visit the antenatal clinic for the second time. You will probably be offered a serum (blood) screening test. Amniocentesis (see page 37) can be done now if there is a chance of the baby having an abnormality.

Your growing baby

- The eyebrows and eyelashes are growing, and the baby has fine downy hair on his face and body. This is called lanugo.
- His skin is so thin that it is transparent; networks of blood vessels can be seen underneath.
- Joints have formed in his arms and legs, and hard bones are beginning to develop.
- His sex organs are sufficiently mature for his sex to be evident, but this is not always detectable by an ultrasound scan.
- The baby makes breathing movements with his chest.
- He moves around vigorously, but you probably won't be able to feel his movements yet.
- His heart is beating about twice as fast as your own; the doctor or midwife can hear it with a sonicaid (a special listening device) after approximately week 14.

See also:
Amniocentesis *pages 36–7*
Eating healthily *pages 50–3*
Relaxation and breathing *pages 48–9*
Skin colour *page 21*
Smoking *page 13*
Supplements *page 52*
Ultrasound *page 36*

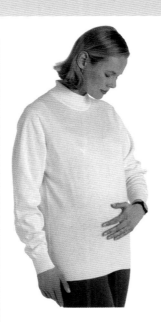

Mixed feelings

You and your partner are bound to have mixed emotions about the pregnancy, so don't be surprised if as well as feeling elated and excited, you sometimes feel low. Try to tolerate and understand any negative feelings – they will probably fade after the birth.

Common worries

The best way to dispel any worries you may have about your baby or parenthood is to talk about them frankly with your partner. It also helps to find out as much as you can about pregnancy, so you understand the changes taking place.

You

It's only natural for your feelings of excitement and anticipation to be clouded sometimes by more negative thoughts. You may worry about loving the baby, but once he's born and you get to know each other, love will grow. You may also feel depressed about your changing shape, and even resent the baby for putting your body through such strains. But most adverse bodily changes disappear after birth, and with some gentle exercising your shape will return.

Your partner

Up to now your partner may have felt left out, and perhaps jealous of all the attention the baby is receiving. However, he should now start to feel positive and excited as your baby becomes a reality and he gets more involved in your pregnancy. If he is worried about whether his income will be enough to support you all, try to plan and budget.

Single mothers

If you're single and anxious about labour and birth, find out about antenatal classes where you can meet people in a similar situation as well as learn and practise techniques, such as good breathing, so you can feel more confident and in control when the time comes. Surround yourself with friends and family, who will act as your support network. You can even get in touch with organizations that offer support and practical advice throughout pregnancy and after the birth.

"How can I be sure the baby will be all right?" Q&A

The chances of the baby being abnormal are very small. Most abnormalities occur in the first few weeks, and usually end in an early miscarriage. By week 13, the baby is fully formed and from then on very little can go wrong. If you check that your lifestyle involves nothing that could harm him, you can reduce the risk still further.

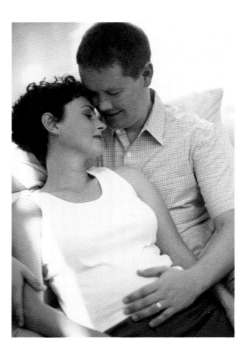

week 20

You will probably have a strong sense of well-being and may look and feel radiant during the middle months of pregnancy. If you're feeling well, it's often a good idea to take a holiday. By now you will be able to feel the baby move, and a second ultrasound scan will check that he is growing normally.

Your nipples *become darker during pregnancy*

Position of the baby in the womb

Changes in you

● Skin pigmentation may be more noticeable, but will fade after birth.
● Your breasts may produce colostrum, a thin cloudy substance that provides all your baby needs in the first days after birth.
● You may be suffering from some of the common problems of pregnancy, such as bleeding gums and an increase in vaginal discharge. The joints and ligaments of your body have relaxed, so you are more likely to suffer from back trouble and other aches and pains.

Your breasts *will have probably increased dramatically in size by now*

Baby at week 20

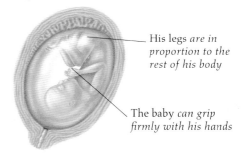

His legs *are in proportion to the rest of his body*

The baby *can grip firmly with his hands*

The top *of the womb is level with your navel*

Your weight gain
at around week 20 of pregnancy

During this month you should gain about 0.5kg (1lb) a week. Take extra care to eat healthily now: the next few weeks is the period of maximum growth for the baby. Model's weight gain to date: 3kg (6½lb)

Your baby
Length 25cm (10in)
Weight 340g (12oz)

You will first feel *your baby's movements as a faint fluttering inside your abdomen, like bubbles rising*

What to do
- Make sure you are holding yourself well, and that you avoid overstretching or straining your back. Wear low-heeled shoes.
- Take the practical steps suggested on pages 40–2 to relieve any other discomforts that you may have.
- Start to think about essential clothes and equipment for the baby.

"Is a long journey advisable?" Q&A

There's usually no reason why you shouldn't travel in pregnancy, but preferably not on your own, especially on a long car journey. Wear loose, comfortable clothes, and break the journey up by walking around for a few minutes at least every two hours, to help your circulation. Stay hydrated and carry healthy snacks to maintain blood sugar levels. Always remember to take your maternity notes with you.

Your growing baby
- Hair appears on the baby's head.
- Teeth are developing.
- Vernix, the white and greasy substance that protects the baby's skin in the womb, forms.
- The baby's arms and legs are well developed.
- Your own antibodies will be transferred to the baby through your blood to help him resist disease in the first weeks after birth.
- The baby is very active; you should have felt his movements for the first time as a faint fluttering. He may even react to noises outside the womb, but don't worry if he doesn't move around much – it's fairly common for babies to have a quiet period now.

See also:
Common complaints *pages 40–2*
Eating healthily *pages 50–3*
Essentials for the baby *page 27*
Protecting your back *page 44*

Looking good

You may look and feel your best during the middle months of pregnancy, with lustrous hair, rosy cheeks, and healthy skin, but not everyone blooms; the high hormone levels can have less flattering effects on your skin, nails, and hair, though any adverse changes usually disappear after giving birth.

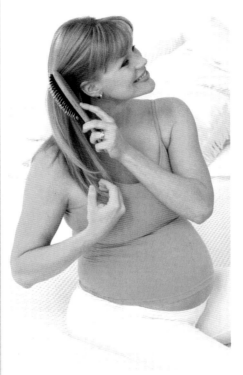

Your hair
Your hair may seem thicker during pregnancy. This is due to higher hormone levels causing the hair to stay in its active growing phase for longer.

Hair
Thick, shiny hair is often a bonus of pregnancy. However, not all hair improves, and greasy hair may become more oily, and dry hair, drier and more brittle, so that you may seem to lose more hair than usual. Facial and body hair also tends to darken.

What to do
If your hair is dry and splits easily, use a mild shampoo and conditioner, and don't brush it too often or too vigorously. Wash greasy hair frequently to keep it shiny. As hair texture is so unpredictable during pregnancy, avoid having your hair coloured too often – colouring it occasionally throughout your pregnancy should be fine. However, if you have any concerns about the chemicals, it is best to check with your health professional first.

Skin texture
Your skin will probably improve in pregnancy: the blemishes disappear, and skin texture becomes smooth and silky. However, you may find that your skin becomes very dry, or greasy, and perhaps spotty.

What to do
Cleanse your skin thoroughly. If it is dry, gently rub moisturizer over the dry areas, and add bath oil to your bath water. Use as little soap as possible.

Skin colour
An increase in skin pigmentation is normal during pregnancy. Moles, birthmarks, scars, and especially freckles usually darken and grow in size, and a brown line often appears on the stomach. You may also notice a brownish patch, or "butterfly mask", across your face and neck. Don't worry, as this disappears soon after the birth.

What to do
Avoid strong sunlight as this makes pigmentation worse, but if you have to go out in the sun, use sun cream with a strong UV filter, cover up exposed skin, and wear a hat. Don't bleach the "butterfly" mask; if you want to disguise it, use a skin-blemish covering stick.

Nails
You may notice that your nails split and break more easily than usual.

What to do
Wear protective gloves for household chores and gardening.

week 24

This is often the best month of pregnancy. You will probably look well and feel happy and contented. If you have not been gaining weight very rapidly so far, you may put on a lot this month. You will start to appear visibly pregnant.

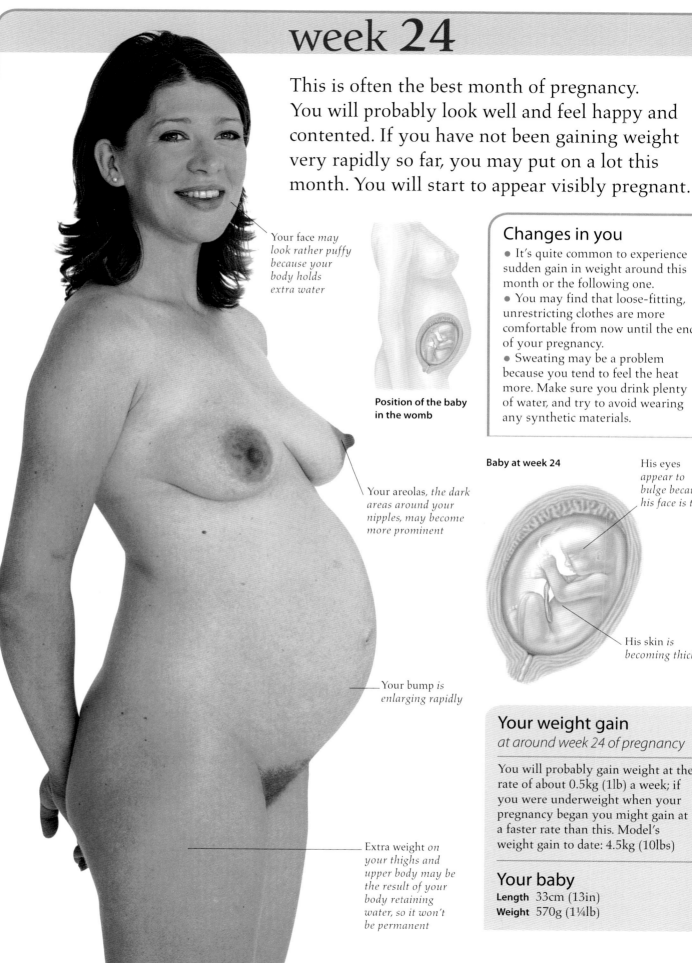

Your face *may look rather puffy because your body holds extra water*

Position of the baby in the womb

Your areolas, *the dark areas around your nipples, may become more prominent*

Your bump *is enlarging rapidly*

Extra weight *on your thighs and upper body may be the result of your body retaining water, so it won't be permanent*

Changes in you

● It's quite common to experience sudden gain in weight around this month or the following one.
● You may find that loose-fitting, unrestricting clothes are more comfortable from now until the end of your pregnancy.
● Sweating may be a problem because you tend to feel the heat more. Make sure you drink plenty of water, and try to avoid wearing any synthetic materials.

Baby at week 24

His eyes *appear to bulge because his face is thin*

His skin *is becoming thicker*

Your weight gain
at around week 24 of pregnancy

You will probably gain weight at the rate of about 0.5kg (1lb) a week; if you were underweight when your pregnancy began you might gain at a faster rate than this. Model's weight gain to date: 4.5kg (10lbs)

Your baby
Length 33cm (13in)
Weight 570g (1¼lb)

What to do
● If you have flat or inverted nipples and you want to breastfeed, you should be able to do so; talk to the midwife.
● Rest as much as possible during the day.
● Continue to exercise gently, but regularly. Practise relaxation and breathing exercises.
● If you have been working during the past year, ask at the clinic for your maternity certificate, which they will issue to you when you are around six months pregnant. Give this to your employer at least 28 days before you leave work.

"What is the best kind of bra?"
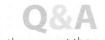
To give your breasts the support they need in pregnancy, choose a bra (preferably cotton) with a deep band under the cups, broad shoulder straps, and an adjustable back that gives you support all the way round. Check your size regularly, as your breasts will continue to swell throughout pregnancy. By full term, you may need a cup two sizes larger than usual. If your breasts become very heavy, wear a lightweight bra at night.

Your growing baby
● No fat has been laid down yet, so the baby is still lean.
● The sweat glands are forming.
● Arm and leg muscles are well developed, and the baby tries them out regularly. He has periods of frenzied activity, when you feel him moving around, alternating with periods of calm.
● The baby can cough and hiccup; you may feel the hiccups as a knocking movement.

See also:
Antenatal exercises *pages 45–7*
Pregnancy clothes *page 25*
Relaxation and breathing *pages 48–9*

The baby in the womb

While your baby is developing physically, he is also becoming an aware, responsive person with feelings. He lies tightly curled up in the womb, cushioned by the amniotic fluid that surrounds him. He is entirely reliant on your placenta for food and oxygen, and for the disposal of his waste products. However, he looks and behaves much the same as a baby at birth.

Sight
His eyelids are still sealed, but by week 28 they become unsealed, and he may see, and open and close his eyes.

Hearing
He can hear your voice, and if he's asleep can be woken by loud music. He may prefer some types of music, and show this by his movements. He jumps at sudden noises.

Facial expressions
He frowns, squints, purses his lips, and opens and closes his mouth. He smiles, too.

Life-support system
The baby is nourished by the placenta and protected by warm amniotic fluid, which can change every four hours. It regulates the baby's temperature, and protects against infection and sudden bumps.

Movements
He kicks and punches, and sometimes turns somersaults.

Sleeping patterns
He sleeps and wakes randomly, and will probably be most active when you are trying to sleep.

Personality
The part of the brain concerned with personality and intelligence becomes far more complex during the seventh month, so your baby's personality may soon be developing.

Sucking, swallowing, and breathing
He sucks his thumb, and swallows the warm water (the amniotic fluid) that surrounds him, passing it out of his body as urine. Sometimes he drinks too much of the fluid and hiccups. He makes breathing movements with his chest, practising for life outside the womb.

Taste
His taste buds are forming, and by week 28, he can respond to sweet, sour, and bitter tastes.

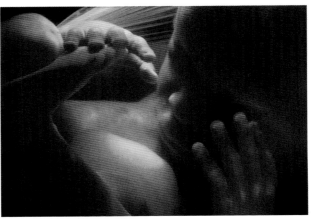

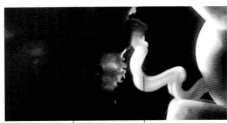

The placenta supplies all the nutrients the baby needs; almost anything entering your body, good or bad, is filtered through to him.

The umbilical cord, a rope of three blood vessels, links the placenta to the baby.

week 28

With only three months of pregnancy left to go, you may be starting to feel large and clumsy, and perhaps forgetful. During the last months your baby lays down fat stores. He is very active, and you may even be able to see him moving around.

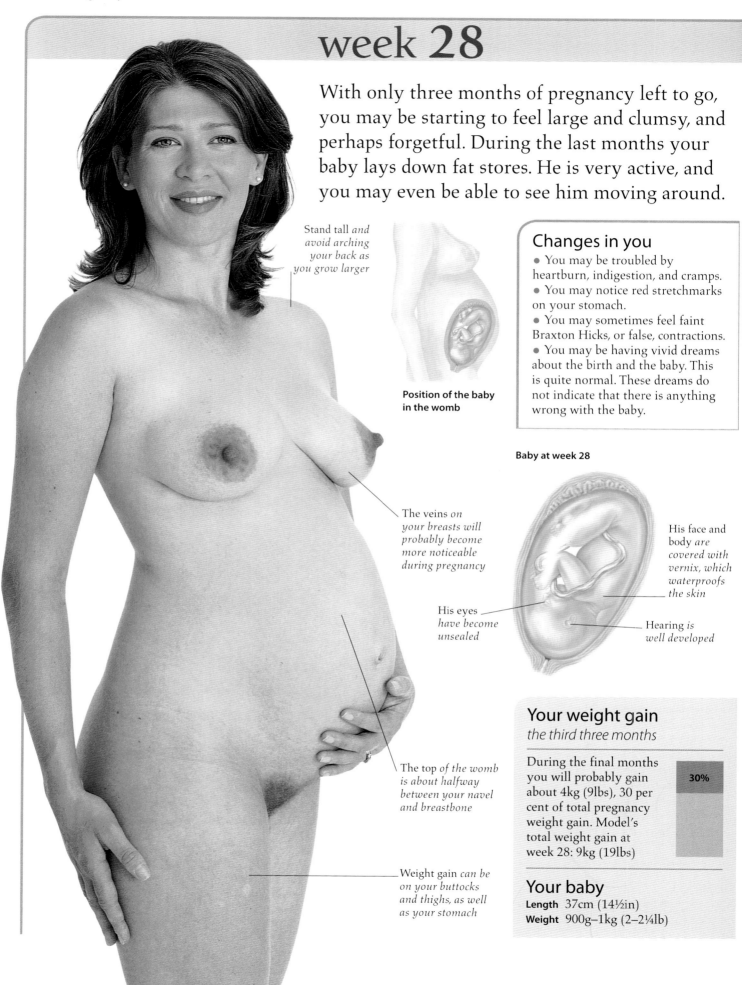

Stand tall *and avoid arching your back as you grow larger*

Position of the baby in the womb

Changes in you
- You may be troubled by heartburn, indigestion, and cramps.
- You may notice red stretchmarks on your stomach.
- You may sometimes feel faint Braxton Hicks, or false, contractions.
- You may be having vivid dreams about the birth and the baby. This is quite normal. These dreams do not indicate that there is anything wrong with the baby.

Baby at week 28

The veins *on your breasts will probably become more noticeable during pregnancy*

His face and body *are covered with vernix, which waterproofs the skin*

His eyes *have become unsealed*

Hearing *is well developed*

The top *of the womb is about halfway between your navel and breastbone*

Weight gain *can be on your buttocks and thighs, as well as your stomach*

Your weight gain
the third three months

During the final months you will probably gain about 4kg (9lbs), 30 per cent of total pregnancy weight gain. Model's total weight gain at week 28: 9kg (19lbs)

30%

Your baby
Length 37cm (14½in)
Weight 900g–1kg (2–2¼lb)

What to do

● Make sure you are getting enough rest in the day, and have as many early nights as possible. If you are still at work, put your feet up during the lunch hour and rest when you come home.

● Let your employer know in writing when you intend to stop work, and if you're planning to go back to your job after the baby is born. Find out your employer's policy about returning to work. Depending on your type of work, how far you have to travel, and your budget, you may want to remain working for a while longer.

● Visit the antenatal clinic for a routine check-up, and optional screening for anaemia and atypical red cell alloantibodies.

● If you're planning a trip involving air travel, check with your doctor, the airline, and your insurance company.

Your growing baby

● His skin is red and wrinkled, but fat starts to accumulate beneath it.

● There have been dramatic developments in the thinking part of the brain, which becomes bigger and more complex. A seven-month-old baby can feel pain, and responds in much the same way as a full-term baby.

● The baby has far more taste buds than he will have at birth, so his sense of taste is acute.

● His lungs are still not mature, and need to develop a substance called surfactant, which stops them collapsing between each breath.

● The baby's heartbeat can be heard distinctly, using either a fetal stethoscope or a Doppler ultrasound device.

● A baby born now could survive, given special care.

See also:
Common complaints *pages 40–2*
Protecting your back *page 44*
Stretchmarks *page 42*

Your pregnancy wardrobe

Up to five or even six months of your pregnancy, many of your normal clothes may be wearable if they fit loosely or you use a little creativity. However, a few new outfits may greatly improve your morale and you don't have to buy special maternity wear. Look for clothes that are attractive, comfortable, and easy to care for.

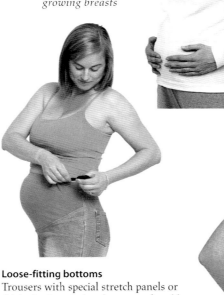

Comfortable tops
Go for stretchy fabrics in soft natural fibres.

Choose a style with plenty of room across the chest to accommodate your growing breasts

Loose-fitting bottoms
Trousers with special stretch panels or thick elastic waistbands are comfortable and unrestricting; they are convenient because they expand as your bump grows.

A versatile fabric will stretch to fit your changing shape

Dressing up
A simple dress can look casual, but is also easy to dress up. Check that there's enough length in the hem so the dress hangs evenly as you grow larger. Maternity dresses are usually 2.5cm (1in) longer at the front to allow for this.

What to choose

You tend to feel the heat more during pregnancy, so look for lightweight, loose-fitting clothes, made of cotton or other natural fibres. If it's cold, put on several layers. Avoid anything that is tight around the waist or that restricts blood flow in your legs, such as tight knee-high socks.

Comfortable, low-heeled shoes are essential, although completely flat heels are best avoided. You probably won't be able to wear lace-ups soon, as you will have difficulty bending down to tie them.

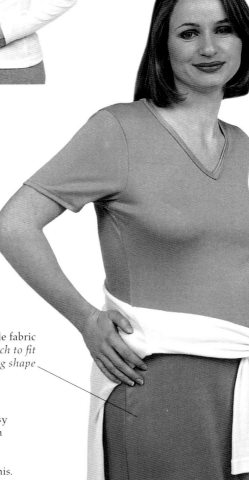

week 32

You need all the rest you can get, so try to lie down in the middle of the day. You will probably be feeling weary of your pregnant state. Now is the time to start going to parentcraft classes, which will run until the end of your pregnancy.

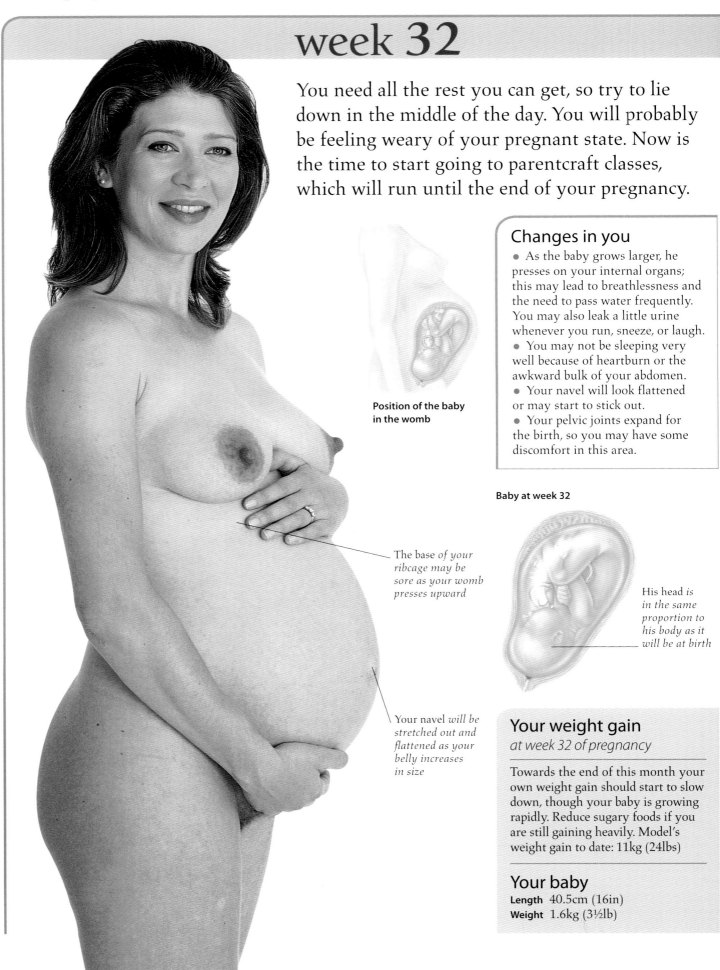

Position of the baby in the womb

Changes in you

- As the baby grows larger, he presses on your internal organs; this may lead to breathlessness and the need to pass water frequently. You may also leak a little urine whenever you run, sneeze, or laugh.
- You may not be sleeping very well because of heartburn or the awkward bulk of your abdomen.
- Your navel will look flattened or may start to stick out.
- Your pelvic joints expand for the birth, so you may have some discomfort in this area.

Baby at week 32

The base *of your ribcage may be sore as your womb presses upward*

His head *is in the same proportion to his body as it will be at birth*

Your navel *will be stretched out and flattened as your belly increases in size*

Your weight gain
at week 32 of pregnancy

Towards the end of this month your own weight gain should start to slow down, though your baby is growing rapidly. Reduce sugary foods if you are still gaining heavily. Model's weight gain to date: 11kg (24lbs)

Your baby
Length 40.5cm (16in)
Weight 1.6kg (3½lb)

What to do

- Break up the day by putting your feet up for an hour or two.
- If you have difficulty sleeping, practise relaxation techniques before going to bed, and try sleeping on your side, with one leg bent and supported on a pillow. Try not to worry if you still can't sleep; it's very normal to be wide awake at night during this stage of pregnancy.
- Keep up with your pelvic floor exercises; especially if you are suffering from leaking urine.
- Start attending antenatal classes if they haven't begun already.
- Have another antenatal check-up, which will include a thorough review of screening tests performed at 28 weeks.

"I'm worried about harming the baby during intercourse. Is there any danger of this?" Q&A

This is a common worry but an unnecessary one if your pregnancy is normal. The baby is cushioned by the bag of fluid surrounding him, so he cannot be harmed when you make love. The doctor or midwife will tell you if there is any danger, such as a low-lying placenta.

Your growing baby

- The baby looks much the same as he will at birth, but his body still needs to fill out more.
- He can now sense the difference between light and dark.
- Because there is less room in the womb, he will probably have turned into a head-down position by now, ready for birth.

See also:
Antenatal classes *page 17*
Breathlessness *page 40*
Frequent urination *page 41*
Pelvic floor *page 45*
Relaxation techniques *pages 48–9*

Essentials for your baby

Buy the following basic equipment and clothing for your new baby, then add anything else you need when he's born.

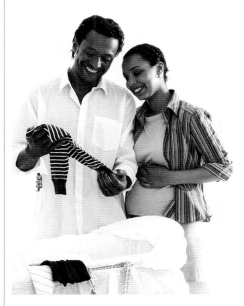

Equipment

Buy new equipment if you can. Check second-hand items carefully to ensure they are safe. You will need:
- a carrycot, a cot, or Moses basket
- appropriate bedding
- a soft cellular blanket
- an infant car seat, if you have a car
- a baby bath
- two soft towels
- changing mat
- nappies and changing equipment
- bottle-feeding equipment (if you are going to bottle-feed and as a back-up if you are breastfeeding).

Clothes

It's important to remember that your baby will grow quickly during the first few months, so buy only the minimum of first size (newborn) clothes. Three or four nighties, stretchsuits, and wide or envelope-necked vests, plus two cardigans should see you through the first few weeks. Babies lose heat easily from their heads, so a soft-knit hat is essential.

Enjoying sex

Making love is often particularly enjoyable during pregnancy because you become aroused more easily as a result of the increase in hormone levels, and there are no worries about contraception.

Other ways of loving

There may be times when you lose interest in sex, especially in the first and last weeks. This doesn't mean that you have to stop showing your loving feelings for each other. Even if you feel too tired or heavy to make love, you can find other ways of showing your affection, such as kissing, cuddling, stroking, and touching.

A change of position

In the last weeks of pregnancy, you may find the traditional man-on-top position rather uncomfortable. Experiment with other positions; perhaps sitting on your partner's lap, kneeling with him behind, or both lying side by side.

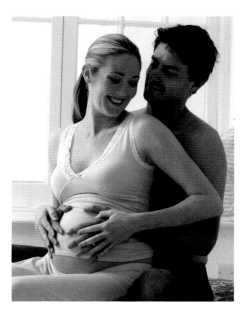

week 36

By now you may have stopped work. You may be longing for the pregnancy to be over, yet feel apprehensive about the birth and becoming a parent. The baby takes up all the space in the womb, so he kicks and punches rather than shifts his whole body.

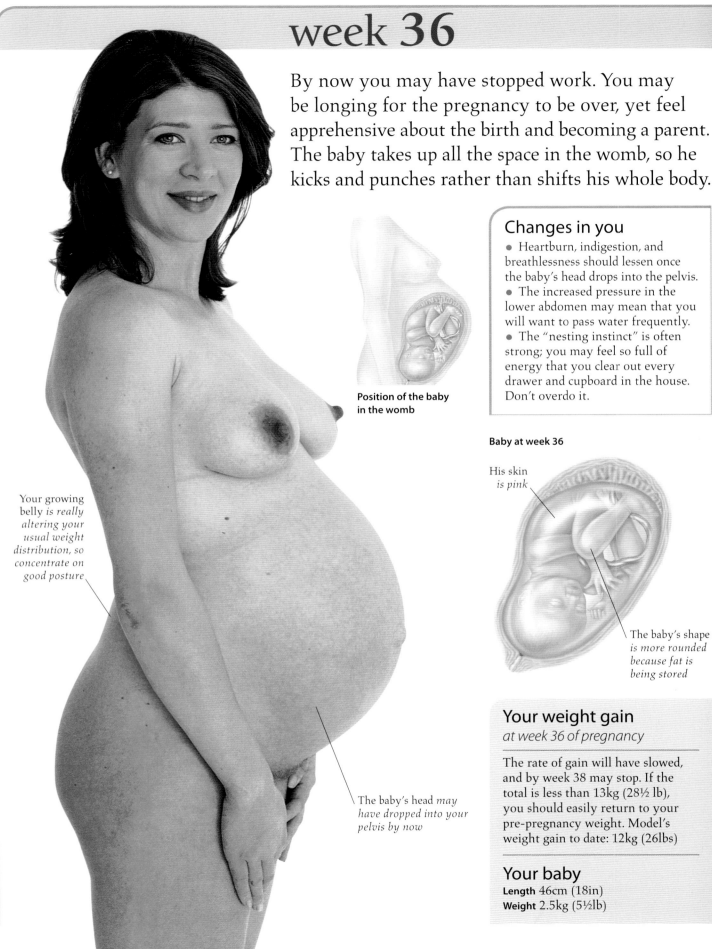

Your growing belly is really altering your usual weight distribution, so concentrate on good posture

The baby's head may have dropped into your pelvis by now

Position of the baby in the womb

Changes in you
- Heartburn, indigestion, and breathlessness should lessen once the baby's head drops into the pelvis.
- The increased pressure in the lower abdomen may mean that you will want to pass water frequently.
- The "nesting instinct" is often strong; you may feel so full of energy that you clear out every drawer and cupboard in the house. Don't overdo it.

Baby at week 36

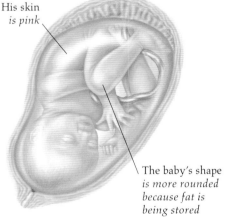

His skin is pink

The baby's shape is more rounded because fat is being stored

Your weight gain
at week 36 of pregnancy

The rate of gain will have slowed, and by week 38 may stop. If the total is less than 13kg (28½ lb), you should easily return to your pre-pregnancy weight. Model's weight gain to date: 12kg (26lbs)

Your baby
Length 46cm (18in)
Weight 2.5kg (5½lb)

What to do

- Put your feet up whenever you can to guard against swollen ankles and varicose veins.
- Visit the clinic. The midwife will check the position of the fetus, and offer an external cephalic version to a woman with a breech presentation.
- If you are having your baby in hospital, take a tour of the delivery room and maternity wards.
- Buy your nursing bras.
- Stock the food cupboards for when you return from the hospital.
- Pack your suitcase for hospital; if you are having a home birth, assemble all the things you need.

"Should I have my partner with me during labour?"

Labour can be a long process, and a rather lonely one unless you have someone to share it with, and a natural choice is your partner, whose presence can be beneficial for both. But if this isn't possible, having a relative or a friend as a companion can be just as reassuring.

Your growing baby

- If this is your first baby, his head will probably have descended into the pelvis ready for birth.
- Soft nails have grown to the tips of his fingers and toes.
- In a boy, the testicles should have descended.
- The baby will gain about 28g (1oz) every day from now onwards.

See also:
Plan for baby's arrival *page 27*
Frequent urination *page 41*
Preparing for the birth *pages 54–5*
Protecting your back *page 44*
Relaxation techniques *pages 48–9*
Swollen ankles *page 42*
Varicose veins *page 42*

Resting in later pregnancy

During the last weeks, you will probably get tired very easily. You may not be sleeping as well as usual, and you will also feel exhausted by the extra weight you are carrying around.

Avoid tiring yourself

Put your feet up whenever you need to during the day. Think of quiet things to do when you rest: practise relaxation exercises, listen to soothing music, read a book, or perhaps knit something for the baby. It also helps if you try to do things at a slower pace than usual, so that you don't over exert yourself.

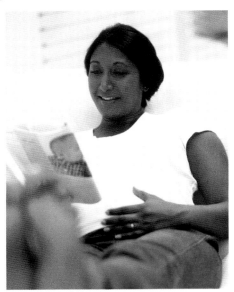

Your nursing bra

If you want to breastfeed, you will need at least two plain cotton nursing bras with firm support straps. To make sure these are the right size, it's best to buy them no earlier than week 36.

What to look for

There are two main types of bra: one has flaps, which open to expose the nipple and some of the surrounding breast; the other fastens at the front, so you can expose the whole breast. The front-opening kind is best, as it allows the baby to feel and fondle the breast while he's sucking. It also allows the milk to flow freely.

Measuring up

Take the measurements while wearing one of your ordinary pregnancy bras.

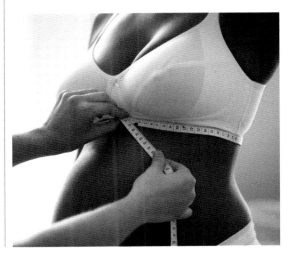

1 Measure around your body below your breasts. Add 12cm (5in) to get your final chest measurement.

2 Measure around the fullest part of your breasts. If this equals your chest measurement, you need an A cup. If it is 2.5cm (1in) more, you need a B cup. If it is 5cm (2in) more, you need a C cup. Alternatively, you can opt to get fitted in shops specializing in maternity bras. In fact, professional fitting is often the best option.

week 40

By this stage you will feel very ungainly and will be bumping into objects because of your size. You will be impatient to give birth, but also excited and relieved that you are nearly there. Rest as much as possible, and enjoy these last baby-free days.

Changes in you
- You will have a feeling of heaviness in your lower abdomen.
- Your cervix will be softening in preparation for labour.
- Braxton Hicks contractions may be so noticeable that you think you are in labour, but they won't be regular.

Your weight gain
at week 40 of pregnancy

In the final two weeks, you may actually lose a little weight. This is a sign that your baby is fully mature, and you can expect labour to start within 10 days. Model's weight gain is negligible from week 36 onwards.

Your baby
Length 51cm (20in)
Weight 3.4kg (7½lb)

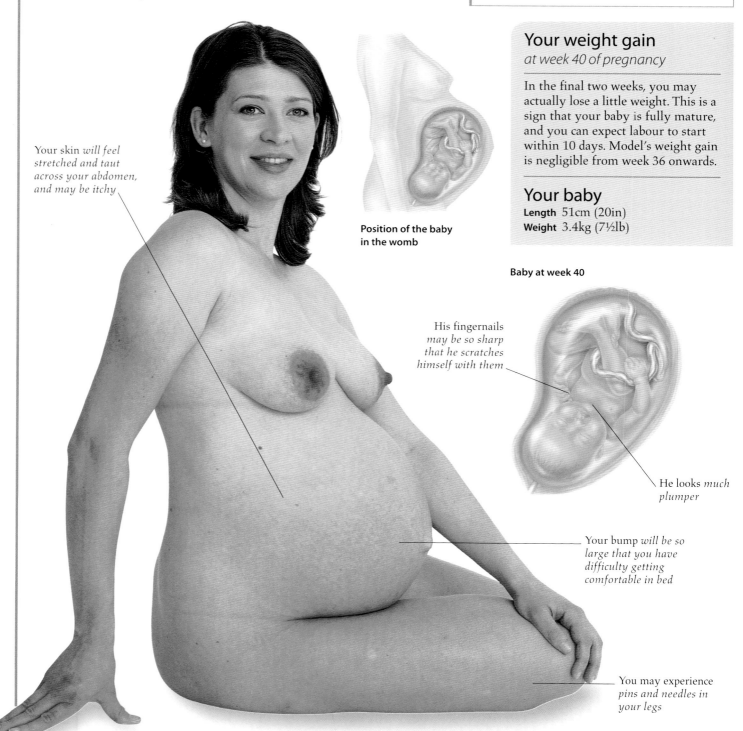

Your skin *will feel stretched and taut across your abdomen, and may be itchy*

Position of the baby in the womb

Baby at week 40

His fingernails *may be so sharp that he scratches himself with them*

He looks *much plumper*

Your bump *will be so large that you have difficulty getting comfortable in bed*

You may experience *pins and needles in your legs*

What to do

- If you don't feel at least 10 movements from your baby in the day, ask your midwife to check his heart rate as he may be distressed.
- If the Braxton Hicks contractions are stronger and more frequent, practise your breathing.
- Don't worry if your baby doesn't arrive on time – it will happen, it always does. It's perfectly normal for a baby to be born two weeks either side of the expected delivery date.

Total weight gain

The average amount of weight gain during pregnancy varies between 10 and 12kg (22 and 27lbs), but you may put on more or less weight. The total weight gain is made up as follows:

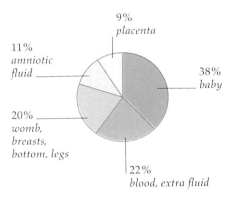

9%
placenta

11%
amniotic
fluid

38%
baby

20%
womb,
breasts,
bottom, legs

22%
blood, extra fluid

Your growing baby

- Most of the lanugo hair (soft prenatal hair) has disappeared, though there may still be a little over his shoulders, arms, and legs.
- He may be covered in vernix, or just have traces in skin folds.
- A dark substance called meconium gathers in the baby's intestines; this will be passed in his first bowel movement after birth.
- If this is your second or later baby, his head may engage now.

See also:
Braxton Hicks contractions *page 56*
Breathing techniques *page 49*

Becoming a mother

After all the weeks of preparation and planning, you are fully ready to give birth. Afterwards, you can hold your baby in your arms. You will probably feel overwhelmingly protective towards this tiny person, who is dependent on you for everything.

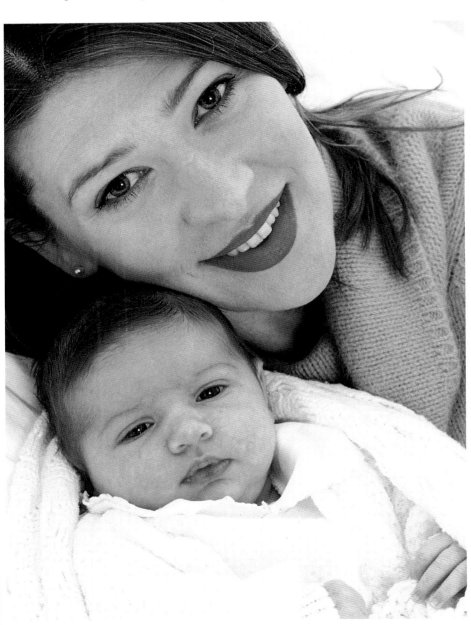

The first weeks

Life in the early weeks following the arrival of your baby revolves around him and his needs, whether he needs feeding, nappy changing, or comforting. But once you get to know each other, and you become more adept at handling your baby and understanding what he requires, both of you will become more settled and life will fall into some sort of routine once again.

Antenatal care

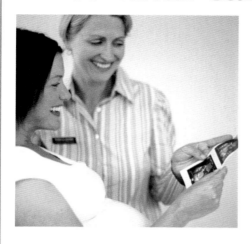

Having a baby nowadays is very safe. This is largely because of the availability of antenatal care, a system of checks and tests at regular intervals throughout pregnancy designed to confirm that all is well with you and your baby. It is important for antenatal care to start early in pregnancy, as the first set of checks provides a baseline for assessing any changes later on. Ask your doctor about the available choices once the pregnancy is confirmed, and he can make the arrangements.

Where to have your baby

Providing you have a normal pregnancy, an important decision you will need to make is where to have your baby. Most babies today are born in a hospital, with medical staff available round the clock. In some areas you may be able to choose to have your baby in a midwifery-led unit. It may also be possible to have your baby at home. Your doctor or midwife will make arrangements for your antenatal care according to your choice of where you want to have your baby.

Hospital birth

Type of antenatal care: If you are having your baby in a hospital unit, you will either have "full care" at a hospital antenatal clinic or "shared care", with a few appointments at a hospital clinic and most at your GP's surgery or local health centre.

Birthing procedure: A hospital has all the equipment and expertise needed for pain relief, for monitoring the baby's progress, for intervening in the birth to help you and the baby if necessary, and for providing emergency care for you both. After the birth, the duration of your stay in hospital varies, but it may be possible for you to go home the same day. Staying in hospital for several days is rarely an option, but you will get support and advice from your community midwife, who will visit you at home.

Because the hospital staff is a team, there is no guarantee that you will see the same doctor at each antenatal clinic. Neither can you be sure which midwife will deliver your baby, so you don't have a chance to build up a relationship with her before your labour.

It can be very noisy in a hospital ward, as well as daunting to be in unfamiliar surroundings. But most hospitals hold antenatal classes (see page 17), and if you go along to these you will be encouraged to look around the delivery room and maternity wards in advance to familiarize yourself with them.

Facilities vary among hospitals, so it's definitely worth seeing what your local hospital has to offer before you decide. Some offer birthing suites that are more like home, and some have birthing pools that may make labour more comfortable.

Midwifery-led units

Type of antenatal care: If you are having your baby in a midwifery-led unit or at home, a midwife will probably provide all or most of your antenatal care, with possibly some hospital visits for tests (such as ultrasound scans).

Birthing procedure: These units, also known as birthing centres, are run by midwives and offer a more homely environment. They may be located either within the main hospital maternity unit or as a stand-alone unit in the local district or community hospital. These units are designed to deal with normal pregnancies and deliveries in a low-tech and informal environment. However, these small units do not have the full medical facilities of a hospital.

Home birth

Type of antenatal care: If you are considering having your baby at home, make sure you secure the services of a trained independent midwife, who will carry out all your antenatal checks, and guide you through your labour and delivery.

Birthing procedure: If you are healthy, have had a normal pregnancy, and feel you would be more relaxed and able to cope during labour in your own familiar surroundings, you may be able to have your baby at home. A home birth is likely to be more suitable if you have had one or more previous pregnancies that were free of complications. Even then, no two pregnancies can be guaranteed to follow the same pattern. Do bear in mind that if there are complications, and you have to go into hospital, there will be extra travel time before you and your baby get emergency treatment. Pain relief at home is limited and epidurals are not available. A few independent midwives specialize in home births. Ask your doctor or midwife for more information.

Questions to ask

Hospital policies vary, so discuss any issues that are important to you with the staff at the clinic. It's natural to have pre-conceived ideas about labour and birth, but the reality is often quite different. However sure you are that you don't want pain relief, keep an open mind and ask for it if you need it. This list covers some questions you might like to ask.

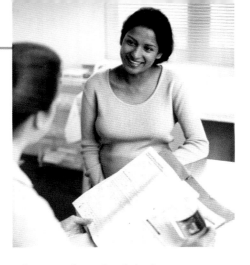

About labour

Can my partner and/or a friend stay with me throughout labour?

Will I be able to move around as I please during labour?

What is the hospital policy on pain relief, routine electronic monitoring, and induction (see pages 64, 65, and 66)?

What kind of pain relief (see pages 64 and 65) will I be offered?

About the birth

Can I give birth in any position I choose to? Are chairs, large cushions, birthing balls, and birth stools available?

Will I be able to use a birthing pool (see page 58)?

What is the hospital policy on episiotomies, Caesareans, and syntometrine (see pages 63, 66, and 67)?

What types of birthing rooms are available?

About after the birth

How long will I stay in hospital after delivery?

Will I be able to have my baby with me all the time, including nights?

Is there open visiting for my partner?

Is there a special care baby unit in case my baby needs treatment?

Does the hospital's policy support (and give advice on) breastfeeding?

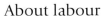

Your maternity records

The results of the clinic tests, and any other details about your pregnancy, are noted on patient-held records, which you are given at your first visit. Keep this on you at all times – if you have to see another doctor the file provides a record of everything he or she will need to know. Make sure that you understand what is written down; ask if you don't.

AFP	Alpha fetoprotein	**MSU**	Mid-stream urine sample
Alb	Albumin (a protein) found in urine	**NAD**	Nothing abnormal discovered
BP	Blood pressure	**NE**	The baby's head has not engaged
Br	The baby is bottom down (Breech)	**Oedema**	Swelling present
C/Ceph or Vx	The baby is in the normal (head down – Vertex) position	**Para O**	A woman who has had no other children
CS	Caesarean section	**Presentation**	Which way up the baby is
E/Eng	The baby's head has engaged	**Primigravida**	First pregnancy
EDD/EDC	Estimated date of delivery/confinement	**Relation of PP to brim**	Relation of the part of the baby to be born first to the brim of the pelvis
Fe	Iron supplements	**Rh+**	Rhesus blood group positive
FH	Fetal heart		
FHH or FH√	Fetal heart heard	**Rh-**	Rhesus blood group negative
FHNH	Fetal heart not heard		
FMF	Fetal movements felt	**SFD**	Small for dates
Fundus	Top of the womb	**TCA**	To come again
Hb	Haemoglobin levels in the blood	**TBA**	To come into hospital; or, to be arranged
H/T	High blood pressure	**Tr**	A trace found
LFTS	Liver function tests	**U/S**	Ultrasound
LMP	Last menstrual period	**VE**	Vaginal examination
LSCS	Lower segment caesarean section		

Abbreviations are used to describe the way the baby is lying in the womb. These are some of the positions:

LOL: left occipito-lateral

ROL: right occipito-lateral

LOA: left occipito-anterior

ROA: right occipito-anterior

LOP: left occipito-posterior

ROP: right occipito-posterior

Your antenatal appointments

Your first antenatal check-up takes place at about 10 weeks, and you will be asked to go two or three times until 28 weeks. Visits become more frequent after this: every two weeks until you are 36 weeks pregnant, and every week in the last month. Routine tests are carried out by the midwife at every visit to check that the pregnancy is progressing normally. Write down questions you have beforehand.

Blood tests
first visit
Some blood will be taken from your arm to check:
● your main blood group and your rhesus blood group (see page 38)
● that you are not anaemic (see page 38); your blood will be tested for this again at about 32 weeks
● that you are immune to rubella (see page 10)
● that you do not have a sexually transmitted disease, such as syphilis, which must be treated before week 20 if it is not to harm the baby, or hepatitis
● for sickle cell trait, if you and your partner are of West Indian or African descent, and thalassaemia, if your families come from the Mediterranean, South Asia, or the Middle and Far East. These forms of anaemia are inherited, and if untreated, could put the baby's health at risk.

General examination
first visit
The doctor or midwife may examine you physically if you have any medical problems. Your breasts may be checked for lumps and inverted nipples (see page 23). You will probably be asked about your dental health, and encouraged to go for a check-up, as increased blood flow to the gums can cause gum problems.

Weight
first visit
You will be weighed at your first visit, as part of the general examination. Don't worry if you lose weight during the first three months because of morning sickness, as this is quite common. If you gain weight suddenly in late pregnancy, this can be a sign of pre-eclampsia (see page 38).

Urine sample
every visit
Most clinics test a sample of urine at your first visit and, from the 28th week onwards, at each visit. The sample will be tested for:
● traces of sugar
● traces of protein, which may indicate the possibility of pre-eclampsia (see page 38) in later pregnancy
● bacteria (germs) – in case you have an asymptomatic urine infection. This can cause problems in later pregnancy. It can be easily treated with antibiotics.

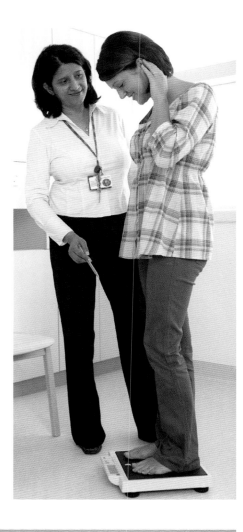

Initial talk

At the first visit, the doctor or midwife will ask some questions about you and your partner to find out whether there is anything that could affect the pregnancy or your baby. Antenatal procedures may vary from place to place, but you can expect to be asked about:
● personal details, such as your date of birth, and what work you and your partner do, and your address. Remember to give the address where you will be staying after the birth, since, in practice, many couples spend the first weeks with family, leaving health visitors unable to contact mother and baby
● your country of origin, as some forms of anaemia are inherited and affect only certain ethnic groups (see above)
● your health: any serious illnesses or operations you may have had in the past, whether you are currently being treated for any disease, and whether you have any allergies, or are taking any drugs
● your family's medical history: whether there are twins or any inherited illnesses in your or your partner's family
● the type of contraceptives you used before you became pregnant, and when you stopped using it
● your periods: when they began, whether they are regular, when the first day of your last period was, and how long your cycle is
● any previous pregnancies, including miscarriages and terminations.

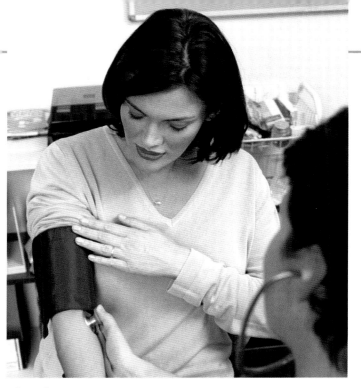

collect more water in their bodies than they would otherwise, but excessive swelling may be a sign of pre-eclampsia (see page 38). Your legs will also be checked for varicose veins (see page 42).

Feeling the abdomen
every visit
The doctor or midwife will gently feel your abdomen to check the position of the top of the womb, which gives her a good idea of the rate of the baby's growth. Later in your pregnancy, checks will be made to ensure that your baby has turned the right way round (head first), and, in the final weeks, that the head is dropping into your pelvis (engaging).

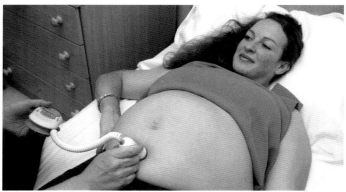

Blood pressure
every visit
Blood pressure may be slightly lower in pregnancy, and it is measured regularly to detect any sudden rises and keep it under control. Normal blood pressure is about 120/70, and there will be cause for concern if your blood pressure rises above 140/90. Raised blood pressure can be a sign of a number of problems, including pre-eclampsia (see page 38).

Legs, ankles, and hands
every visit
The doctor or midwife will look at your lower legs, ankles, and hands, and feel them to check there is no swelling or puffiness. A little swelling in the last weeks of pregnancy is normal, especially at the end of the day, since during pregnancy women normally

Listening to the baby's heartbeat
every visit (after week 14)
From early in pregnancy, this may be done with a sonicaid (see above), which amplifies the baby's heartbeat so you can hear it too.

Screening and diagnostic tests in pregnancy

During your pregnancy you will probably be offered tests to look for conditions that might cause your baby to have a disability. Some of these tests are offered as a routine part of antenatal care and others when it is thought that there is a chance of an abnormality. The object of the tests is to detect any serious problem as early as possible so that the pregnancy can, if you wish, be safely terminated. The most likely outcome is that they will give you the reassurance that your baby is normal.

Your choice
You don't have to have any of these tests if you don't want to, and indeed you may prefer not to if you are certain that, whatever the outcome, you would never consider terminating the pregnancy. Even so, you might want to be prepared for a baby with a disability before the birth and, if the condition is treatable, to discuss and plan the treatment in advance.

Types of tests that you may be offered
Screening tests
A screening test will not detect any abnormality. It will only show whether you are more likely to have a baby with a particular disability. If the results show you are in a "high risk" group ("screen positive"), you will be offered a diagnostic test, but this does not mean there is anything wrong with your baby.

Diagnostic tests
If a screening test shows you are "high risk", you may be offered a diagnostic test that will give you a firm answer and show whether or not your baby has a particular abnormality. All diagnostic tests, except an "anomaly" ultrasound scan, involve taking samples from inside your uterus, and they carry an increased risk of miscarriage. If you are unsure whether to agree to a test or want to discuss it further, do ask.

Ultrasound scan

An ultrasound scan is a test you will be offered routinely at some stage of your pregnancy. Your first ultrasound scan, when you actually see your baby on the screen, turns your pregnancy into a fascinating reality. A thin layer of gel is rubbed over your stomach and a hand-held instrument, a transducer, is passed gently over it. This beams and receives sound waves that are built into an image of your baby on the screen.

The scan is painless and takes about 15–45 minutes. Ultrasound scans are safe. Unlike X-rays and other imaging tests, ultrasound does not use radiation. It has not been found to cause any problems or complications.

Early scan

If you have a history of miscarriage, or have had any pain or bleeding, you may be offered a very early scan, at 6–11 weeks. This will confirm that the pregnancy is safely established, and may also detect an ectopic pregnancy. If you have an early scan, the transducer may be placed in your vagina, but there is no risk that this will cause a miscarriage.

Dating scan

You will be given a dating scan when you are between 10 and 14 weeks pregnant to help date your pregnancy accurately.

18–20 week anomaly scan

This scan is offered routinely to confirm the date of the pregnancy, to make sure the baby's growth is normal, and that his heart, brain, other organs, spine, and limbs are all developing normally. It will also show any condition that might complicate the delivery.

Further scans

You may be offered additional scans later in pregnancy if you are expecting twins, or if your doctor thinks that your baby is not growing properly. A scan within the last six weeks of pregnancy may be offered to check on the "lie" of the baby and the position of the placenta.

Nuchal translucency scan
(11–14 weeks)

In some areas (it's offered in some NHS antenatal classes), you will be offered a special scan to help calculate the risk of Down's syndrome. This scan measures fluid accumulation at the back of the baby's neck. All babies have some fluid there between 11 and 13 weeks, but most babies with Down's have an increased amount. This test result, combined with the mother's age and the results of blood-screening, will help calculate the risk of Down's, and to decide whether the mother should be offered a diagnostic test.

Doppler ultrasound scan
(as necessary)

A Doppler scan is an ultrasound scan used to examine blood flow to the baby through the umbilical cord. If a baby is not growing at the expected rate, this scan may be given to check that the placenta is working properly and the baby is getting enough oxygen. During labour it may also be used to monitor the baby's heart rate.

Serum screening test

You may be offered a blood test to assess your risk of having a baby with Down's syndrome and other abnormalities.

The triple test
(about 15 weeks)

This measures three blood chemicals, AFP, estriol, and HCG (human chorionic gonadotrophin). The test is carried out to assess the risks of a neural tube defect, Down's syndrome, and other chromosomal abnormalities. Some hospitals measure only two of these markers (the double test).

HIV testing
(Booking visit)

You may be offered a test for HIV (the Human Immunodeficiency Virus). The virus can be transmitted to your baby during pregnancy, at the birth, or even during breastfeeding. Your baby can be infected even if you have no symptoms. However, if your doctor knows that you are HIV+ve, precautions can be taken to minimize the risk of the infection being passed to your baby during the birth. It is worth having the test even if you do not think that you or your partner are particularly at risk.

Hepatitis B testing
(Booking visit)

This test may be offered to look for evidence of the hepatitis B virus. The virus can be fatal if passed on to a baby, but this can be prevented by giving antibodies.

Amniocentesis
(weeks 15–20, usually at week 16)

Amniocentesis can be used to detect some abnormalities in the baby, such

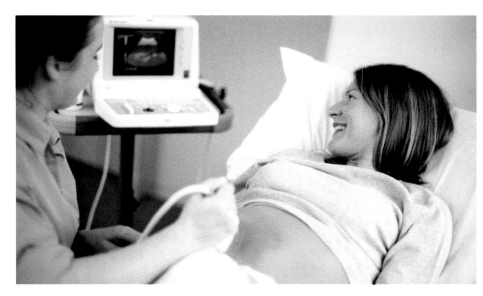

Ultrasound scan
It can be very exciting to see your baby on the ultrasound monitor, and it will reassure you that your baby's development is normal.

as Down's syndrome. It is not offered routinely as there is a risk of miscarriage in about one woman in 100. You may be offered the test if:
- you are over 35, when there is a higher risk of a Down's baby
- you have a family history of an inherited disease
- your screening test was positive.

An ultrasound scan is done to check the position of the baby and the placenta. A hollow needle is inserted through the wall of the stomach into the womb, and a sample of the fluid that surrounds the baby, and which contains some of her cells, is taken. The cells are then tested for abnormality. The test results can take three weeks.

Chorionic villus sampling (CVS)
(10–14 weeks)
Some inherited disorders can be detected by examining a small piece of the tissue that forms part of the placenta. The sample can be obtained either through the vagina, or by inserting a needle directly into the uterus through the abdominal wall, guided by an ultrasound scan. The test carries a slightly greater risk than amniocentesis but the results are available more quickly.

Cordocentesis
(18–22 weeks)
If amniocentesis and CVS tests are inconclusive, cordocentesis may be used to diagnose some blood disorders. Cordocentesis may also be used to treat congenital heart defects and respiratory disorders while the baby is still in utero.

Table of screening and diagnostic tests

Time	Test	What for	Disadvantages
Booking visit	HIV test (diagnostic test) Hepatitis B test (diagnostic test)	The presence of antibodies to the HIV virus Evidence of hepatitis B virus	A positive test will cause alarm Post-test counselling offered to all women when they receive test result
10–14 weeks	Chorionic villus sampling (CVS) (diagnostic test)	Down's syndrome Some blood disorders Baby's sex	You may find the procedure uncomfortable and worrying. Increased risk of miscarriage – about 2 per cent
11–14 weeks	Nuchal scan (screening test)	Down's syndrome	A "high risk" result may cause unnecessary anxiety
11–14 weeks	Double, triple, or quadruple test (screening tests)	Down's syndrome Chromosomal abnormalities	A "high risk" result may cause unnecessary anxiety A few "low risk" women will have affected babies
15–20 weeks	Amniocentesis (diagnostic test)	Down's syndrome Chromosomal abnormalities Some inherited disorders	The procedure may be worrying and can be a bit uncomfortable Increased risk of miscarriage (0.5–1 per cent)
18–20 weeks	Ultrasound fetal anomaly scan (diagnostic test)	Confirms dates of pregnancy Checks for fetal abnormality	Accuracy of the result depends on the skill of the radiographer, how good the equipment is, and how the baby is lying
18–22 weeks	Fetal blood sampling (cordocentesis) (diagnostic test)	Chromosomal and blood disorders	Not commonly done Carries risk of miscarriage of 1–2 per cent Results take 3–4 days

Special care pregnancies

Nearly all pregnancies are normal and straightforward, but there may be circumstances that make your doctor think there is greater risk of complications, and hence you need to be monitored closely during pregnancy. This could be because you have a general medical condition, or perhaps you are expecting twins. Sometimes symptoms develop that also warn the doctor that special care is needed.

Anaemia

Many women are slightly anaemic before pregnancy, and this is usually due to an iron deficiency. It's important to correct this in order to cope with the increased demands of pregnancy, and any bleeding during labour.

Treatment Try to prevent the problem by eating a varied diet, with plenty of iron-rich foods. However, you should avoid liver and liver products in pregnancy (see page 52). If blood tests at the clinic show that you are anaemic, the doctor may prescribe iron supplements. Take iron tablets directly after a meal, with fluid, as otherwise they can cause constipation, diarrhoea, or nausea.

Diabetes

Diabetes must be carefully controlled during pregnancy, and your blood-sugar level constantly monitored. If this is done, there's no reason why the pregnancy shouldn't be straightforward.

Anaemia Eating foods that are a good source of iron, such as spinach, will help to guard against the problem.

Treatment It's imperative that your blood-sugar level remains stable, so the doctor may adjust your insulin intake for the pregnancy, and you should pay special attention to diet. You will also need to visit the antenatal clinic more often. Some women find a mild form of the disease appears for the first time during pregnancy, which nearly always disappears soon after delivery.

Incompetent cervix

In a normal pregnancy, the cervix (neck of the womb) stays closed until the beginning of labour. But if miscarriages frequently occur after the third month of pregnancy, it could be because the neck of the womb is weak and so it opens up, allowing the baby to pass through.

Treatment Your doctor may suggest a small operation to stitch the cervix firmly closed at the beginning of pregnancy. The stitch is then removed towards the end of pregnancy, or as labour starts.

Pre-eclampsia

This is one of the more common problems in late pregnancy. Warning signs are: raised blood pressure above 140/90; excessive weight gain; swollen ankles, feet, or hands; and protein in the urine. If you develop any of these symptoms, the doctor will monitor you very carefully.

If high blood pressure is untreated, it could progress to the extremely dangerous condition called eclampsia, where fits occur.

Treatment At the moment there is no effective way to prevent pre-eclampsia. If the signs are severe, you will be admitted to hospital even though you might be feeling fine. If your blood pressure is high, you may be given a drug to lower it. Labour may be induced (see page 66), especially in late pregnancy.

Rhesus-negative mother

Your blood is tested at the first clinic visit to see if it is rhesus positive or rhesus negative. About 15 per cent of people are rhesus negative, and if you are one of these you will only have a problem in pregnancy if you give birth to a rhesus positive baby. Your blood groups will be incompatible, and although this won't harm a first baby, you could have problems with later pregnancies.

Treatment A protective vaccination called anti-D is given to all rhesus-negative women antenatally, usually at 28 and 34 weeks. It is also given after any bleeding and after the birth of a rhesus positive baby to prevent problems in future pregnancies.

"Small for dates" babies

A baby who doesn't grow properly in the womb and is small at birth is called a "small for dates" baby. This may happen because the expectant mother smokes or eats a poor diet, or because the placenta

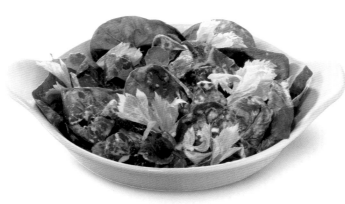

Emergency signs

Call for emergency help immediately if you have:
- a severe headache that won't go away
- misty or blurred vision
- severe, prolonged stomach or back pains
- vaginal bleeding
- a leakage of fluid, which suggests your waters have broken early
- frequent, painful urination (drink plenty of water in the meantime).

Consult your doctor within 24 hours if you have:
- swollen hands, face, and ankles
- severe, frequent vomiting
- a temperature of 38.3°C (101°F)
- no movement or fewer than 10 kicks from your baby for 12 hours after week 28.

Miscarriage

A miscarriage is the ending of a pregnancy before 24 weeks, and up to one in five pregnancies end in early miscarriages and bleeding. Most miscarriages occur in the first 12 weeks, often before the woman even knows she is pregnant, and usually because the baby is not developing normally. Bleeding from the vagina accompanied by lower backache and severe stomach cramps are usually the first signs. You should call your doctor straightaway if this happens.

Threatened miscarriage

If the bleeding is mild and painless, and occurs around the time of a missed period, you may not necessarily miscarry. You will be given an ultrasound scan (see page 37), which will show whether the fetus is alive.

True miscarriage

If the bleeding is heavy and you are in pain, it probably means that the baby has died.

You may have to go into hospital, so that your womb can be cleaned out under general anaesthetic.

Your feelings

Even if you lose the baby early in pregnancy, you will feel an intense sense of loss. You'll probably feel very emotional, and this will be made worse by the hormonal changes that take place after a miscarriage. Other people don't always understand that you need to mourn the loss of your baby. Worrying about whether you can ever have a normal, healthy baby is common. You may feel guilty, too, though don't blame yourself – it really isn't your fault. You can try for another baby as soon as you like, although some doctors suggest waiting until one menstrual cycle has passed. Unless you have had several miscarriages, there is no reason why you shouldn't experience a successful pregnancy the next time.

pregnancy, call your doctor without delay. Before 24 weeks, it can be a sign of an impending miscarriage. After this time, it may mean that the placenta is bleeding. This can happen if the placenta has started to separate from the wall of the womb (placental abruption) or if the placenta is too low down in the womb and covers, or partially covers, the cervix (placenta praevia).
Treatment The placenta is the baby's lifeline, so if the doctor thinks that there is a risk to it, you will probably be admitted to hospital straightaway, where the position of the placenta can be checked. You may stay in hospital until after the birth. If you have lost a lot of blood, you may be given a blood transfusion, and the baby will probably be delivered as soon as possible by induction or Caesarean section (see pages 66 and 67). But if bleeding is only slight and occurs several weeks before the baby is due, the doctor may decide to wait for you to start labour naturally while keeping you under close observation.

is inefficient (usually when the mother has a general medical condition, such as diabetes).
Treatment If tests show your baby is small, you will be monitored closely throughout pregnancy to check his health, and whether the flow of blood to the placenta is adequate. If the baby stops growing, or appears to be distressed, then he will be delivered early, either through induction or Caesarean section (see pages 66 and 67).

Twins

Your pregnancy and labour will progress normally, although you will have two second stages in labour, and there is a greater chance that you may go into labour prematurely. There's a greater likelihood of complications such as anaemia and pre-eclampsia, and of the babies lying abnormally in the womb. You may also find that all the common disorders

of pregnancy are exaggerated, especially in the last few months.
Treatment Regular visits to the antenatal clinic are essential if you are expecting two or more babies, so that any complications can be spotted immediately. A multiple pregnancy puts greater strain on your body than usual, so watch your posture and rest as much as possible, especially in

the last few weeks. To avoid problems with your digestion, eat smaller amounts of fresh, unprocessed food often. You may be more comfortable lying on one side rather than on your back. Using pillows to support the awkward bulk may also help.

Vaginal bleeding

If you notice bleeding from your vagina at any time in

Twins
You may find this position more comfortable to rest in.

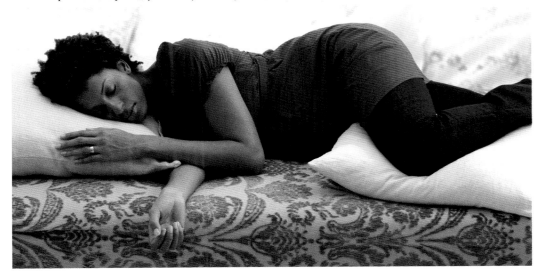

Common complaints

You may suffer from a variety of discomforts in pregnancy, which, although worrying at the time, are perfectly normal. Many are caused by hormonal changes, or because your body is under extra pressure. A few symptoms, however, should be taken very seriously, so call the doctor if you have any of the complaints that have been highlighted in the box on page 38.

Complaint	Symptoms	What to do
Bleeding gums ❶ ❷ ❸ The gums become softer and more easily injured in pregnancy. They may become inflamed, allowing plaque to collect at the base of the teeth. This can lead to gum disease and tooth decay.	Bleeding from the gums, especially after brushing your teeth.	• Floss and brush your teeth thoroughly after eating. • See your dentist. Treatment is free during pregnancy, but you should avoid X-rays or any dental procedures under general anaesthetic wherever possible.
Breathlessness ❸ Late in pregnancy, the growing baby puts pressure on the diaphragm and prevents you from breathing freely. The problem is often relieved about a month before the birth, if the baby's head engages. Breathlessness can also be caused by anaemia.	Feeling short of breath and panting excessively when you exert yourself.	• Rest as much as possible. • Try crouching if there's no chair around until your breathing slows down. • At night, use an extra pillow. • If the problem is severe, consult your doctor or midwife.
Constipation ❶ ❷ ❸ The pregnancy hormone progesterone relaxes the muscles of the intestine, which slows down bowel movements, making you more likely to become constipated. Approximately 30 to 40 per cent of pregnant women suffer from constipation at some point during pregnancy.	Passing hard, dry stools at less frequent intervals than usual.	• Eat plenty of high-fibre foods and drink lots of water. Go to the lavatory whenever you need to. • Exercise regularly. • Take any iron supplements you have been prescribed on a full stomach, with plenty of fluid. • See your doctor if the problem persists. • Avoid laxatives. • Camomile, fennel, and ginger herbal supplements may help.
Muscle cramps ❸ May be caused by calcium deficiency.	Painful contractions of muscles, usually in the calves and the feet, and often at night. Commonly started by a leg stretch with the toes pointed down.	• Massage the affected calf or foot. • Walk around for a moment or two once the pain has eased to improve your circulation. • See your doctor who may prescribe calcium and vitamin D supplements. • Eat plenty of calcium-rich foods, and include garlic in your diet. Drink more water.
Feeling faint ❶ ❸ Your blood pressure is lower in pregnancy, so you are more likely to feel faint.	Feeling dizzy and unstable. Needing to sit or lie down.	• Try not to stand still for too long. • If you suddenly feel faint, sit down and put your head between your knees until you feel better. • Get up slowly from a hot bath, or when sitting or lying down. Turn on to one side first, if lying on your back.

Complaint	Symptoms	What to do
Frequent urination ❶ ❸ Caused by the womb pressing on the bladder. The problem is often relieved in the middle months of pregnancy.	You need to pass water often.	• If you find yourself getting up in the night to go to the lavatory, try drinking a little less in the evenings. • See your doctor if you feel any pain or burning sensation when passing urine, as you could have an infection.
Heartburn ❸ The valve at the entrance to your stomach relaxes in pregnancy because of hormonal changes, so stomach acid passes back into the oesophagus (the tube leading to your stomach).	A strong burning pain in the centre of the chest.	• Avoid large meals and highly spiced or fried foods. • At night, try a warm milk drink, and raise the head of the bed or use extra pillows. • See your doctor, who may prescribe a medicine to treat stomach acidity. • Camomile or peppermint tea may give relief.
Leaking urine ❸ Caused by weak pelvic floor muscles (see page 45) and the growing baby pressing on your bladder.	Leakage of urine whenever you run, cough, sneeze, or laugh.	• Pass water often. • Practise your pelvic floor exercises regularly. • Avoid constipation and heavy lifting.
Morning sickness ❶ Often one of the first signs of pregnancy, which can occur at any time of day. Tiredness can make the problem worse. Nausea usually disappears after week 12, but can sometimes return later.	Feeling sick, often at the smell of certain foods or cigarette smoke. Most women find there is a particular time of day when this happens.	• Eat a couple of plain biscuits first thing in the morning. • Avoid foods and smells that make you feel sick. • Have small, frequent meals throughout the day. • Drink an infusion of ginger or camomile tea.
Piles ❷ ❸ Pressure from the baby's head causes swollen veins round the anus. Straining to empty the bowels will make the problem worse. Mild piles usually disappear, without treatment, after the baby is born.	Itching, soreness, and possibly pain or bleeding when you try to pass stools.	• Avoid constipation. • Try not to stand for long periods. • An ice pack (frozen peas tied in a polythene bag) held against the piles may ease any itching. • If piles persist, tell the doctor or midwife who may give you an ointment. • Try camomile, dandelion root, nettle, and liquorice (safe in moderation) herbal supplements.
Rash ❸ Usually occurs in women who are overweight and who perspire freely. Can be caused by hormone changes.	Red rash, which usually develops in sweaty skin folds under the breasts or in the groin.	• Wash and dry these areas often. Use unperfumed soap. • Soothe the skin with calamine lotion. • Wear loose cotton clothes.
Sleeping difficulty ❶ ❷ ❸ You may have a problem because the baby is kicking, you keep on needing the lavatory, or the size of the bulge makes it difficult to get comfortable in bed. Your doctor will be reluctant to prescribe sleeping pills.	Having trouble going to sleep in the first place, and finding it hard to get to sleep after waking. Some women find they have very frightening dreams about the birth or the baby. Don't worry about dreams, they do not reflect what will happen.	• Reading, gentle relaxation exercises, or a warm bath before bedtime may help. • Experiment with extra pillows. If you sleep on your side, put a pillow under the top thigh. • Drink camomile tea or limeflower tea before bedtime. • Ask your partner for a head and neck massage, which may relieve tension.

❶ ❷ ❸ The numbers in circles after each complaint relate to the third of pregnancy in which you are most likely to suffer from the problem.

Complaint	Symptoms	What to do
Stretchmarks ❷ ❸ These form if your skin stretches beyond its normal elasticity. Excess weight gain can also cause them. The marks seldom disappear altogether, but they may fade to thin silvery streaks after pregnancy.	Red marks that sometimes appear on the skin of the thighs, stomach, or breasts in pregnancy.	● Avoid putting on weight too rapidly. ● Rubbing moisturizer into the skin may feel cool and soothing, although creams and ointments won't prevent or heal stretchmarks. ● Try a light massage of lavender and neroli essential oils in a carrier oil.
Sweating ❷ ❸ Caused by hormone changes, and because blood flow to the skin increases in pregnancy.	Perspiring after very little exertion, or waking up in the night feeling hot and sweaty.	● Wear loose cotton clothes. ● Avoid synthetic materials. ● Drink plenty of water. ● Open a window at night.
Swollen ankles and fingers ❸ Some swelling (oedema) is normal in pregnancy, as the body holds extra water. This is usually no cause for concern.	Slight swelling in the ankles, especially in hot weather and at the end of the day. This shouldn't cause pain or discomfort. You may also notice stiff, swollen fingers in the morning, and that your rings don't fit.	● Rest often with your feet up. ● Try gentle foot exercises. Hold your hands above your head; flex and stretch each finger. ● See your doctor or midwife. More marked swelling could be a warning sign of pre-eclampsia (see page 38).
Thrush (Candida) ❶ ❷ ❸ Hormone changes in pregnancy increase the chances of getting thrush. It is important to treat this before the baby is born, as it can affect his mouth and make feeding difficult.	A thick white vaginal discharge and severe itching. There may also be soreness and pain when you pass water.	● Stop using soap if you are sore. ● Insert a little live yogurt into the vagina with your finger. ● Avoid all nylon underwear, tight trousers, and vaginal deodorants. ● See your doctor who will probably prescribe cream or pessaries. ● Add a few drops of tea tree oil to a cup of cool water, and apply to the vaginal area.
Tiredness ❶ ❸ Caused by the extra demands that pregnancy makes on your body. Sometimes tiredness can be made worse as a result of worrying too much.	Feeling weary, and wanting to sleep in the day. Needing to sleep longer at night or even suffering from insomnia.	● Rest as much as possible and practise relaxation exercises. ● Go to bed earlier. ● Don't over-exert yourself. ● Olive Bach Flower Remedy is good for general exhaustion.
Vaginal discharge ❶ ❷ ❸ You may notice some increase in the amount of mucus produced by the vagina because of the hormone changes during pregnancy.	Slight increase in clear or white discharge, without soreness or pain.	● Avoid vaginal deodorants and perfumed soap products. ● Wear a light sanitary pad. ● See your doctor if you have any itching, soreness, coloured or smelly discharge.
Varicose veins ❶ ❷ ❸ You are more likely to have them later on in pregnancy, if you are overweight, or if they run in your family. Standing for too long, or sitting cross-legged, can worsen the problem.	Aching legs; the veins in the calves and the thighs become painful and swollen.	● Rest often with your feet up. Try raising the foot of your bed with pillows under the mattress. ● Support tights may help. Put them on before getting up in the morning. ● Exercise your feet. ● Apply a witch hazel compress to the legs.

Keeping fit and relaxed

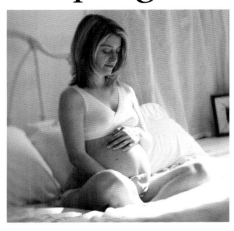

Pregnancy, labour, and birth will make great demands on your body, so the more you can prepare yourself physically, the better you will feel. You will also find it easier to regain your normal shape after the birth. Relaxation exercises are just as important – they will help you cope effectively during labour, and they are invaluable for relieving stress and increasing blood flow to the placenta. Begin exercising as soon as the pregnancy is confirmed, or earlier if you wish.

Exercising sensibly

If you have always enjoyed sport, you can usually carry on during pregnancy, but remember that there are provisos. Pregnancy is not the time to launch into a fitness blitz – just continue with what your body is used to. If you want to keep on going to your dance or exercise class, make sure that the teacher knows you are pregnant. Don't exercise to the point where you get very tired or out of breath.

Avoid any contact sports or sports where there is a danger of hurting your abdomen, such as riding, skiing, and water-skiing. Be extra careful in the first weeks and towards the end of pregnancy, as you may overstretch your ligaments.

Swimming
This is excellent and perfectly safe throughout pregnancy; the water supports your body.

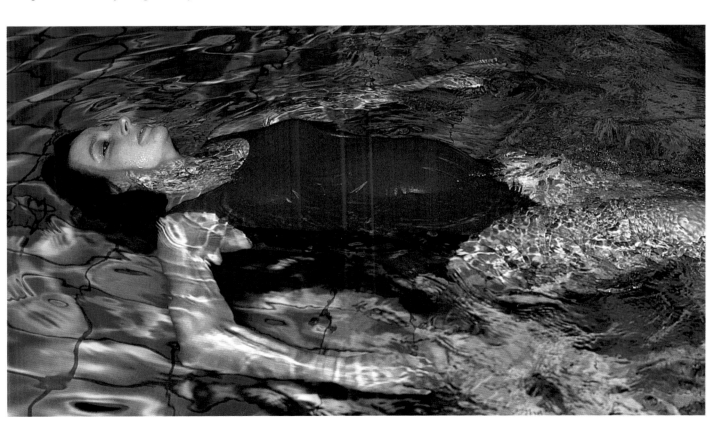

Looking after your body

During pregnancy, it's important to hold yourself well and avoid strain on your back. A good posture becomes increasingly important. You're far more likely to suffer from backache as the weight of the baby pulls you forwards, and so there is a tendency to lean slightly backwards to compensate. This strains the muscles of the lower back and pelvis, especially towards the end of pregnancy.

Be aware of your body, whatever you are doing. Avoid heavy lifting, and try to keep your back as long as possible. Wear low heels, as high heels tend to throw your weight even further forwards.

Protecting your back

To avoid back trouble, it's important to be aware of how you use your body when going about everyday activities, such as lifting a child or carrying heavy bags. The hormones of pregnancy stretch and soften the muscles of the lower back, so they are more easily strained if you bend over, get up too suddenly, or lift something the wrong way. You may need to support the small of your back when you are sitting or lying down.

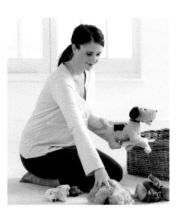

Working at a low level
Do as much as you can at floor level, kneeling down to garden or clean instead of bending over. If you have younger children, have them climb up to your lap for a cuddle instead of lifting them from the floor.

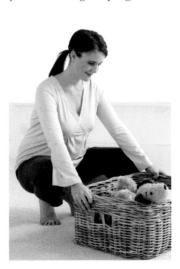

Lifting and carrying
When lifting an object, bend your knees and keep your back as straight as possible, bringing the object close in to your body. Try not to lift something heavy from up high, as you may lose your balance. If you're carrying heavy bags, divide the weight equally on each side. Ask for help whenever possible. This is no time to be proud.

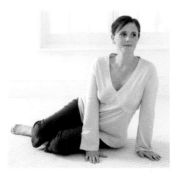

Getting up from lying down
Always turn on your side when you have been lying down. Then move into a kneeling position. Use the strength of your thighs to push yourself up; keep your back straight. During pregnancy you might suffer from bouts of dizziness due to the hormones, so always get up slowly from either sitting or lying down.

Standing well

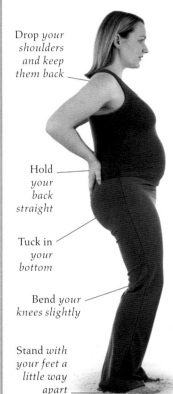

Drop *your shoulders and keep them back*

Hold *your back straight*

Tuck in *your bottom*

Bend *your knees slightly*

Stand *with your feet a little way apart*

Getting it right
You can check that you are standing the right way in front of a full-length mirror. Lengthen and straighten your back, so that the weight of the baby is centred and supported by your thighs, buttocks, and stomach muscles. Try to drop your shoulders to prevent tension in your neck. Distribute your weight evenly on both legs. Lift your chest and ribs and tighten your stomach muscles. This will help prevent backache, and tone up your abdominal muscles, making it easier for you to regain your figure after the birth.

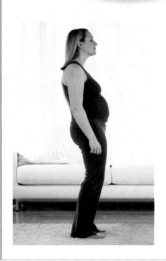

Bad posture
This is an example of posture commonly adopted during pregnancy. As the baby grows, its weight throws you off-balance, so you may over-arch your back and thrust your abdomen forwards. Take extra care to maintain good posture as a bad posture can lead to discomfort and can strain the lower back, and can even cause injury.

The pelvic floor

This is a hammock of muscles that supports the bowel, bladder, and womb. During pregnancy, the muscles go soft and stretchy, and this, together with the weight of the baby pushing down, weakens them, making you feel heavy and uncomfortable. You may also leak a little urine whenever you run, sneeze, cough, or laugh. So, to improve pelvic muscle tone, prevent incontinence, and aid the process of labour, it's essential to strengthen the pelvic floor.

Do this when:

- waiting for a bus or train
- ironing or cooking
- watching TV
- having intercourse
- you have *emptied* your bladder.

Strengthening the pelvic floor

Lie on your back, with your knees bent and your feet flat on the floor. Tighten the muscles, squeezing as if stopping a stream of urine. Imagine you are trying to pull something into your vagina, drawing it in slightly, then pausing, then pulling, until you can go no further. Hold for a moment, then let go gradually. Repeat 10 times. Practise this exercise often – at least three or four times a day. Once you've learned it, you can do it anytime, anywhere, lying down, sitting, or standing. You will also find it useful in the second stage of labour, when knowing how to relax the muscles can reduce the risk of a tear, by easing the passage of the baby through the pelvis.

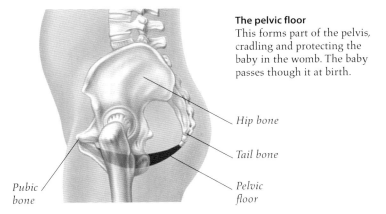

The pelvic floor
This forms part of the pelvis, cradling and protecting the baby in the womb. The baby passes though it at birth.

Hip bone

Tail bone

Pubic bone

Pelvic floor

Pelvic tilt

This exercise helps you move the pelvis with ease, which is good preparation for labour. It also strengthens the stomach muscles and makes the back more flexible. The pelvic tilt is especially helpful if you suffer from backache. You can do the tilt in any position; remember to keep your shoulders still.

Do this when:

- lying on your back
- standing or sitting
- kneeling
- dancing to music.

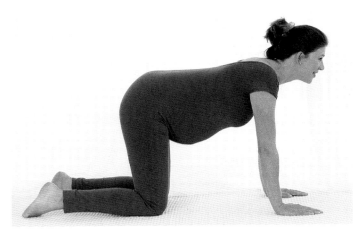

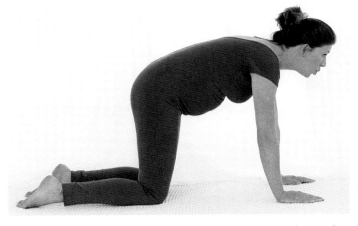

1 Kneel on the floor on your hands and knees. Make sure that your back is flat (you can use a mirror to check this). Your hands should be directly under your shoulders.

2 Pull in your stomach muscles, tighten your buttock muscles, and gently tilt the pelvis forwards, breathing out as you do so. Your back should jump up. Hold this position for a few seconds, then breathe in and let go. Repeat this step several times, so that your pelvis is rocking in and out of the position.

Tailor sitting

Tailor sitting strengthens the back and makes your thighs and pelvis more flexible. It will also improve the blood flow in the lower part of the body, and will encourage your legs to flop apart during labour. The main position below is far easier than it appears. This is because your body becomes more supple during pregnancy.

Thigh strengthener

Sit with your back straight, the soles of your feet together, and your heels touching also. To get used to the position, try to spend 10 minutes sitting like this 2–3 times a day while reading, meditating or simply relaxing. Grasp your ankles, and press your thighs down with your elbows. Hold them there for 20 seconds. Do this several times once you're comfortable. Breathe normally throughout.

Warning

When you are doing any exercise remember these guidelines.
• Don't push yourself beyond your own limits or exhaust yourself.
• If you feel any pain, stop.
• Try not to lie flat on your back in late pregnancy.

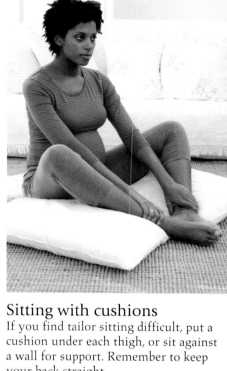

Sitting with cushions

If you find tailor sitting difficult, put a cushion under each thigh, or sit against a wall for support. Remember to keep your back straight.

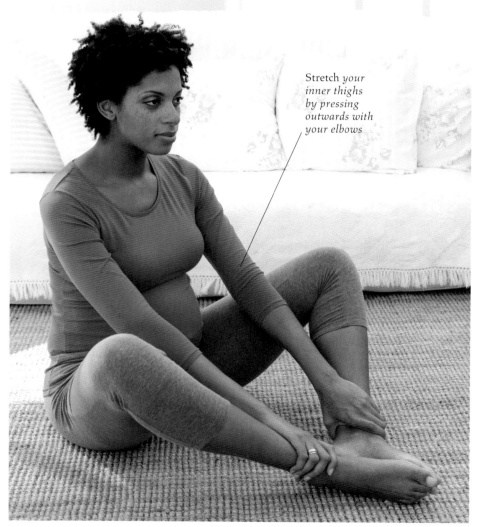

Stretch *your inner thighs by pressing outwards with your elbows*

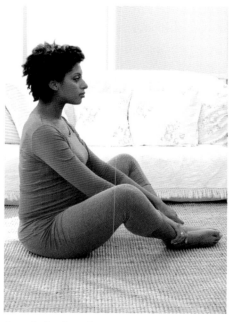

Straight back

Sit up straight and don't bend your back or slump. Look straight ahead, not down at your legs. You may use a wall to support your back if you have difficulty in keeping your back straight.

Squatting

Squatting makes your pelvic joints more flexible, and strengthens the back and thigh muscles. It can also protect your back if you squat down instead of bending over, and is comfortable if you experience backache. Squatting is also a good position to take up during labour.

You may find it difficult to do a full squat at first, so try holding on to a firm support, such as a chair or window ledge, and place a rolled-up rug or blanket under your heels. Get up slowly or you may feel slightly dizzy.

Do this when:
- picking up an object
- taking something from a low drawer
- on the telephone
- there's no chair around
- listening to music.

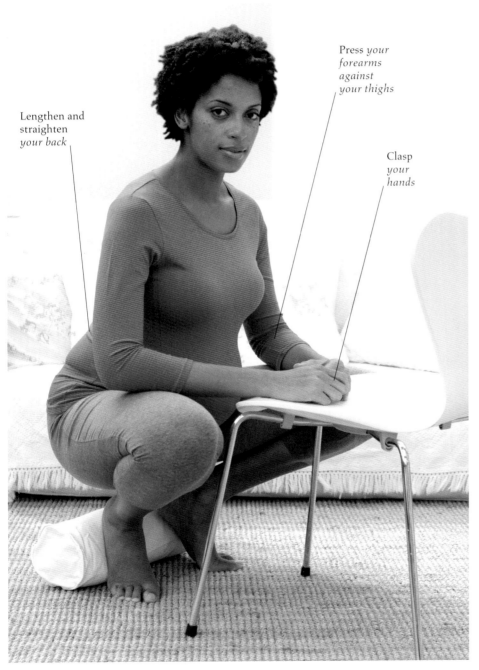

Lengthen and straighten *your back*

Press *your forearms against your thighs*

Clasp *your hands*

With a chair
Stand facing a chair with your feet slightly apart. Keeping your back straight, open out your legs, and squat down, using the chair to support you. Stay in this position as long as it is comfortable to do so. If you find it difficult to keep your feet flat on the ground, place a folded blanket under your heels.

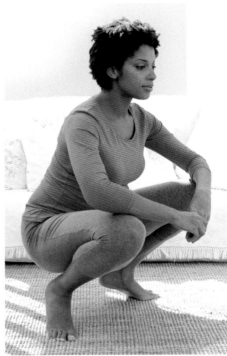

Unsupported
Keeping your back straight, open out your legs and squat down, turning your feet out slightly. Try to keep the balls of your feet flat on the ground, and stretch your inner thighs by pressing outward with your elbows. Stay in this position as long as you find it comfortable.

Relaxation and breathing

These relaxation and breathing exercises are among the most beneficial that you can learn to prepare yourself for childbirth. They are invaluable during labour. Proper breathing will help relax the muscles of your body, which will help you cope with painful contractions, and in doing so, you will conserve vital energy. Practise them regularly so that they become a natural response during labour. These exercises will also help you unwind any time you feel tense or anxious during your pregnancy.

How to relax
At first it's best to practise the following exercises in a warm and quiet room where you won't be disturbed. Later you should find it easy to relax anywhere.

Relax your body
Make yourself comfortable. Lie on your back, propped up by pillows, or on your side, with one leg bent and supported on cushions. Now, tense and relax each muscle of your body in turn, starting with the toes and working upwards. After doing this for several minutes, let your body go limp.

Lying on your side
You may be more comfortable, especially during later pregnancy, lying on your side with one leg bent and supported on cushions. Don't place too many pillows under your head because this is bad for your spine.

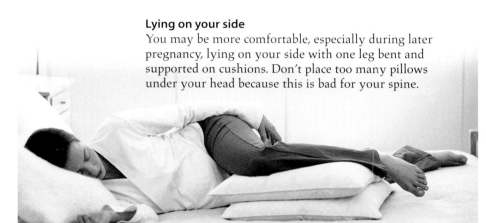

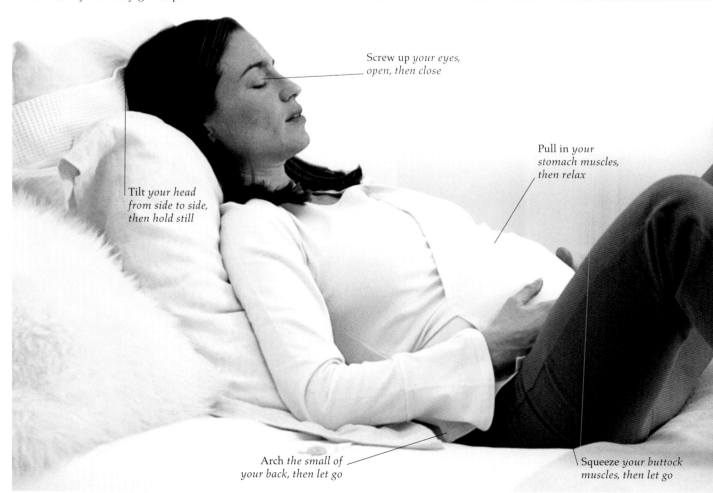

Screw up *your eyes, open, then close*

Tilt *your head from side to side, then hold still*

Pull in *your stomach muscles, then relax*

Arch *the small of your back, then let go*

Squeeze *your buttock muscles, then let go*

Your partner's role
Lean back against your partner so he can support your weight and cuddle you.

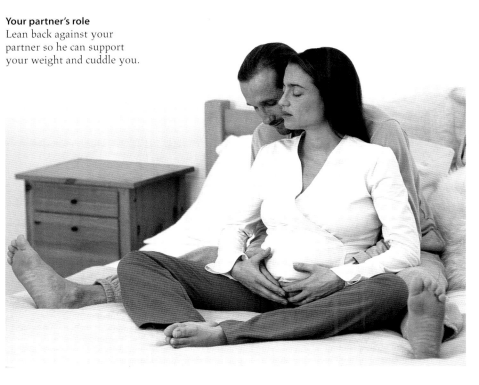

Relax your mind
While relaxing your body, try to calm and empty your mind. Breathe slowly and evenly, sighing each breath out gently. Do not breathe too deeply. Alternatively, repeat a word or sound silently to yourself or concentrate on some pleasant or peaceful image. Try not to follow any thoughts that arise.

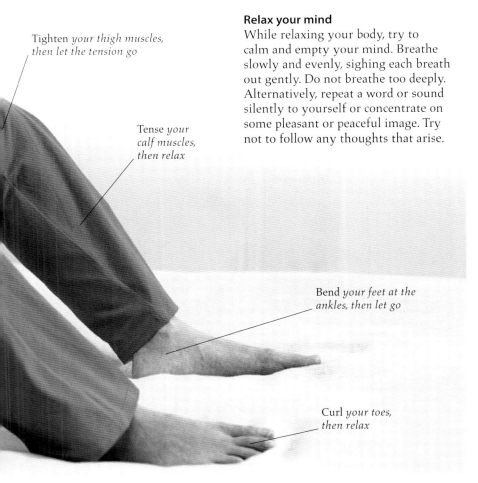

Tighten *your thigh muscles, then let the tension go*

Tense *your calf muscles, then relax*

Bend *your feet at the ankles, then let go*

Curl *your toes, then relax*

Breathing for labour
Practise the different levels of breathing on a regular basis in the weeks leading up to labour. Controlled breathing will help you remain relaxed and calm during labour, and can even control your body during contractions.

Joined breathing
Practising breathing exercises with your partner, a friend, or a family member will help you feel supported. Sit together in a comfortable position so that both of you have your hands over the baby. Take steady breaths focusing primarily on your birthing muscles and try not to tense any other part of your body unnecessarily.

Light breathing
This level of breathing will help you at the height of a contraction. Breathe in and out of your mouth, taking air into the upper part of your lungs only. A partner or friend should put her hands on your shoulder blades and feel them move. Practise making the breaths lighter and lighter, but take an occasional deeper breath when you need one.

Panting
After the first stage of labour, you will want to push, even though the cervix may not be fully opened. You can resist this by taking two short breaths, and then blowing a longer breath out: say "huff, huff, blow" to yourself.

Deep breathing
This helps to calm you at the start and end of contractions. Sit as comfortably as possible. Breathe in deeply through the nose, right to the bottom of your lungs. Your partner or friend should place her hands just above your waistline and feel your ribcage move. Concentrate on breathing slowly and gently out. Let the next in-breath follow naturally.

Warning
Try not to lie flat on your back in the late stages of pregnancy as you can restrict the flow of oxygen to the baby in this position, and you may also feel faint.

Eating for a healthy baby

A baby has only one source of food – you. During pregnancy more than at any other time it is essential that you have as varied and balanced a diet as possible. You do not need to plan this specially, nor do you have to eat for two. Choose from the selection below to ensure that you get all the nutrients you need. Once you are, or know you want to become, pregnant think about how many healthy foods you eat regularly. Do you eat or drink anything that may harm the baby?

Essential nutrients

Calcium

This is important to ensure the healthy development of your baby's bones and teeth, which start to form from around week eight. You will need about twice as much calcium as normal. Good sources include cheese, milk, yogurt, and leafy, green vegetables. However, dairy products are also high in fat so, if possible, choose low-fat varieties, such as skimmed milk. Get the extra calcium you need in a day from: 85g (3oz) hard cheese, 170g (6oz) sardines, 7 slices of bread, or 2 glasses of milk.

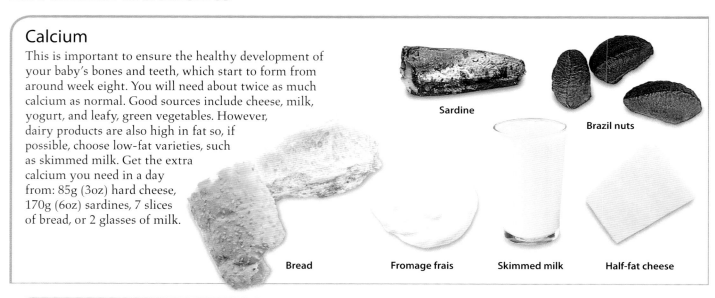

Sardine

Brazil nuts

Bread

Fromage frais

Skimmed milk

Half-fat cheese

Protein

Try to eat a variety of protein-rich foods because your needs increase during pregnancy. Fish, meat, nuts, pulses, and dairy foods all supply protein, but animal sources can also be high in fat so limit your intake of these, and choose lean cuts of meat whenever possible. Avoid lightly cooked or raw eggs and make sure all eggs you buy are fresh.

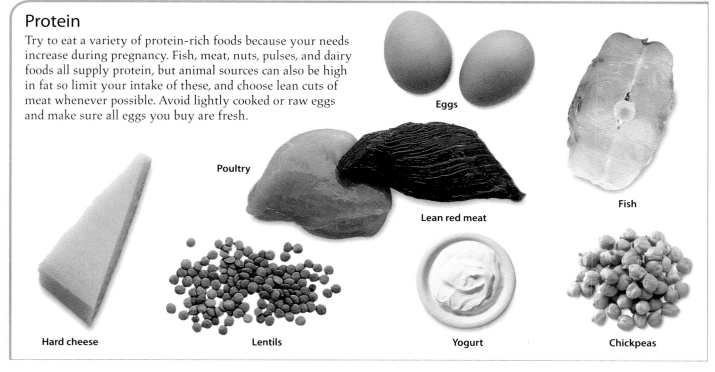

Eggs

Fish

Poultry

Lean red meat

Hard cheese

Lentils

Yogurt

Chickpeas

Vitamin C

This will help build a strong placenta, enable your body to resist infection, and aid the absorption of iron. It is found in fresh fruit and vegetables, and supplies of the vitamin are needed daily as it cannot be stored in the body. A lot of vitamin C is lost by prolonged storage and cooking so only eat fresh produce, and steam green vegetables or eat them raw.

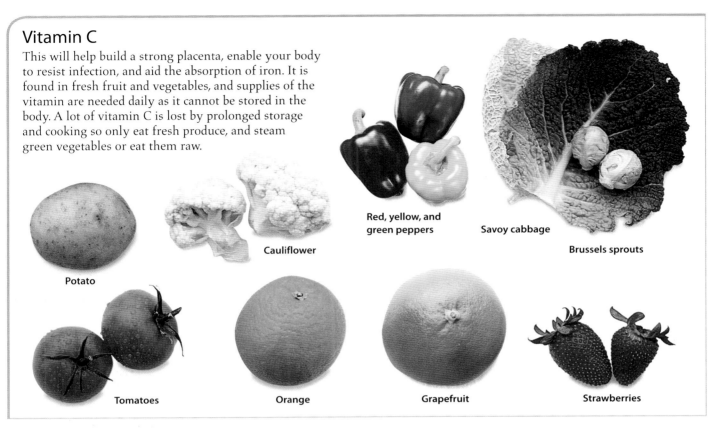

Potato

Cauliflower

Red, yellow, and green peppers

Savoy cabbage

Brussels sprouts

Tomatoes

Orange

Grapefruit

Strawberries

Fibre

Foods rich in fibre should form a large part of your daily diet since constipation (see page 40) is common in pregnancy and fibre will help prevent this. Fruit and vegetables are important sources as you can eat a lot of them every day. Don't rely too heavily on bran because it can hinder the absorption of other nutrients – there are plenty of better sources.

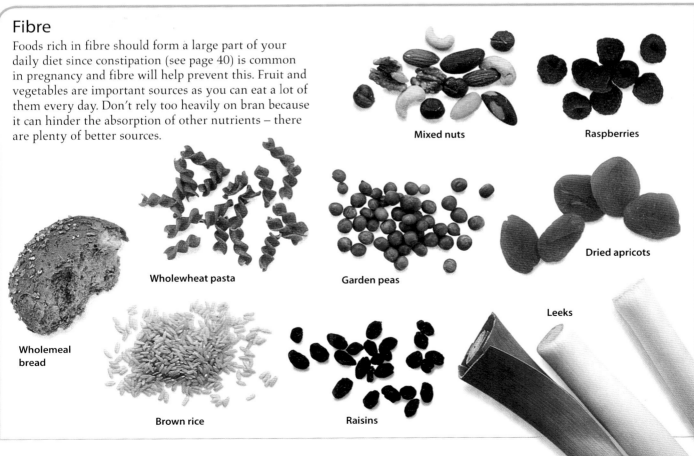

Mixed nuts

Raspberries

Wholewheat pasta

Garden peas

Dried apricots

Wholemeal bread

Brown rice

Raisins

Leeks

Folic acid

Folic acid is a B vitamin that is needed for the development of the baby's central nervous system, especially in the first few weeks (see page 11). During the first three months of pregnancy you need as much as three times the amount of folic acid than normal. Folic acid is destroyed by over-cooking and by prolonged storage, but not by freezing. So, if you can't buy fresh vegetables daily, buy frozen ones instead. Look out for bread and cereals fortified with folic acid – they usually provide between 30 and 100 mcg of folic acid in an average portion. But you cannot get enough folic acid from even the healthiest diet alone – it's essential to take a folic acid supplement as well.

Foods high in folic acid (50–100 mcg/serving) include: cooked black-eyed beans, brussels sprouts, beef extract, yeast extract, cooked kidney, kale, spinach, granary bread, spring greens, broccoli, green beans, wholemeal bread, hazelnuts.

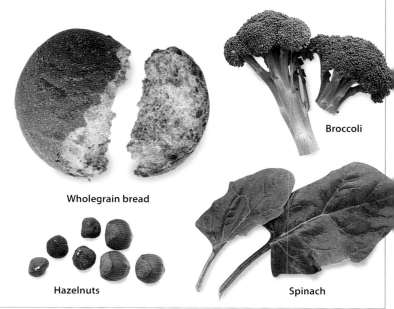

Broccoli

Wholegrain bread

Hazelnuts

Spinach

Iron

Lean red meat and oily fish, such as sardines, are the most easily absorbed sources of iron. Baked beans, spinach, black-eyed beans, wholemeal bread, cereals, and pulses are all iron-rich too, though they are not quite as readily absorbed. Iron is absorbed more easily in the presence of vitamin C, while tea and coffee inhibit iron absorption. So try to avoid drinking tea or coffee with iron-rich foods, especially if you are a vegetarian and cannot eat the most easily absorbed sources of iron – drink blackcurrant or orange juice instead. Avoid liver because it is too rich in vitamin A, which can be harmful in high doses.

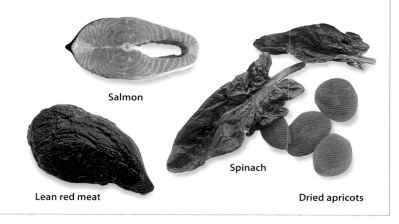

Salmon

Spinach

Lean red meat

Dried apricots

Vegetarian diet

If you eat a variety of protein-rich foods and fresh fruit and vegetables every day, you should provide the baby with all the nutrition she needs to grow. The only nutrient you may lack is iron. This is because the body has great difficulty absorbing iron that comes from plant sources, so you may be given supplements of the mineral to compensate. If you are vegan and don't eat any dairy foods, you may be prescribed calcium, and vitamins D and B12.

Salt

Pregnant women used to be advised to restrict the amount of salt in their diet, as it was believed that too much salt was related to problems such as excess swelling and pregnancy-induced high blood pressure. But it is now thought that there is little evidence to justify such advice.

Fluid

This is essential during pregnancy for keeping your kidneys healthy and avoiding constipation. Water is best.

Top 10 foods

These 10 types of foods are excellent sources of at least one nutrient. Try to eat some of them once a day:
- Cheese, milk, yogurt: *calcium, protein.*
- Dark green, leafy vegetables: *vitamin C, fibre, folic acid.*
- Lean red meat: *protein, iron.*
- Oranges: *vitamin C, fibre.*
- Poultry: *protein, iron.*
- Raisins and prunes: *iron.*
- Sardines: *calcium, protein, iron.*
- White fish: *protein.*
- Wholemeal bread: *protein, fibre, folic acid.*
- Wholewheat pasta and brown rice: *fibre.*

Taking supplements

Folic acid supplements are recommended from the time you stop using contraception until the 12th week of pregnancy. Iron supplements may be prescribed if you are anaemic. If you eat a varied diet with lots of fresh foods, these are probably the only supplements you will need. Avoid supplements containing vitamin A.

Protecting your baby

As the nutrients from your food can cross the placenta to the baby, so can many harmful substances that we regularly eat and drink.

Processed foods

Avoid processed convenience foods, such as processed meals and packet mixes. Processed foods often have sugar and salt added, and they may contain a lot of fat, as well as preservatives, flavourings, and colourings. Read the labels carefully, and choose additive-free products.

Cook-chill foods

Avoid hot canteen foods, pre-cooked supermarket meals, and ready-to-eat poultry (unless served piping hot). These foods may contain bacteria that can be passed to your baby and put her life at risk.

Cheese

Unpasteurized milk and dairy products, and soft matured cheeses, such as Brie made from both pasteurized and unpasteurized milk, can be harmful because of the risk of listeria infection, so it's best to avoid them. Listeriosis may be a cause of recurrent miscarriage.

Coffee, tea, and hot chocolate

Caffeine, a substance found in all these drinks, may affect your baby's growth if taken in high levels. Try to have no more than three cups of caffeine-containing drinks a day, and if possible, cut them out altogether. Drink plenty of water instead.

Herbal teas

If you want to drink herbal teas in pregnancy, it is sensible to check first with your doctor or health advisor. Most pre-packaged teas won't harm the baby but some may have unwanted effects, such as having a stimulating effect on the uterus.

Sugar

Sugary foods, such as cakes, biscuits, jam, and fizzy drinks, are low in essential nutrients, and can make you put on excess weight during your pregnancy. During pregnancy, sugar is rapidly absorbed into the blood and requires a large release of insulin to maintain normal levels. It is therefore best to try to get your energy from starchy carbohydrates, such as wholemeal bread and pasta, and cut down on sweet things.

Alternatives to alcohol

Any alcohol that you drink during pregnancy is passed through the placenta into your baby's bloodstream, and can be harmful. So it's best to cut out alcohol altogether. Even beers and wines that claim to be alcohol free or low in alcohol are not necessarily free from undesirable additives and chemicals.

Essential fatty acids (EFA)

Long chain, polyunsaturated fatty acids are vital for the development of your baby's brain, nervous system, and retina. The fetus relies on an efficient supply from the mother across the placenta, and your baby receives this after birth, from breast milk. Essential fatty acids aren't synthesized by the body, so it's important to include EFA-rich foods in your diet, especially during pregnancy. Oily fish, such as salmon, tuna, and mackerel, are by far the richest source but they do contain pollutants, so you are advised to eat no more than two portions a week and to avoid large predator fish such as swordfish, shark, and marlin, which may contain high levels of mercury. Nuts, seeds, wholegrain cereals, and dark green, leafy vegetables are other sources of essential fatty acids.

Genetically modified foods

At present there is not enough evidence to be certain that genetically modified foods are safe. Neither is there enough evidence to show that they could be harmful for either you or your baby.

Genetic engineering is not a precise process. No-one can be sure that the inserted gene will not interact with other genes or that it will have precisely and solely the action it is expected to have. For example, many vegetables, including potatoes and tomatoes, have poisonous ancestors. The fact that the modern potato is not poisonous does not necessarily mean that it has lost the toxic gene, only that the gene is not at present being expressed. There is at least a theoretical possibility that genetic engineering of a potato might reactivate a dormant ancestral gene for toxicity.

It is likely to be some time before there is evidence to prove conclusively whether or not GM foods are safe, so if you are at all concerned, the best thing is to play safe and avoid them.

Cravings

It's common in pregnancy to find that you suddenly develop a taste for certain foods, such as pickled onions or ice cream. You can go ahead and indulge yourself within reason, provided it isn't too fattening, and doesn't cause indigestion.

Practical preparations

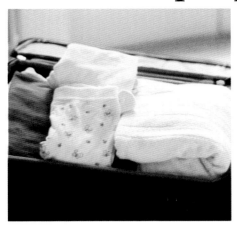

About a month before your delivery date, check that everything is ready for the baby and buy food and other essentials to make life easier for you after the birth. Now is the time to pack for hospital, or to think about what you need if you are having a home birth. Some hospitals provide a list of what to take with you, and even some of the items on it, so check with your hospital before you start making your arrangements. Keep your bag packed and near the door.

Helpful things for labour

All the items below may be useful in labour and immediately after birth. Pack them separately as you will probably need them in a hurry.

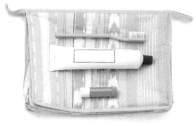

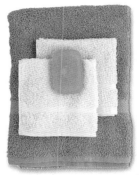

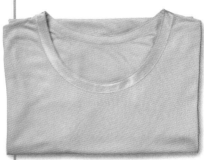

Baggy T- shirt or an old nightdress
You will also need a front-opening nightdress for after the birth.

Spongebag, toothbrush and paste, lipsalve

Thick socks
You may become cold in the later stages of labour.

Small natural sponge
Moisten it, and suck on it if your mouth is dry.

Dark-coloured towel, two face flannels, soap

Deodorant

Also

- your maternity notes
- a hot-water bottle
- books, magazines, MP3 player, or a personal stereo
- camera or video equipment
- mobile phone and mobile phone charger
- food and drink for your partner
- anything else that you have practised with at antenatal classes and would like to use during labour, such as a bean bag or birthing ball – check availability with your hospital first.

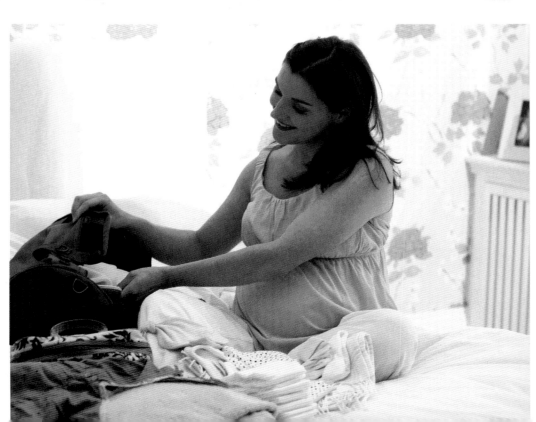

Home birth

There are several preconditions for a home birth (see page 32), so talk to your midwife if you are thinking about one. This includes a warm room, with easy access to hot water, a lavatory, and a telephone. You should also be within easy reach of a hospital, in case any kind of complications arise.

What you will need:
- bed with a firm mattress
- two clean surfaces nearby, one for equipment, the other for the midwife's examination of the baby after birth
- clean towels, sheets, and blankets
- plenty of cushions and pillows
- plastic sheets to protect the bed and the surrounding floor
- one medium-sized plastic bowl
- large rubbish bags
- two packets of stick-on sanitary pads, one superabsorbent
- baggy T-shirt or nightdress
- front-opening nightdress, bra, pants
- nappy, vest, stretchsuit or nightie, and blanket for the baby.

Making the bed

Put a clean undersheet on the bed. Cover this with a plastic sheet and another clean undersheet, which can be taken off after birth, leaving the bed freshly made underneath.

For after the birth

You will need a few essentials after the birth, but your partner can bring these along later if you go into labour unexpectedly. The hospital will probably provide all you need for the baby during your stay.

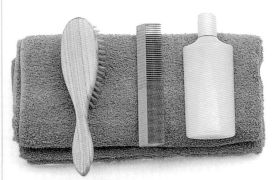

Brush, comb, shampoo, towel

Breast pads
Slip these inside your bra to absorb leaking milk. Shaped ones are best.

Also

- tissues
- face wash
- hairdryer, for drying your stitches, as well as your hair
- big plastic bags for dirty washing.

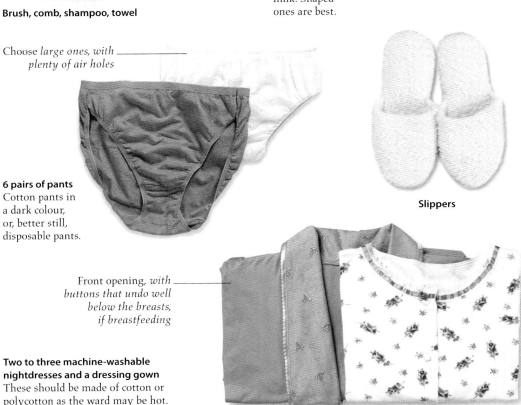

Choose *large ones, with plenty of air holes*

6 pairs of pants
Cotton pants in a dark colour, or, better still, disposable pants.

Front opening, *with buttons that undo well below the breasts, if breastfeeding*

Two to three machine-washable nightdresses and a dressing gown
These should be made of cotton or polycotton as the ward may be hot.

Slippers

Coming home

You will need to leave out a set of clothes for your partner to bring when it's time for you to leave hospital. Don't choose anything too tight fitting; you will not be back to your pre-pregnancy size. The baby needs clothes for coming home in, too, so set aside these things:

- two nappies (don't forget baby cleaning equipment)
- vest
- stretchsuit or nightie
- cardigan and hat
- blanket (for cold weather).

Labour and birth

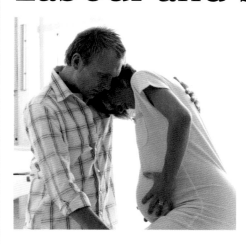

At last, the labour is beginning. You will feel excited, yet apprehensive, about how your labour will progress. You will feel more confident if you have prepared yourself well so that you understand what is happening to your body at each stage of labour. Giving birth can be an immensely fulfilling experience, and keeping calm and relaxed is key. Practise your relaxation and breathing techniques beforehand to help you stay calm during the contractions and cope with the pain.

Knowing you are in labour

You may worry that you won't recognize labour when it comes. This is most unlikely. Although it is possible to confuse the first labour contractions with the contractions that may occur in the last weeks of pregnancy, you will probably be able to tell if labour is imminent, as it is heralded by a number of signs.

Signs of labour

A show
The plug of thick, blood-stained mucus that blocks the neck of the womb in pregnancy usually passes out of the vagina, either before or during the early stages of labour.
What to do The show may happen a few days before labour starts, so wait until you have regular pains in your stomach or back, or your waters break, before ringing the hospital or midwife.

Your waters break
The bag of fluid that surrounds the baby can break at any time during labour. It may be a sudden flood, but it's far more common to notice a trickle of fluid as the baby's head has often engaged – this stems the tide.
What to do Call the hospital or midwife at once. You need to go to hospital even if you don't have any contractions, as there is a risk of infection. In the meantime, wear a sanitary towel to absorb the flow.

Contractions
These may start off as a dull backache, or you may have shooting pains down your thighs. As time goes on, you will probably have contractions in your stomach, rather like bad period pains.
What to do When the contractions seem to be regular, time them. If you think you are in labour, call the hospital or midwife. Unless contractions are coming frequently (every five minutes), or are very painful, there is no need to go to hospital immediately. A first labour usually lasts about 12 to 14 hours, and it is often better to spend several hours of this time at home. Remain calm. Perhaps relax in a warm bath if your waters haven't broken, or eat a light snack. The hospital will probably suggest you wait until the contractions are strong and occurring every five minutes or so before you leave home.

False starts
Throughout pregnancy, the womb contracts. In the last weeks, these Braxton Hicks contractions become stronger, so you may think you are in labour. But true labour contractions occur very regularly, and grow stronger and more frequent, so you should be able to tell when the real thing begins. Occasionally contractions start and then die away. Keep moving – in time they will get going again.

Timing contractions

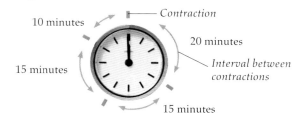

10 minutes

Contraction

20 minutes

15 minutes

Interval between contractions

15 minutes

Time contractions over an hour, noting the length of each one. They should become stronger and more frequent, and last for at least 40 seconds as labour becomes established. The diagram shows the kind of intervals between contractions you may have in early labour.

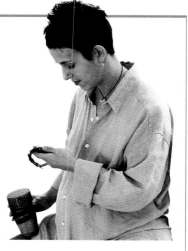

The first stage

During this stage, the muscles of your womb contract to open up the cervix (neck of the womb) to allow the baby to pass through at birth. It takes an average of 10 to 12 hours for a first baby.

Don't be surprised if at some time in the first stage you suddenly feel panic-stricken. You may even find yourself rushing around trying to finish last-minute tasks. However well-prepared you are, the feeling that your body has been taken over by a process that you can't control can be frightening. Stay calm and try to go with your body. It is now that you will most appreciate having your partner or a good friend by your side, especially if they know about labour and have gone to antenatal classes.

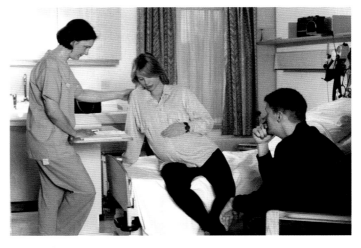

During admission
A midwife will review your maternity notes and ask you about your contractions.

Admission to hospital

At the hospital, a midwife will carry out several routine admission procedures. Your partner can stay with you during this process. If you are having the baby at home, your community midwife will probably prepare you for the birth in much the same way.

The midwife's questions

The midwife will check your notes and will ask if you think your waters have broken and whether you have had a show. She will also ask you about your contractions: when they started, how frequent they are, what they feel like, and how long each one lasts.

Checking you

After you have changed into the hospital gown or your own clothes for the birth, the midwife will take your blood pressure, temperature, and pulse, and may give you an internal examination to check how far the neck of the womb has opened.

Checking the baby

The midwife will check the baby's position by feeling your abdomen, and she will listen to his heartbeat with a sonicaid. She may attach a heart monitor to you for 20 minutes or so, to record the baby's heartbeat and make sure that he is getting enough oxygen during contractions.

Group B streptococcal infection

About 10 per cent of women are carriers of Group B streptococcus, a bacterium that can cause serious infections in newborn infants, particularly those whose birthweight is low. The risk of infection is increased if the membranes rupture before contractions have begun. If you are a known carrier, or if you go into premature labour, or your membranes rupture before labour begins, you may be given an antibiotic during labour to protect you and your baby from infection.

Internal examinations

The midwife may give you regular internal examinations to check the position of the baby and how much the cervix is dilating (opening up). Ask if you are not told – it is encouraging to find that the cervix is widening, but this may not happen at a steady rate.

The examination is usually done between contractions, so tell the midwife if you feel one coming. Try to relax as much as possible, and take slow deep breaths to minimize any discomfort. You can also use the gas and air inhaler.

The cervix in labour

This is normally kept closed by a ring of muscles. Other muscles run from the cervix up and over the womb. These contract during labour, drawing the cervix into the womb, and then stretching it so it is wide enough for the baby's head to pass through. The tough cervix is gradually softened by hormone changes.

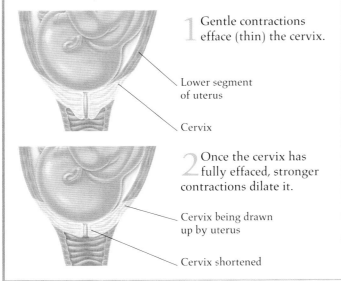

1 Gentle contractions efface (thin) the cervix.

Lower segment of uterus

Cervix

2 Once the cervix has fully effaced, stronger contractions dilate it.

Cervix being drawn up by uterus

Cervix shortened

Positions for the first stage

Try a variety of positions during the first stage of labour as different positions will probably be comfortable at different times. Practise these positions beforehand so that you can follow your body's natural cues with ease.

Your birth partner

If you do not have a partner, or if he cannot be at the birth, choose your mother, sister, or a friend to be with you. Research shows that effective labour support can actually shorten labour and reduce the risk of complications.

Stay upright

As far as possible, try to maintain an upright position. This keeps pressure on the base of the uterus and helps to stimulate strong contractions.

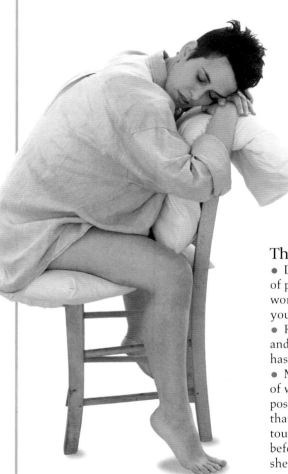

Early labour
During early contractions, support yourself on a nearby surface, such as a wall, chair seat, or the hospital bed.

The birth partner's role

- During contractions give her plenty of praise, comfort, and support. Don't worry if she becomes annoyed with you; you are important.
- Remind her of the relaxation and breathing techniques she has learned.
- Mop her brow, give her sips of water, suggest a change of position, or do anything else that helps. Learn what sort of touch and massage she likes beforehand, but remember that she might not feel like having a massage during the birth. Always take your cues from her.
- Act as a mediator between her and the hospital staff, letting them know, for example, if she decides she needs pain relief.

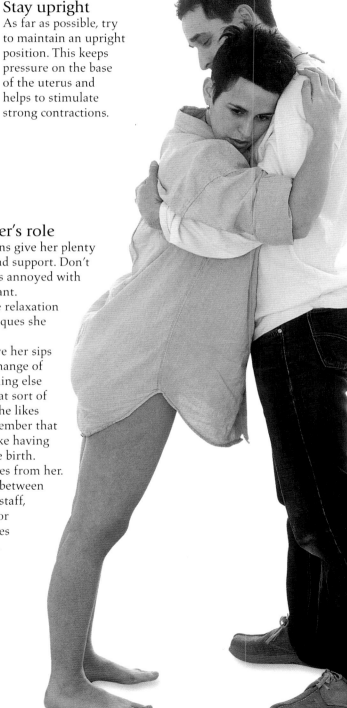

Water births

Immersion in water, warmed to body-heat temperature, can help you to relax and ease pain during labour. Some hospitals provide birthing pools, and it is also possible to hire a portable pool for a home birth. If you decide that you want to use a birthing pool in labour, it is essential for you to have a midwife with water-birth experience.

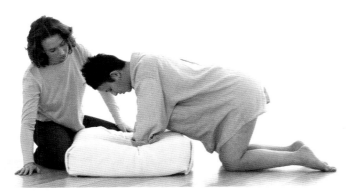

On all fours

Kneel down on your hands and knees on the floor (you may find a mattress more comfortable), and tilt your pelvis to and fro. Do not arch your back. Between contractions, relax forwards and rest your head in your arms.

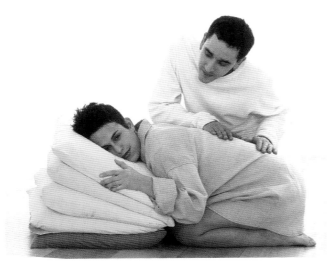

Lower back massage/kneel forwards

This will relieve your backache. Your partner should massage you at the base of your spine, using the heel of his hand to make firm, circular movements. Kneel down with your legs apart and relax on a pile of cushions. Sit to one side between contractions.

Breathing for the first stage

Deep even breaths	Light breaths	Deep even breaths

IN

OUT

Peak

Length of contraction

At the beginning and end of a contraction, breathe deeply and evenly, in through the nose, and out of the mouth. When the contraction peaks, try a lighter, shallower kind of breathing – in and out breaths both through your mouth. Don't do this for too long as you will begin to feel dizzy.

Birthing balls

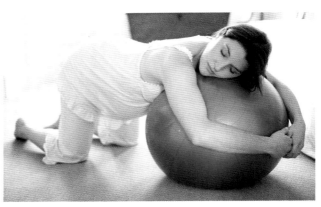

A birthing ball can help you find a comfortable, supported position during contractions. You may want to kneel and lean over it, or sit on it and lean forward over a stack of pillows on your bed so that you are virtually lying down and yet can still rock your hips backwards and forwards. This can be especially helpful during backache labour (see below). You can still use the birthing ball during fetal monitoring. Some hospitals also offer birthing balls when they administer light epidural anaesthesia.

Ways to help yourself

- Keep moving between contractions; this helps you cope with the pain. During contractions, take up a comfortable position.
- Try to stay as upright as possible, so the baby's head sits firmly on the cervix, making your contractions stronger and more effective.
- Concentrate on your breathing. This will calm you and take your mind off a contraction.
- Relax between contractions (see pages 48–9) to save energy for when you need it.
- Sing, or even moan and groan, to release pain.
- Look at a fixed spot or object to help take your mind off a contraction.
- Take one contraction at a time, and don't think about the contractions to follow. Perhaps see each contraction as a wave, which you have to ride over to reach the baby.
- Pass water often, so your bladder doesn't get in the way of the baby.

Backache labour

When the baby is facing towards your abdomen instead of away from it, her head tends to press against your spine, causing backache. To relieve pain:
- during contractions lean forwards with your weight supported, such as on all fours, to take the baby's weight off your back; rock your pelvis to and fro, and move around between contractions
- ask your partner to massage your back.

Transition

The most difficult time in labour is often at the end of the first stage, when contractions are strongest. They last about a minute and may be only a minute apart, so there is little time to rest after one ends before the next is upon you. This phase is known as transition. You will be tired, and may feel tearful, excitable, or just bad-tempered. You may also lose all sense of time and doze off between contractions. Feeling sick, vomiting, and shivering are common in this phase.

Eventually, you may experience a strong urge to push. However, if you start to push too early, before the cervix is fully dilated, it can become swollen. It's important that you tell the midwife when you first feel the urge to push. She will probably examine you to determine whether your cervix is fully dilated. If it is not, she may ask you to pant during contractions (see box, above right) to help you resist the urge to push until the cervix has dilated to about 10cm (4in). If you wish to change position at this stage, kneeling down and leaning forwards with your head resting on your arms and your bottom in the air can help you resist the urge to push.

If your waters have not yet broken, they will almost certainly do so during transition. You may feel a gush or only a trickle when this happens. Without the amniotic sac, the baby's head presses directly on the bottom of the uterus, and labour often speeds up.

Breathing for transition

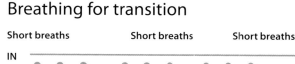
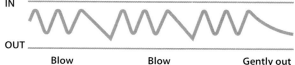

If you want to push too early say "huff, huff, blow" to yourself, taking two short in- and out-breaths, blowing a longer out-breath. When the need to push fades, breathe out slowly and evenly.

The birth partner's role

- Try to relax her, encourage her, and wipe away any perspiration; if she doesn't want to be touched, stay back.
- Breathe with her through contractions.
- Put thick socks on her feet if they start to shake, and gently hold them still.

The cervix in labour

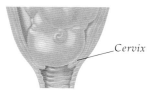
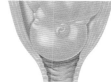

Cervix

At 7cm (2¾in), the midwife feels the cervix well stretched out around the baby's head.

When the midwife can't feel the cervix (at about 10cm/4in), you are fully dilated.

The second stage

Once the cervix has dilated and you can push, the second stage of labour has begun. You can now add your own efforts to the powerful contractions of the womb, and help push the baby out. If the baby is lying in a slightly different position you may not feel this urge to push, but the midwife will guide you so that you push when it is most needed. She will also help you find the most comfortable position in which to push. Even though the contractions are stronger, they don't feel as bad as before. This stage usually lasts about an hour for a first baby.

Breathing for the second stage

When you want to push (this may happen several times during a contraction), take a deep breath and hold it for a short time as you bear down, if this helps the push; it's important to do what your body tells you. Between pushes, take a few deep calming breaths to relax.

Positions for delivery

Try to remain as upright as possible when you are pushing during the second stage of labour, so you are working with gravity rather than against it. This will help the delivery process.

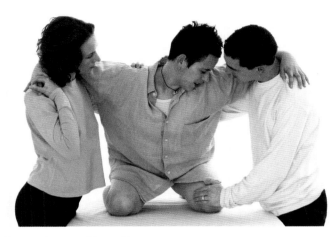

Squatting and kneeling

Squatting is an excellent position for delivery, because it opens the pelvis wide and uses gravity to help push out the baby. But unless you have practised it beforehand (see page 47), you may find it tiring after a while. If your partner sits on the edge of a chair with his legs apart, you can squat between his knees, resting your arms on his thighs for support.

Kneeling may be less tiring than squatting (see above), and is also a good position to push from. A helper on each side will make you feel more stable. You may also find kneeling down on all fours comfortable; keep your back straight.

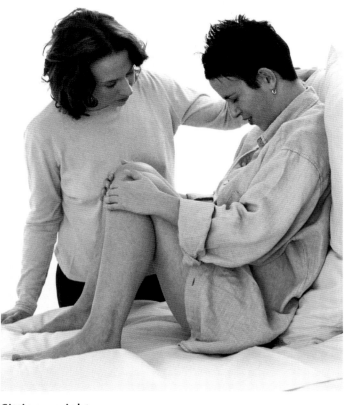

Sitting upright

A common delivery position is to sit on the bed propped up by pillows, a beanbag, or a wedge. Keep your chin down, and grip your knees as you push. Relax between contractions.

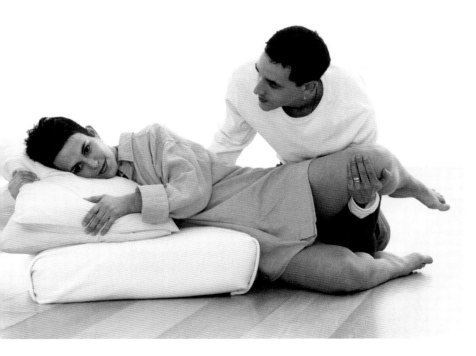

Side lying

A side lying position is good if you need to slow labour down. Your partner can support your upper leg.

Ways to help yourself

- Push steadily during a contraction.
- Try to relax the muscles of your pelvic floor (see page 45).
- Keep your face relaxed.
- Don't worry about trying to control your bowels, or leakage from the bladder.
- Rest between contractions, so you save all your energy for pushing.

The birth partner's role

- Try to relax her between the contractions, and give encouragement.
- Tell her when you can see the baby's head emerging.

The birth

The climax of labour has now arrived. After all your hard work, you can actually touch your baby's head for the first time as she emerges. Your partner's company may calm you and give you confidence during the long hours of labour and delivery. If you have both been to childbirth classes you have trained together for this moment. He can support you and remind you of breathing and relaxation techniques. The sheer force of the muscular contractions can make you feel like you have little control over your body – your partner can help by rubbing your back, sponging your brow, and counting you through the contractions so that you can push with them. His involvement will help him to feel that he is a more integral part of the birthing process. If your partner is not able to be there, you will appreciate the help of a close friend or relative, or even a doula. You will probably feel a great sense of physical relief once your baby is born. There may also be tears of joy, and a feeling of great tenderness towards your baby.

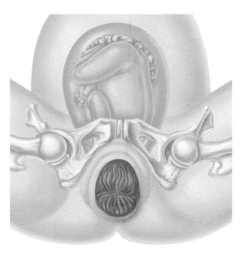

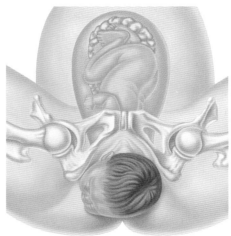

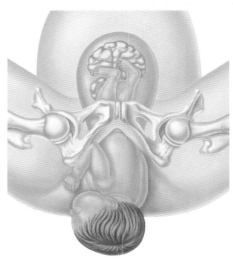

1 The baby's head moves nearer the vaginal opening, until eventually the midwife will be able to see the bulge where it is pressing against the pelvic floor. Soon the head itself will be seen, moving forwards with each contraction, and perhaps slipping back slightly as the contraction fades. Don't be discouraged if this happens – it is perfectly normal.

When the head "crowns" (the top is visible), the midwife will ask you not to push because if the head is born too quickly your skin might tear. So, relax, and pant like a dog for a few seconds. If there is a risk of a serious tear, or the baby is distressed, you will have an episiotomy (see page 66).

As the baby's head widens the vaginal opening, there will be a stinging feeling, but this will only last for a short while, and will soon be followed by numbness because the tissues have been stretched so much.

2 The head is born face down. The midwife will probably check the umbilical cord, to make sure it isn't looped around the baby's neck (if it is, the cord can usually be slipped over the head when the body is delivered). Then, the baby turns her head to one side so that it is in line with her shoulders. The midwife cleans her eyes, nose, and mouth, and, if necessary, sucks out any fluid from her upper air passages through a tube.

3 The body comes sliding out within the next two contractions. The midwife will usually deliver her on to your stomach, still joined to the cord. Your baby will probably look rather blue at first, covered in vernix, with streaks of blood on her skin. She may be crying. If she is breathing normally, you can hold her at once, otherwise the midwife may clear her airways again and, if required, give her oxygen.

"I'm very worried about permanently damaging myself during the birth of my baby. Is there any danger of this occurring?"
You won't damage yourself as you push during the birth. The vaginal walls are elastic, and made of folds, so they can stretch to allow the baby through.

"Should I breastfeed my baby immediately after the birth?" Q&A
Try offering your baby the breast and leave the decision up to her. Although there won't be any milk yet, a newborn baby's urge to suck is often strong, and she will find the sucking comforting.

The third stage

During, or just after, the birth you will probably be given an injection in your thigh, of a drug called syntometrine, which makes the womb contract strongly, and delivers the placenta immediately. Otherwise, you can lose more blood and there is a risk of haemorrhaging if you wait for the placenta to be expelled naturally. If you are concerned about this, talk to the midwife beforehand.

To deliver the placenta the midwife puts her hand on your stomach and gently pulls the umbilical cord with her other hand to help the placenta come away. Later, she will check the placenta to ensure it is complete.

After the birth

You will be cleaned up, and stitched if necessary. The midwife will weigh and measure the baby and check if all is well. The baby may be given vitamin K to prevent a rare bleeding disorder. The umbilical cord will probably be clamped and cut soon after the delivery, especially if syntometrine has been given. Your hormone levels will drop markedly the minute your baby is born and the placenta is delivered because the placenta was the hormone production factory in your body.

The Apgar score

Immediately after birth, the midwife will assess the baby's breathing, heart rate, skin colour, movements, and response to stimulation, and give her an Apgar score of between 0 and 10. Most babies score between 7 and 10. The test is done again about five minutes later, so even if the score was initially low, it should have improved the second time around.

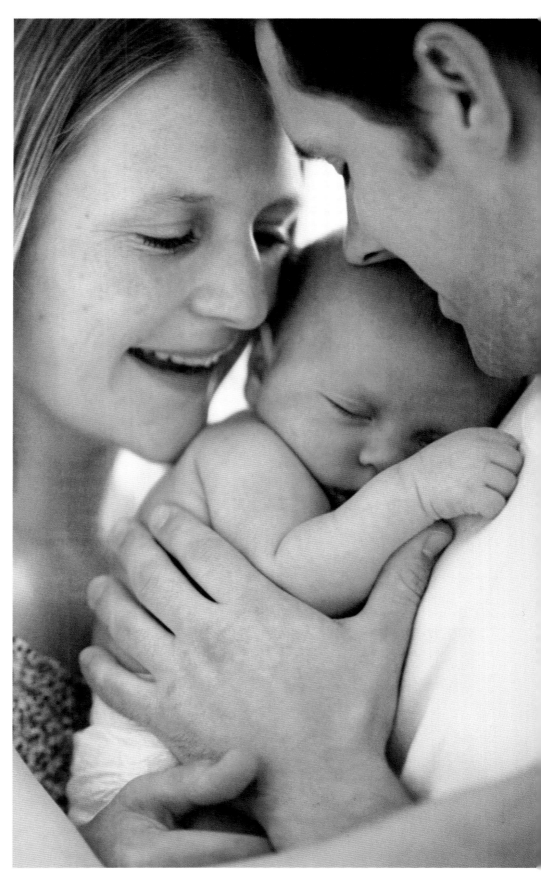

Becoming a family
After the birth, you and your partner can relax and spend a few quiet moments with your baby.

Pain relief

Although labour is not usually pain free, the pain does have a purpose: every contraction brings you one step nearer the birth of your baby. However determined you may be not to have pain relief, do try to keep an open mind. Whether you need it or not depends very much on your labour and your ability to deal with pain. You may be able to cope better during labour using the self-help methods on pages 59 and 61. Remember that pain is always worse if you try to fight it. But if the discomfort is more than you can bear, ask for pain relief. There are several options that are available to you.

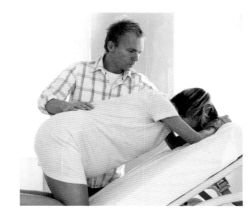

Epidural

An epidural is an anaesthetic that relieves pain by temporarily numbing the nerves in the lower body. It can be especially good in a backache labour. Most hospitals offer epidurals.

The epidural must be timed very carefully, so its effect has worn off by the second stage. Otherwise you will take longer to push the baby out, and this increases the chances of having an episiotomy and an assisted delivery.

What happens

An epidural takes about 20 minutes to set up. You will be asked to tuck your knees up under your chin, so that your back is rounded. The anaesthetic is injected through a tube into your lower back. This is left in place, so that you can be given top-ups as necessary; the anaesthetic wears off in about two hours. You will have a drip in your arm, and be monitored continually. Movements may be restricted but some hospitals offer an epidural that allows you to walk around.

Effects

You If the epidural works properly, you should feel no pain, and remain fully aware of what is happening. Some women feel faint and have a headache that may last for a few hours afterwards. Your legs may feel rather heavy for several hours.
The baby None.

Entonox
(gas and air)

This is a mixture of oxygen and nitrous oxide. Entonox gives effective pain relief to most women. It is easy to administer, quick-acting, and completely safe for your baby.

What happens

You inhale the gas through a hand-held tube, so you control it. It takes about half a minute to reach a peak so you need to breathe deeply when a contraction starts.

Effects

You Entonox may not provide enough pain relief. You may feel light-headed or sick while inhaling the gas.
The baby None.

Pethidine

This is given by injection early in the first stage of labour. The pain-relief effect is small but it will help to calm and relax you during labour.

What happens

Pethidine will probably be given by injection in your buttock or thigh. It takes about 20 minutes to work and its effect lasts about two to three hours.

Effects

You It makes some women feel out of control, confused, or "high", while others feel relaxed and drowsy. You may experience vomiting.
The baby If given too close to the birth, it can slow the baby's breathing and make her sleepy.

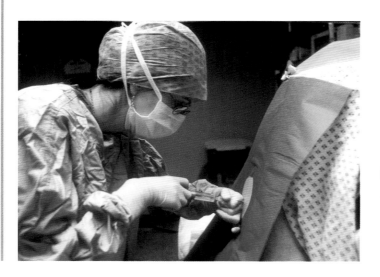

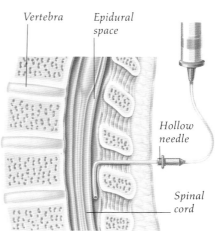

Vertebra *Epidural space*

Hollow needle

Spinal cord

Giving the anaesthetic A hollow needle is inserted between the vertebrae of your spine. A fine tube is passed through the needle, and local anaesthetic fed directly into this. The picture (far left) shows a woman in labour being administered an epidural.

TENS

This treatment lessens pain and stimulates the body's natural system of pain relief by delivering impulses of electrical current into your body. It helps to practise with the TENS machine in the last month before the birth. If your hospital doesn't have one to lend you, ask your local branch of the NCT if they can help.

What happens
Four pads containing electrodes are stuck on your back, over the nerves that supply the womb. These pads are joined by wires to a hand-held control with which you regulate the strength, frequency, and duration of the electric current to suit yourself.

Effects
You TENS can lessen the pain considerably for some women, especially if used from early labour. If labour is very painful, TENS probably won't be sufficient.
The baby None.

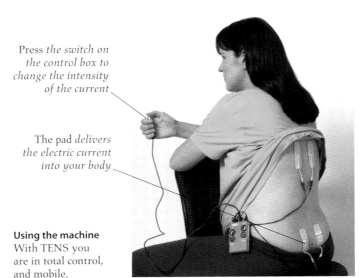

Press *the switch on the control box to change the intensity of the current*

The pad *delivers the electric current into your body*

Using the machine
With TENS you are in total control, and mobile.

Monitoring

Throughout labour your baby's heartbeat will be monitored to make sure she is coping well during the entire process and that any signs of distress can be detected as early as possible. This will be done with the help of a sonicaid or an electronic fetal monitor.

Sonicaid
The midwife places the instrument on your stomach at regular intervals throughout labour to listen to the baby's heartbeat.

Electronic fetal monitoring (EFM)
This is a way of recording the baby's heartbeat and your contractions using sophisticated electronic equipment. Some hospitals routinely monitor women throughout labour, others only at intervals unless:
- your labour is induced (see page 66)
- you are having an epidural
- you have a problem or condition that puts you or your baby at risk
- the baby is distressed at any time.

EFM is not painful. The procedure is perfectly safe for both you and your baby. If your doctor or midwife suggests continual monitoring it is probably because they believe it is in the best interests of your baby.

Your baby's heart rate is monitored with a small plastic circular device. One or two elastic belts are placed around your abdomen to secure the monitors. You should be able to stand, sit, or squat with the monitors in place, and some hospitals even have monitors that allow you to walk around and be monitored by radio signals.

How Electronic Fetal Monitoring works

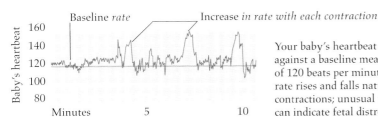

Baseline *rate*   Increase *in rate with each contraction*

Your baby's heartbeat is recorded against a baseline measurement of 120 beats per minute. The heart rate rises and falls naturally with contractions; unusual variations can indicate fetal distress.

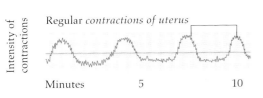

Regular *contractions of uterus*

A separate reading records the frequency and duration of each contraction. This can detect infrequent or irregular contractions and can be useful with an epidural when you can't feel contractions.

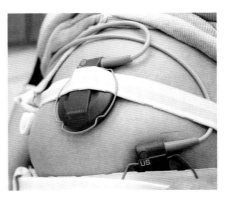

Continuous monitoring
Two monitors strapped to your stomach continuously monitor the baby's heart rate and your contractions.

Special procedures

Episiotomy	Assisted delivery	Induction
This small cut widens the vaginal opening and prevents a tear. Some hospitals perform episiotomies more often than others, so speak to your midwife about the trends in your hospital.	Sometimes the baby has to be helped out with forceps or by suction (vacuum). Forceps are used only when the cervix is fully dilated, and the baby's head has engaged, although suction may be used occasionally before full dilation, if labour is prolonged.	If you are induced, labour is started artificially. Hospital policies on induction vary from place to place, so find out from your hospital how long you can wait before being induced.
When used An episiotomy may be needed if: ● the baby is breech, premature, distressed, or has a large head ● you have an assisted delivery ● you are having difficulty controlling your pushing ● the skin around your vaginal opening hasn't stretched enough.	**When used** You may have an assisted delivery if: ● you cannot push the baby out, perhaps because he has a large head ● you or the baby show signs of distress during labour ● your baby is breech or premature; the forceps protect his head from pressure in the birth canal.	**When used** Labour may be induced if: ● it is more than two weeks past the baby's due date and he shows signs of being distressed, or the placenta starts to fail ● you have high blood pressure, or another problem or condition that puts you or the baby at risk.
What happens Your pelvic floor area will probably be numbed with an injection of local anaesthetic, and a small cut will be made from the bottom of the vagina, usually slightly out to one side, at the peak of a contraction. Sometimes there is no time for an injection but the stretching of the tissues also numbs them, so you shouldn't feel any pain. Stitching up after an episiotomy or a tear may take some time, as the different layers of skin and muscle have to be carefully sewn together. It can be painful, too, so ask for more anaesthetic if you need some. The stitches are soluble and do not have to be removed.	**What happens** ● You will probably be given an injection of local anaesthetic into your pelvic floor area, and an episiotomy. The doctor uses the forceps or a vacuum to deliver the head. You can help by pushing. The rest of your baby's body is delivered normally. **Forceps** These form a cage around the baby's head, protecting it from pressure and damage. **Vacuum** A small plastic cup, connected to a vacuum pump, is passed into the vagina and attached to the baby's head. The baby is gently pulled through the birth canal as you push.	**What happens** Induction is always planned in advance, and you will probably be asked to go into hospital the night before. Labour may be induced in three ways: **1** Inserting a pessary into the vagina containing a hormone (prostaglandins) that softens the cervix. This is done in the evening or very early morning. You may go into labour within an hour or so, but the pessary is not usually very effective on its own in a first pregnancy. **2** Breaking your waters. If labour still has not started within eight to 12 hours, the doctor makes a small hole in the bag of waters surrounding the baby. Most women don't feel any pain. Contractions nearly always start soon afterwards. **3** Giving you a hormone (syntocinon) that makes the womb contract. This is fed through a drip in your arm at a controlled rate. Ask for the drip to be inserted into the arm you use least.
Effects Some discomfort and soreness is normal after an episiotomy, but the pain can be quite severe, especially if an infection develops. The wound should heal within 10 to 14 days, but if you are sore after this time, go to see your doctor. There is usually less pain with a natural tear.	**Effects** ● If forceps are used to deliver your baby, they may leave pressure marks or bruises on either side of the baby's head. However, these are harmless and will disappear within a few days of the birth. ● The vacuum cup will cause slight swelling, and later a bruise, on the baby's head. This gradually subsides.	**Effects** Induction by pessary is preferable as you avoid having your waters broken and you will still be able to move around freely. With the drip in particular, your contractions may be stronger and more painful, with shorter intervals between them than in labour that has started naturally. Your mobility is restricted.

Breech birth

A breech baby is born bottom first. In a breech birth, the baby's head will be more vulnerable to pressure as it passes along the birth canal. This is because the birth canal has not been sufficiently stretched by the buttocks. About four in 100 births are breech.

As the largest part of the baby (the head) is born last, this is usually measured by ultrasound towards the end of pregnancy to check that it is small enough to fit through your pelvis.

Labour with a breech baby can be more prolonged and difficult than a head down presentation, and must always take place in hospital. You will need an episiotomy, and forceps are commonly used. It is the policy of many hospitals to deliver all breech babies by a Caesarean section.

Twins

It is essential to have twins in hospital. Forceps delivery or a Caesarean section may be necessary and the babies may be small and need special care afterwards. You will be advised to have an epidural (see page 64) too to relieve the pain.

There is only one first stage, but you will have two second stages as you push one baby out, and then the other usually 10 to 30 minutes after the first.

Caesarean section

With a Caesarean birth, the baby is delivered abdominally. You may know you are going to have a Caesarean in advance, or it may be an emergency operation because of problems in labour. If a Caesarean is planned you can have it under an epidural or spinal anaesthesia (see page 64), so you are awake throughout and can hold your baby straightaway. This may also be possible if you are told in labour you need the operation, but rarely a general anaesthetic is necessary.

It's only natural to feel disappointed, and perhaps cheated of a normal delivery, if you need a Caesarean. But these feelings can be minimized if you prepare yourself thoroughly, and seek support from your birth partner. Ask your hospital if your birth partner can be with you throughout.

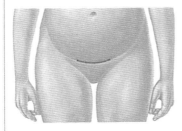

The incision
The "bikini" cut is usually made horizontally, just above the pubic hairline, and it is almost invisible when it heals.

Stitching the wound
You or your partner can hold the baby, while the doctor stitches you up.

What happens

A drip will be put in your arm, and a tube inserted into your bladder. You will be given the anaesthetic. If you are having an epidural, a screen will be set up between you and the surgeon. The cut is usually made horizontally, and the surgeon drains away the amniotic fluid. The baby is lifted out, sometimes with forceps. You can hold him as the placenta is delivered. The start of surgery to the birth usually takes about five minutes. A further 20 minutes or so are spent stitching you.

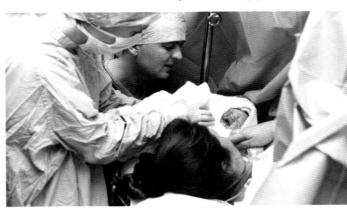

After the operation

You will be encouraged to walk soon after the birth, and will probably be asked to wear special support stockings to prevent the development of a blood clot. The incision will be painful for a few days, so ask for pain relief. Moving around won't open it up. When walking, stand tall, and cup your hands over the wound. Approximately two days after the operation, begin gentle exercise (see page 72), and a day or so later, when the dressing is removed, you can have a bath. The stitches will be removed five days after birth, unless soluble, and you'll feel much better after a week. Avoid straining yourself for at least six weeks. The scar fades, usually in three to six months.

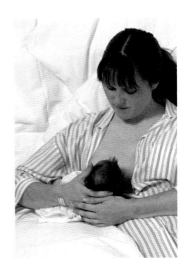

Breastfeeding after a Caesarean section
Support your baby on one or two pillows beside you, so he is not resting on the wound.

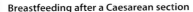

Your new baby

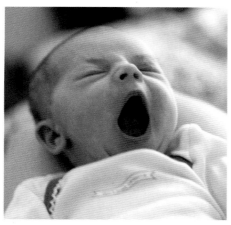

Your baby will probably look very different from what you expected. He may seem smaller than you imagined, the shape of his head may seem strange, and you are bound to notice spots, blotches, and changes of colour – this is all perfectly normal. Ask your midwife if anything worries you. You may love your baby immediately. But if you don't feel this strongly at first, allow yourself time. Once you start caring for your baby, the bond will deepen, and love will grow naturally.

First impressions

Don't be dismayed if your baby doesn't look perfect – few babies do at birth. You may notice the following imperfections, but most of these will disappear within two weeks. Below and facing is a rundown of how different parts of your baby's body may appear after birth.

Head

A cone-shaped head is usually caused by the pressure of birth. The head should look normal within two weeks.
On the top of the head is a soft spot (fontanelle), where the bones of the skull have not yet joined together. They should fuse by the time the child is 18 months old.

Eyes

True eye colour may not develop until the baby is about six months old.
Puffy eyelids are usually caused by the pressure of birth, but ask the doctor to check your baby's eyes, as it could be an infection.
Squinting is common in the first months.

Tongue

This may seem anchored to the floor of the mouth and might look slightly forked when the baby sticks the tongue out. The tip will grow forwards in the first year.

Hands and feet

These may be bluish because the baby's circulation is not working properly. If you move your baby into another position, they should turn pink.
The fingernails are often long at birth; carefully trim using special baby scissors.

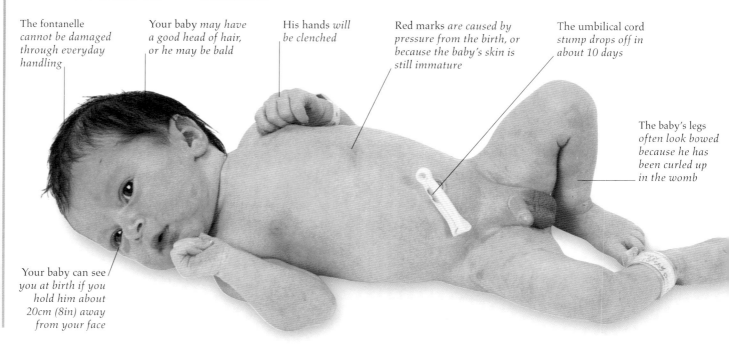

The fontanelle *cannot be damaged through everyday handling*

Your baby *may have a good head of hair, or he may be bald*

His hands *will be clenched*

Red marks *are caused by pressure from the birth, or because the baby's skin is still immature*

The umbilical cord *stump drops off in about 10 days*

The baby's legs *often look bowed because he has been curled up in the womb*

Your baby can see *you at birth if you hold him about 20cm (8in) away from your face*

Breasts

Your baby's breasts may be swollen and even leak a little milk. This is normal in both sexes. The swelling should go down within two days; do not squeeze the milk out.

Genitals

These appear large on both male and female babies.
A baby girl may have discharge from her vagina. This is caused by the mother's hormones and will soon disappear.
The testicles of a baby boy are often pulled up into his groin. If worried, see your doctor.

Skin

Spots and rashes are very common, and should vanish of their own accord.
Peeling skin, especially on the hands and feet, should disappear in a couple of days.
Downy body hair (lanugo) may be visible, especially if the baby was born early. This rubs off within two weeks.
Greasy white vernix covers and protects the baby's skin in the womb. It can be wiped off.
Birthmarks usually vanish. These include:
- red marks (stork bites) often found on the eyelids, forehead, and at the back of the neck; they take about a year to go
- strawberry birthmarks, which gradually increase in size; they usually disappear by the time the child is five
- blue patches (Mongolian blue spots), often found on the lower backs of babies with dark skin
- port wine stain, a bright red or purple mark, which is permanent.

Stool

At birth, the baby's bowel contains a dark, sticky substance called meconium.

Checks on the baby

Your baby will be examined several times in the first week. The midwife will weigh him regularly, and check him daily for any problems or signs of infection. She also does one other test, the Guthrie test, see below, when the baby is about six or seven days old. In addition, the baby will be thoroughly examined by a doctor at least once in the first few days. This is a good time to discuss any worries that you may have.

General examination

The doctor will check the baby from head to toe to make sure there is nothing abnormal.

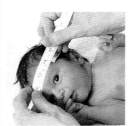

1 The doctor measures the head. He checks the fontanelle, and feels the roof of the mouth to make sure it is complete.

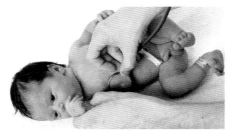

2 He listens to the heart and lungs to see if they are normal. Heart murmurs are common among newborn babies, and do not usually indicate any kind of defect.

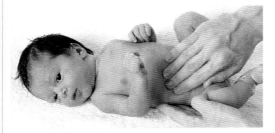

3 By putting his hand on the baby's stomach, the doctor checks that the abdominal organs are the right size. He also feels the pulses in the baby's groin.

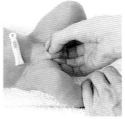

4 The genitals are checked for abnormality. If you have a boy, the doctor checks if both testicles have descended.

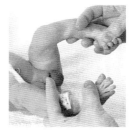

5 He moves the baby's limbs to see that the lower legs and feet are in alignment and legs are the right length.

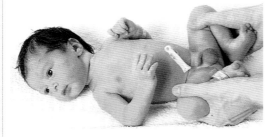

6 The doctor checks the hips for any dislocation, by bending the baby's legs up and gently circling them.

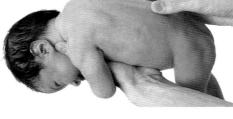

7 He makes sure that all the vertebrae are in place along the spine.

8 The doctor checks the baby's vision and hearing.

The Guthrie test

This test is usually done at home by the midwife six or seven days after birth. A blood sample, taken via a small prick on the baby's heel, is tested for PKU (a rare cause of mental handicap), thyroid deficiency, and other blood disorders.

Babies needing special care

Premature (born before 37 weeks) or small for dates (see page 38) babies need extra care after birth. They are more likely to have problems with breathing, feeding, and maintaining their temperature, and so need special treatment and monitoring. If your baby needs intensive medical care, she will have to spend her first days in an incubator, but once this is no longer necessary, you will be able to give her "kangaroo care", the prolonged skin-to-skin contact that has been found as effective as an incubator in keeping a premature baby warm and safe. Research shows that babies given kangaroo care sleep better and gain weight more quickly, and it even improves the chance of successful breastfeeding.

Getting to know your baby

Even if your baby is in an incubator, she needs as much love and attention as any other baby, so it's important to spend as much time with her as possible, and take part in her daily care. All babies respond to loving handling, and even if she can't be taken out of the incubator and cuddled, you can still talk to her and stroke her through the portholes in the side.

Asking questions

Ask the doctor or nursing staff about anything that worries you. Often parents don't ask questions because their baby looks so frail that they are afraid of the reply. But with modern intensive care, even babies born before 28 weeks can survive.

Feeding

If your baby can suck, you may be able to feed her normally. Otherwise, she will be fed through a tube, which is passed through her nose or mouth and down into her stomach.

Jaundice

Many newborn babies develop very mild jaundice about three days after birth, which turns their skin and the whites of their eyes slightly yellow. This happens because a baby's liver is still immature, and a pigment called bilirubin accumulates in the blood faster than the liver can dispose of it.

Jaundice usually clears up in a few days of its own accord, although the baby may be more sleepy than usual, so wake her up often and encourage her to feed. It also helps if her cot is near a window, so she is exposed to sunlight. Sometimes jaundice has to be treated with a special light (phototherapy). This can usually be done in the postnatal ward, and only in a few severe cases is the baby taken into special care. If the baby is still jaundiced after two weeks, the doctor will refer her back to the hospital for a check up.

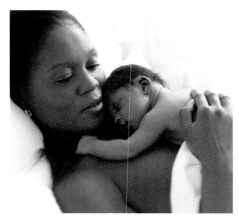

Kangaroo care
You – or even your partner – can give this skin-to-skin contact, either propped up in bed or sitting in a chair, holding your baby against your chest.

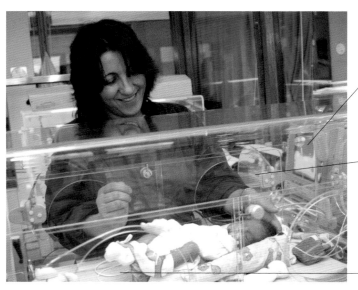

Control, *to regulate the temperature inside the incubator*

Portholes, *so you can touch your baby and talk to her*

Feeding tube, *which passes into the baby's stomach; you can express your own milk to be fed to the baby*

The baby in the incubator
Even with all the extra medical care available in the special care unit, your baby needs just as much love and attention as any normal baby.

Stillbirth

Very rarely, a baby is born dead. The exact cause for stillbirths remains uncertain as it can be a number of different factors. What makes this so hard to bear is that you never knew your child. It's probably a good idea to see her after birth; by holding her, and giving her a name, you can grieve for her as a person, and it's important to do this. You will probably feel angry, and want to know what went wrong, and find something or someone to blame. Shame and guilt are also quite common. But you should know that it is not your fault. Ask your doctor to put you in touch with a group of people who have had a stillbirth.

Getting back to normal

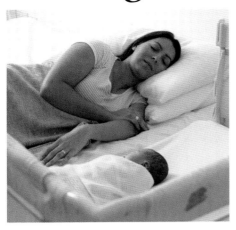

For the first week after delivery try to rest whenever you can. The midwife will visit you at home until the baby is at least 10 days old. She will check your womb, breasts, and any stitches, and will help you with your new baby. You may be rather disheartened when you see your body after birth. Your tummy won't be flat, your breasts will be large, and the tops of your legs will feel heavy. But if you practise your postnatal exercises as soon as possible after birth, you will begin to look and feel better.

How you will feel

As the initial rush of excitement of your baby's birth settles down, you will probably experience some discomfort, and even pain, in the first days. Ask the midwife if anything worries you.

After pains

You may feel cramping pains in your stomach, especially when breastfeeding, as the womb contracts back to its pre-pregnant size. This is a good sign that your body is returning to normal. The pains may last several days.
What to do If contractions are severe, a mild painkiller such as paracetamol may ease them.

Bladder

It's normal to pass more water in the first days, as the body loses the extra fluid gained in pregnancy.
What to do Urinating may be difficult at first because of soreness, but try to do so as soon as possible after birth.
● Get up and about to encourage the urinary flow.
● Soak in a warm bath. Don't worry if you pass urine into the water as urine is sterile; wash yourself well afterwards.
● If you have stitches, try pouring warm water over them as you pass urine to stop your skin stinging.

Bleeding

You may have vaginal bleeding for anything from two to six weeks. This usually stops more quickly if you are breastfeeding. The bright-red discharge is heavy at first, but over the next few days it decreases and gradually becomes brownish. Often the discharge continues until the first menstrual period.
What to do Wear sanitary pads to catch the flow; don't use internal tampons, because they may be uncomfortable.

Bowels

You may not need to empty your bowels for a day or more after the birth.
What to do Get mobile as soon as possible: this will start your bowels working.
● Drink plenty of water and eat high-fibre foods to stimulate your bowels.
● When you want to open your bowels, do so at once, but don't strain too hard.
● It is most unlikely that any stitches will tear when you move your bowels, but holding a clean sanitary pad against the area while you do so may help you feel more confident.

Stitches

These may be very sore for a day or two. Most dissolve in about a week.
What to do The following suggestions will help the recovery process.
● Practise pelvic floor exercises as soon as possible after birth to speed up healing.
● Keep the stitches clean by relaxing in a warm bath. Dry the entire area thoroughly afterwards.

Coping with the blues

Many women feel low a few days after delivery, usually when the milk comes in. One cause is the sudden change in hormone levels, another is the feeling of anticlimax that sometimes occurs after birth. These postnatal blues usually vanish. If you feel depressed for more than four weeks, or your depression is severe, see your doctor or talk to your health visitor.

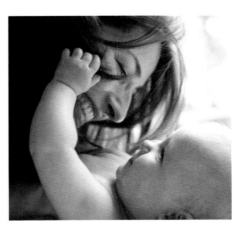

Thinking positively
The sheer pleasure and delight of finally having your newborn baby will probably more than compensate for the after effects of the labour and birth process.

● Soothe soreness by applying an ice-pack to the area.
● Lie down to take pressure off the stitches, or sit on a rubber ring.

Shaping up after birth

With some gentle exercising every day your figure can return to normal in as little as three months after the birth, although your stomach muscles may not be as firm as before. Build up your exercise programme slowly at first as your ligaments are still soft and stretchy, and always stop straightaway if you feel pain or tiredness. It's best to exercise a little, but on a regular basis. You may want to join a local postnatal exercise class.

Warning

If you have had a Caesarean, you won't be ready to start the exercises for your stomach muscles described in *week one* or the *week two* daily routine until much later after birth. Check with your doctor first before practising these exercises, and stop immediately if you feel any pain.

Week one

You can begin to strengthen the stretched, and possibly weakened, muscles of your pelvic floor and stomach from as early as the first day after birth. The pelvic floor and foot pedalling exercises are also good if you have had a Caesarean but delay doing them until you have no more wound discomfort.

Pelvic floor exercise
from day one
Practise gentle squeezing and lifting exercises (see page 45) as often as possible every day to stop yourself leaking urine involuntarily. It's important to do this before you go on to the exercises in week two. If you have had stitches, strengthening the pelvic floor will heal them.

Foot pedalling
from day one
This will guard against swelling in the legs and improve circulation. Lie down and bend your feet up and down at the ankle. Practise hourly.

Stomach toner
from day one
A gentle way to strengthen stomach muscles is to pull them in as you breathe out, hold them in for a few seconds, then relax. Try to do this as often as possible.

from day five after birth
If you feel fine, practise the following exercise twice a day, too:

1 Lie on your back with your head and shoulders supported on two pillows and your legs bent and slightly apart. Cross your arms over your stomach.

2 Lift your head and shoulders, and as you do this, breathe out and press gently on each side of your stomach with the palms of your hands, as if pulling the two sides together. Hold this position for a few seconds, then breathe in, and relax. Repeat three times.

Week two

Introduce the following exercises into your daily routine, and continue for at least three months. Repeat each exercise as many times as is comfortable. Remember to keep practising the exercise for your pelvic floor.

Cat arching exercise

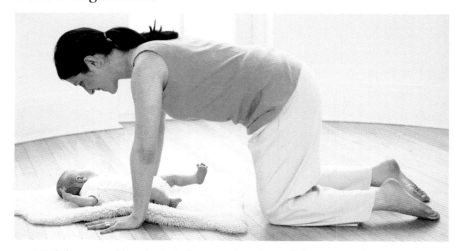

1 With knees and hands slightly apart, kneel on all fours. Your back, head, and neck should be absolutely straight.

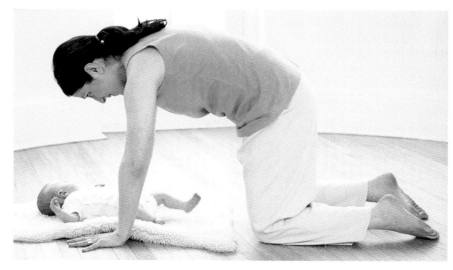

2 Clench your buttocks and arch your back upwards slowly. Your arms should be straight, but remember not to lock your elbows. This exercise helps you to relieve stress from your lower back.

Curl ups

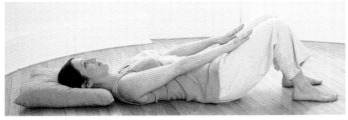

1 Lie flat on your back on the floor, with your knees bent and your feet slightly apart. Rest your hands on your thighs.

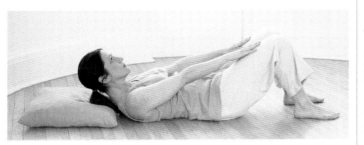

2 Breathe out, and lift your head and shoulders, stretching forwards to touch your knees with your hands. Don't worry if you can't reach far enough at first, you will with practise. Breathe in and relax.

3 When this is easy, try lifting yourself up more slowly and holding the position for longer, placing your hands on your chest as you lift your head and shoulders, or you could clasp your hands behind your head as you lift yourself up.

Side bends

1 With your arms by your sides, stand straight with your feet apart and the palms of your hands resting on the outsides of your thighs.

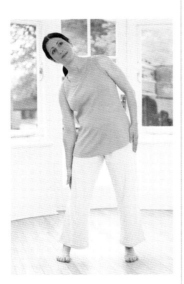

2 Bend sideways slowly at the waist, stretching your leg outwards at the same time. Come back to the initial position and repeat on the other side. Remember to exhale on the effort and inhale when you relax.

Checking your pelvic floor

By three months after birth these muscles should be strong again. Test them by skipping. If any urine leaks, practise the pelvic floor exercises for another month and try again. If leaking is still a problem, see your doctor.

How your body recovers

Your body won't be fully recovered for at least six months after the birth of your baby. However, by the time you visit your GP or the hospital for your six-week check-up, your body should be getting back to normal. Your womb may have shrunk back to its pre-pregnant size and you may have started your periods again. If you have been practising your postnatal exercises regularly, your muscles should be in far better shape.

The six-week check-up

About six weeks after the birth, you will have a check-up at the doctor's surgery. It is a good time to discuss any worries with the doctor or nurse who performs the check-up.

What happens

- Your blood pressure, weight, and a sample of urine will be checked.
- Your breasts and stomach will be examined. The doctor will check if any stitches have healed.
- You may have an internal examination to check the size and position of the womb, and may be given a cervical smear test.
- The doctor will discuss contraception; you can be fitted with a cap or coil or go on the pill.

Your periods

The first period after the birth is often longer and heavier than usual. When it arrives depends on how you are feeding your baby. If you are breastfeeding, your periods may not start until after your baby is weaned. If you are bottle-feeding, the first period usually comes four to six weeks after the birth.

Q&A

"When can we resume our sex life?"

The best time to start making love again is when you both are ready. You may feel too sore and tender to resume sex until after the postnatal check-up, or you may want to try sooner – it's entirely up to you.

When you resume your sex life, take it slowly. Relax as much as you can, and use extra lubrication as your vagina may be slightly drier than normal.

"I'm breastfeeding my baby; do we still have to use contraception?"

Even if you are breastfeeding or haven't started your periods again, you need to use contraception. The doctor or midwife will discuss this with you soon after the birth. If you want to go on the pill, make sure the doctor knows you are breastfeeding; if you previously used a cap, you must have a new one fitted, as your cervix will have changed shape.

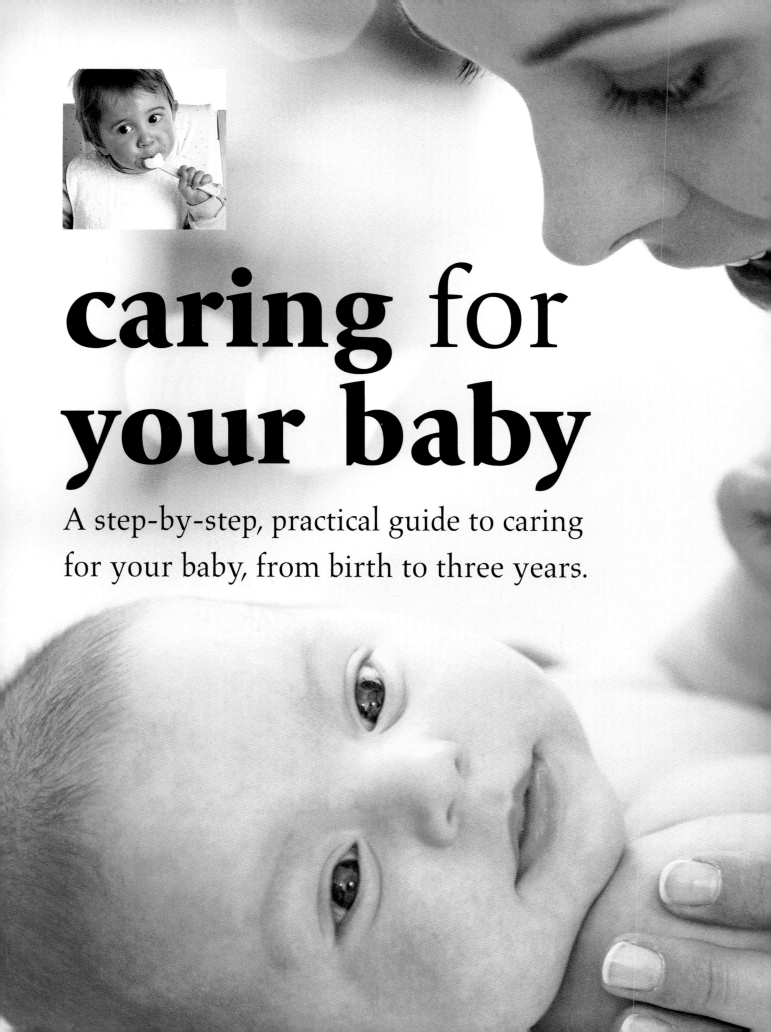

caring for your baby

A step-by-step, practical guide to caring for your baby, from birth to three years.

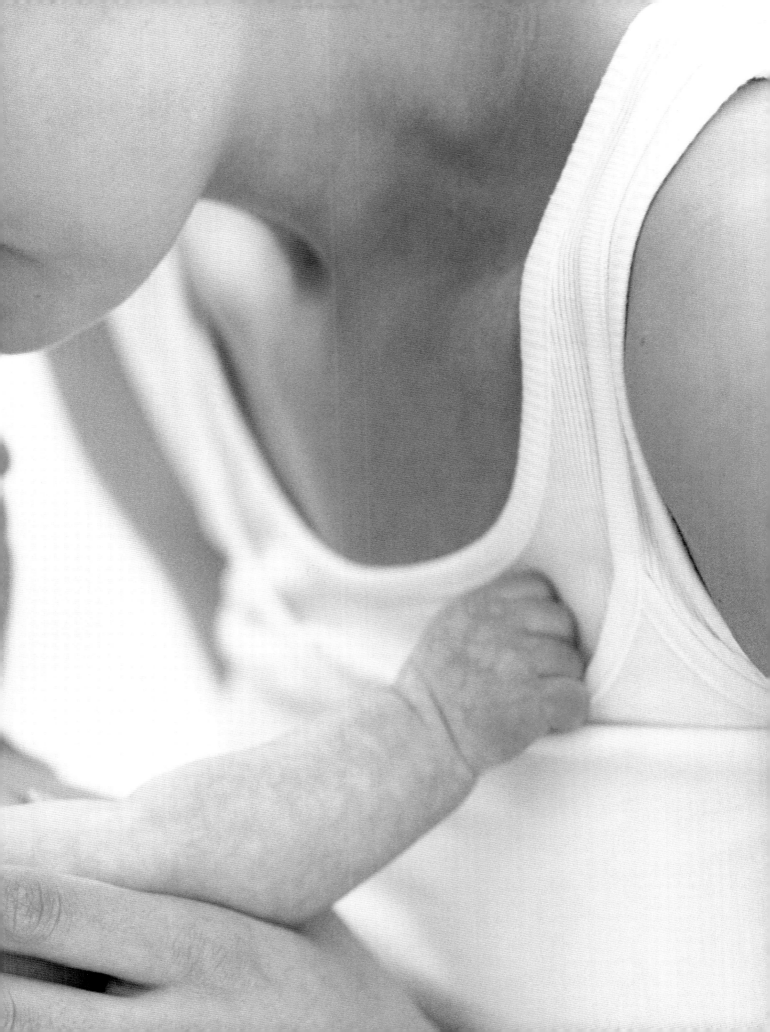

The first weeks of life

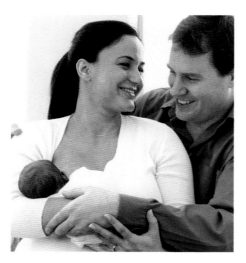

Nothing can prepare you for the reality of having a child. The first weeks of your baby's life will seem like a whirlwind of new experiences as you adapt to being a parent. Looking after a new baby involves providing lots of warmth and attention, and although some of this will be instinctive, some has to be learnt by both of you. The early phase of adjustment won't last long. You'll quickly learn new skills and before long eating one-handed while your baby feeds will be second nature. Here is how one couple and their baby, Amy, coped in the first few weeks.

"The first weeks weren't easy. You think you're a capable, confident person, then you have a helpless baby to look after, and you feel like jelly!"

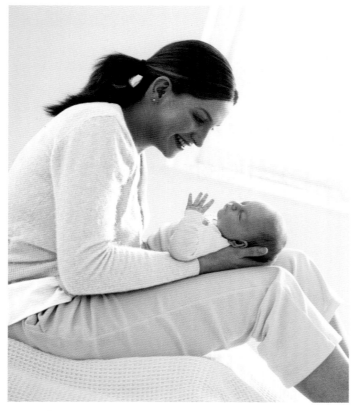

First days at home

Life with your new baby will take you by surprise. Her apparent vulnerability produces powerful feelings within you, while a turmoil of emotions makes you burst into tears for no known reason. You may become distressed by, for example, the television news. Don't fight your feelings; concentrate on the new life that you are nurturing.

Amy at one week

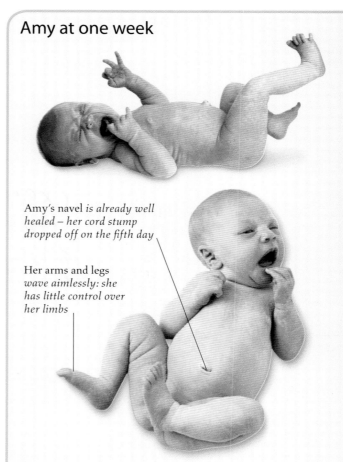

Amy's navel is already well healed – her cord stump dropped off on the fifth day

Her arms and legs wave aimlessly: she has little control over her limbs

She lies curled up just as she was in the womb. Her fists are usually tightly clenched, and when she lies on her back she can't stop her head from lolling to one side. If her hand comes into contact with her mouth she sucks it. As happens with almost all newborn babies, her weight has dropped, from 3.54kg (7lbs 13oz) at birth to 3.4kg (7lbs 8oz) now. She should be back to her birthweight by about 10 days.

Becoming a family

Now there are three of you and everything changes. Your partner is no longer just your lover, he's your companion and ally in this new adventure of parenthood – and the baby is as much his as she is yours. Your tried and tested family relationships will subtly change, too – you're not just a son or a daughter any more, you're a parent with a new life depending on you.

Often it's the new father who is most shell-shocked in the days immediately after the birth. But for a while you'll both be tired, sleep deprived, anxious, and possibly even shorter tempered than usual. Make allowances for each other and try to support and make time for each other, too. It's easy to make your partner feel sidelined and useless at this time if you behave as though the baby's welfare is your exclusive domain. Talk to each other about your feelings and share babycare as much as you can – it will be very much to your advantage if your baby has a hands-on father. At first he may be more nervous than you of handling her floppy little body, but he will soon grow more confident.

Above all, relax and enjoy your baby. New parenthood may seem like an island of anxiety surrounded by good advice, but remember that there are very few absolute rights and wrongs about baby care. Babies can survive inexperienced parents, what they need most if they are to thrive are happy and loving ones. So have the confidence to rely on your own intuition, and do things in the way that seems right to you – the chances are that it will be right for your baby, too.

"The first days were such a tangle of conflicting feelings – elation and overwhelming pride at being a father, anxiety about Ruth, exhaustion from the round-the-clock demands of our new baby, even a tiny regret that our happy, carefree life together seemed to be at an end."

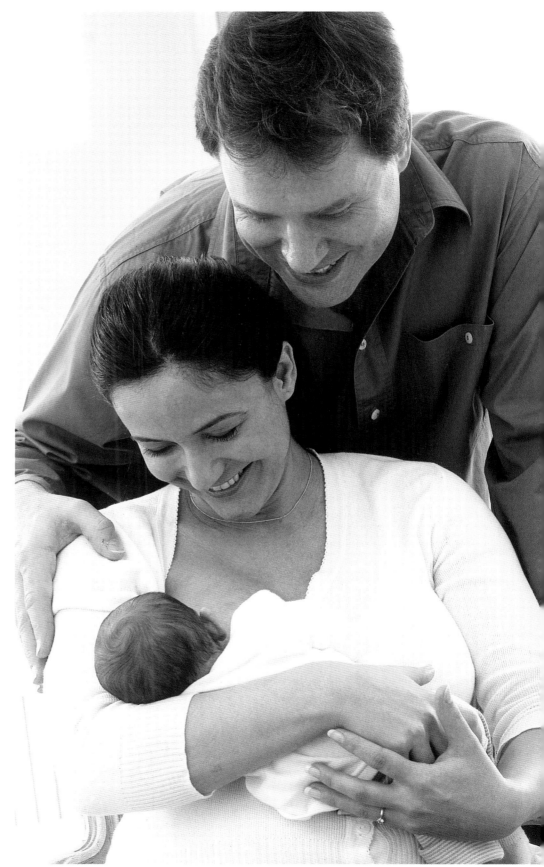

Amy's day

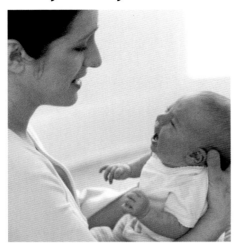

"Amy seemed insatiably hungry and sometimes in the evening she would cry inconsolably for hours at a stretch. I was worried that it was because I hadn't enough milk, but the health visitor assured me that this was probably evening colic and would only last for about three months. Despite the disturbed evenings, this was a huge relief because I loved breastfeeding her and would have been so sad if I'd had to stop. I felt that it was making us really close. Meanwhile, it did at least mean that Tim got to see more of Amy because she was awake so much in the evening when he was home."

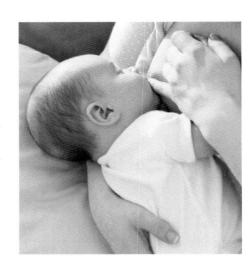

Building a loving relationship

Right from the beginning, your relationship with your new baby is an intense, two-way one that will grow into a real and lasting love. Bring her up close to your face to talk and coo to her – she will look intently back at you, gazing raptly at your face. Eye contact always plays a big part in falling in love, and it is the same with you and your baby. Try sticking the tip of your tongue out when you are looking at each other; she will quickly learn to respond by doing the same – this is real two-way communication. She will reward your efforts to calm her by quietening at the sound of your voice. And when she's miserable, she will want you to hold and comfort her.

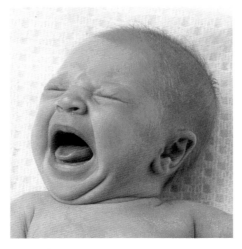

Amy crying
Crying is your baby's way of expressing her need for love and comfort. Always respond – don't leave her to cry.

A typical day at around three weeks old

9:00am	**Ruth is woken** by Amy's crying. She had her last feed at 6am (breaks between feeds at 3 weeks should be 3 hours normally, with one 4 hour stretch at night), then they both fell asleep together. It is time for Amy to have another feed now.	1:00pm	**Ruth has** some lunch and then dozes.
10:00am	**Ruth takes Amy** into the bathroom to change her nappy and clothes, and top and tail her. Then she puts Amy in the carrycot, and chats to her while she dresses herself.	3:00pm	**The health visitor's** ring on the doorbell wakes Ruth. The health visitor wakes Amy to examine her. She weighs Amy and reassures Ruth that Amy is back to her birthweight. She also shows Ruth how to help Amy latch on properly as Ruth's nipples are getting sore.
11:00am	**Amy falls asleep.** Ruth puts the washing in the washing machine, and tidies up, then she puts her feet up, but doesn't sleep.	4:00pm	**The health visitor** leaves, but Amy is cross from being woken abruptly from her afternoon sleep, so Ruth feeds her to soothe her. It doesn't take long before Amy settles down once again.
11:30am	**Amy cries** for a feed, and then dozes off after she is fed. Ruth takes the opportunity to have a nap, too.	5:30pm	**Ruth puts Amy** in her pram, and takes a walk in the fresh air to the station to meet Tim. The movement of the pram soothes Amy, and she drops off to sleep within a few minutes.

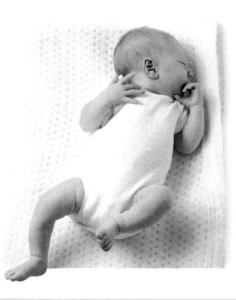

Amy asleep
Newborn babies sleep an average of 16 hours a day, but Amy sometimes slept as little as 10 or 11 hours in total, with a long, stormy period from late afternoon to late at night when she only dozed for very short periods. Within five weeks Amy had adopted a more sociable sleep pattern, with a longer sleep during the night, and an earlier bedtime.

"Rubbing her tummy was a good way to soothe her, provided we rubbed fast and positively – despite my instincts to be very gentle. You soon learn how tough babies are."

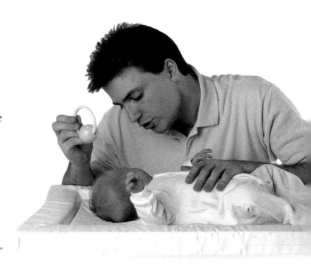

6:15pm	**Home again**, and Amy starts to cry. Ruth feeds her, changes her, then rocks her in her arms. Feeding is the only thing that really soothes Amy at this time of the day, but Ruth is sore so it's painful. After feeding, Ruth leaves her nipples exposed to the air for as long as possible. Tim snatches some sleep.	**10:00pm**	**Amy is still crying;** she will be soothed for a while, then cry again. Tim and Ruth let her suck, walk her around, and push her to and fro in her pram.
		1:00am	**Amy falls asleep** at last. Tim and Ruth are exhausted, and go to bed immediately.
8:30pm	**Tim wakes up,** and he and Ruth take turns to carry Amy around and prepare some food. Amy dozes off for a few minutes at a time, then wakes and cries – so supper is interrupted by short feeds at the breast. Tim helps out as much as possible with the preparation of the food.	**3:00am**	**Amy wakes** and cries, Ruth gets up and feeds her. Tim wakes up too, and helps to rock Amy back to sleep again after her feed.
		7:00am	**The alarm goes off** and Tim gets up to go to work while Ruth tries to snatch some more sleep before Amy wakes for her morning feed.

Involving other family members
Your parents, sisters, brothers, and other members of your family will all be extremely keen to meet the new baby, but don't feel guilty about limiting visitors if you want to.

Getting plenty of rest
Every new mother has to learn how to cope with too little sleep. Plenty of rest whenever you can snatch it is the only answer – and this is especially important if you're breastfeeding your baby. Rest whenever your baby is asleep, even if you don't go to sleep yourself. Your body isn't strong enough yet for strenuous work, and the housework can go undone for now.

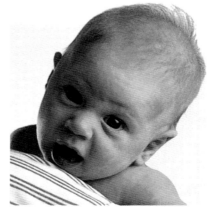

Amy wakeful
Held against your shoulder, your baby has a good view of the world around her, and will enjoy her wakeful times.

Six weeks old

"By six weeks Amy was a real person – nothing like the greedy, screaming bundle she had been only weeks before. She responded to each of us in her own way: her first crooked smiles were just for me, usually when I changed her, but at times only Ruth would do. We were lucky – Amy was very perky, and she helped us to love her. You certainly learn fast when you have a new baby reliant on you for her every need."

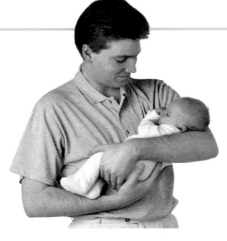

Amy at six weeks

Amy has a range of facial expressions

Amy has much more control over her limbs now, and enjoys the sensation of kicking them around in the air. She's no longer curled up and her fists are unclenched. When she lies on her stomach, she may lift her head momentarily. She doesn't cry as much as she used to – she has a definite wakeful time during the day, when she will sit happily in her bouncing chair and love being entertained by Ruth and the world around her.

She has a round stomach in relation to the rest of her torso

Premature babies

Your baby's first six weeks at home may be especially difficult if she was born prematurely. She may cry incessantly and refuse to be comforted, or be very sleepy and reluctant to feed. In addition to your natural anxiety about your new baby, you may feel rejected by her – she doesn't make you feel that she loves you, so it's that much harder to love her in return. Your pre-term baby will need extra care from you – she loses heat quickly, so you need to keep your home warm, especially when bathing or changing her, and she will need frequent feeding to help her grow. Even though she may have a small appetite and be a troublesome feeder, you should offer her a feed as often as every three hours, letting her take as much as she wants at each feed. Concentrate on giving the care she needs and in time your baby will grow more responsive to you, and you will learn to understand her better. Don't wait longer than four hours between feedings because if you do so your baby may become dehydrated.

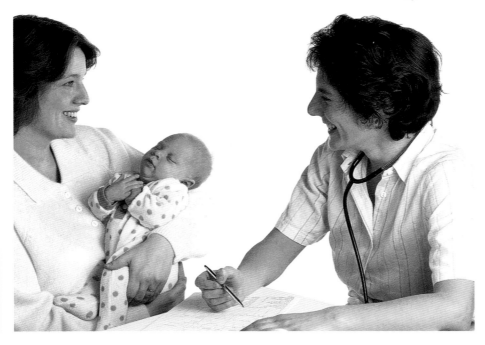

Amy's six-week check-up

The six-week check-up is the first of the major development checks for a new baby. Your doctor or local baby clinic will perform the check in a friendly, informal atmosphere.

1 **General assessment** The doctor discusses Amy's general well-being and demeanour with Ruth. She wakes Amy, and talks to her to assess how she responds to the stimulus of a new face. The doctor is looking for that magical early smile, a sure sign that Amy is developing a normal, sociable personality. She looks at Amy's retina through an ophthalmoscope to check that the retina is healthy, and moves a rattle across her field of vision. Amy follows it with both eyes, demonstrating healthy eyesight with no sign of a squint.

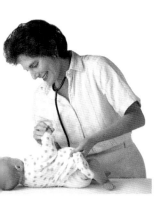

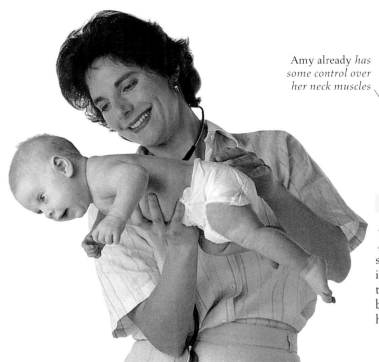

Amy already has some control over her neck muscles

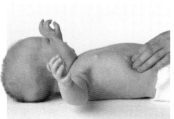

2 **Limbs and muscle tone** The doctor undresses Amy so she can observe her muscle tone and how she moves her limbs.

3 **Head control** The doctor holds Amy in the air to see that she holds her head in line with her body. Then the doctor lays Amy on her back and observes as she pulls her into a sitting position.

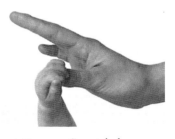

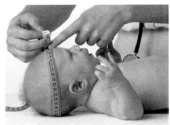

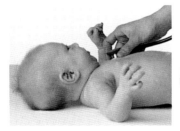

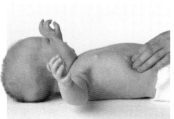

4 **Grasp reflex** A baby at birth can grasp hold of a finger put into her palm and hold on strongly. By six weeks, it's normal for her birth reflexes to begin to disappear, as Amy's have.

5 **Head circumference** Amy has her head measured, to check for normal growth. Her head is now 30cm (15in). The doctor also checks Amy's facial features for shape and symmetry.

6 **Heartbeat** The doctor listens to Amy's heart with a stethoscope to make sure that it has a steady rhythm – about 120 beats a minute is normal for the first year.

7 **Internal organs** A good feel around Amy's stomach reassures the doctor that her liver, stomach, and spleen are all growing normally, and none is too big or in the wrong shape.

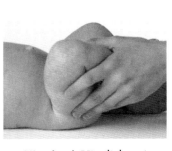

Amy's weight is recorded on her personal chart

9 **Weighing** Amy has been weighed naked at weekly intervals up to now, and will be weighed at every visit to the baby clinic, or whenever Ruth requests. Normal weight gain means a healthy baby. Amy's weight will be plotted on a centile chart to ascertain her growth in comparison to length and weight averages. The chart will be an important record for months to come.

8 **Hip check** Hip dislocation is a possibility still, so the doctor tests the joints' action with her middle fingers as she manipulates Amy's legs. She checks for hip symmetry, too.

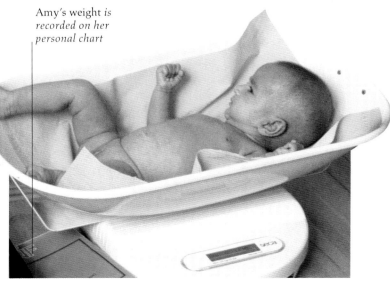

Handling your baby

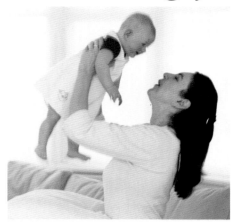

Your baby needs closeness and the comfort of your reassuring voice, so talk to her as you handle her. She cannot hold up her head until she is about eight weeks old, and needs you to support her body. Careful handling won't hurt her, but you may startle her if you pick her up suddenly. By five months she'll enjoy more boisterous games, and may love to be swung above your head or perched on your shoulders. If she's timid, handle her gently until she's more confident.

Picking up a newborn baby

If you are a first-time parent you might find picking up and holding a newborn baby a little daunting at first because your baby seems too delicate to handle. But as long as you provide proper support, you'll find that she's perfectly safe and loves being held.

Always put your baby on her back to sleep. She will be at lower risk of cot death and choking than if she sleeps on her tummy or her side (see page 123). However, when she is awake, she should spend some time each day lying on her front.

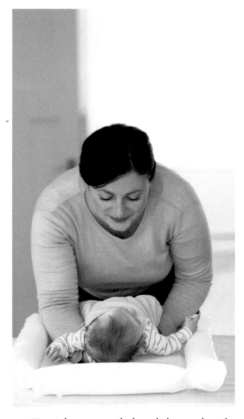

1 To pick up your baby, slide one hand under her lower back and bottom and the other under her head and neck.

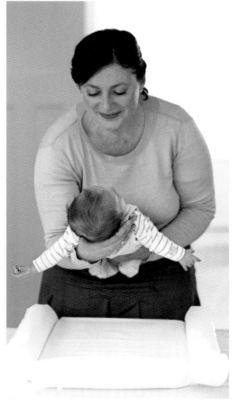

2 Lift her gently and slowly so that her body is supported and her head can't loll back.

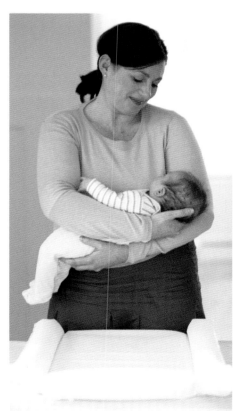

3 Carefully transfer her head to the crook of your elbow or your shoulder so that it remains supported.

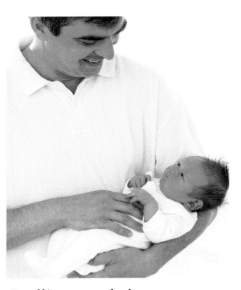

Cradling your baby in your arms

Your baby will feel secure cradled in the crook of your elbow, with her head and limbs well supported.

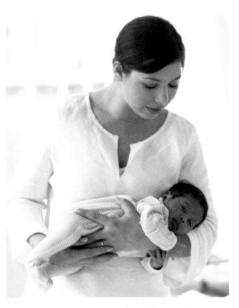

Holding your baby face down

Your baby may like being held face down in your arms, her chin and cheek resting on your forearm.

Holding your baby against your shoulder

Your baby feels secure when held upright like this. Take her weight with one hand under her bottom. Make sure you support her with the other hand.

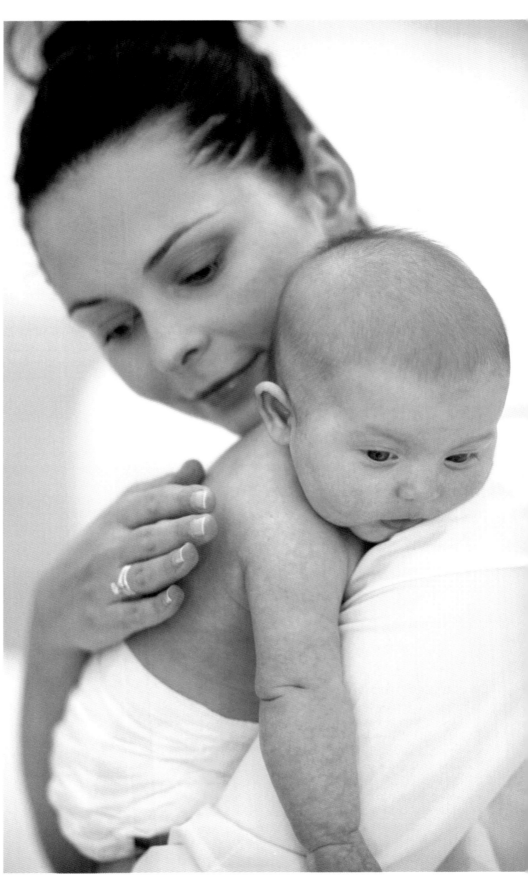

Putting your baby down

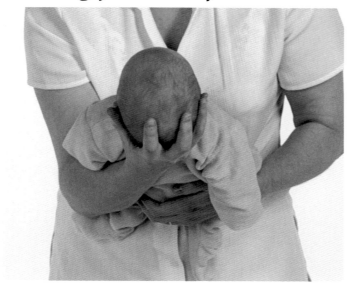

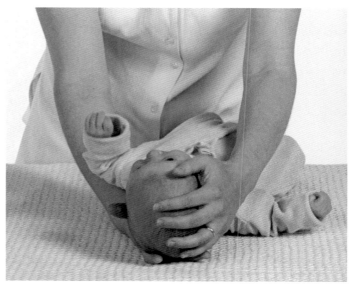

1 Put one hand underneath her head and neck, then hold her under the bottom with the other. Lower her slowly, gently supporting her until the mat or mattress is taking her weight. Make sure her head is fully supported.

2 Slide your nearest hand out from under her bottom. Use this hand to lift her head a little so you can slide out your other hand, and lower her head down gently. Don't let her head fall back on to the surface, or jerk your arm out quickly.

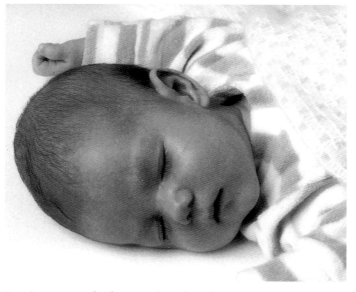

Laying your baby on her back

Recent research has shown that it is much safer for a baby to sleep on her back than on her side or tummy. Babies who sleep on their backs have reduced risk of cot death, although we don't know exactly why (see page 123). And although it used to be thought that if a baby in this position vomited there was a danger that she might choke, childcare experts now believe that babies sleeping on their back have no difficulty turning their heads if they are sick. Once your baby is old enough to begin turning over by herself, she may well turn over during the night. Continue to put her to bed on her back as usual, but don't worry if she turns over later. There is no need to turn her back during the night.

Safety first

You will often want to lay your baby down for a few moments, either for her own amusement, or because you need to do something. Whether in your own home or visiting family or friends, follow the simple precautions given below to ensure that your baby keeps safe and sound at all times:

● Never leave your baby unsupervised – even for a single second – on a bed, sofa, chair, or changing table.
● Never place your baby's chair, basket, or carrycot on a raised surface – only the floor will be completely safe.
● Never put your baby next to a radiator, fire, or open window. She may burn herself or overchill.
● Never leave your baby alone with a dog, cat, or any other animal.
● Never place your baby within reach of unstable furniture or other heavy objects. She may pull them over and seriously hurt herself.
● Leaving your baby's favourite toys with her will keep her entertained – but take care never to leave anything sharp in her reach. Avoid toys that are small enough to fit into her mouth, or heavy enough to hurt her.
● Until your baby is a little older and her immune system has had time to develop, it is a safe practice not to expose her to a large group of people or other small children to minimize the risk of infection.

Using a sling

A sling is an excellent way of carrying your baby around in the first three months. The contact with your body and the motion as you walk will soothe and comfort her. An added advantage is that it leaves your arms free. It's not difficult to put the sling on when there's no one to help you. You can take it off using the same method in reverse.

Putting a sling on

1 Slip the sling straps over your shoulders so that the two metal rings hang down at the front.

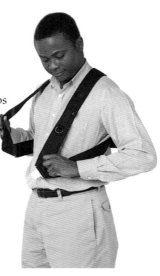

2 Attach the padded triangular section by snapping the circular fasteners on the straps into place.

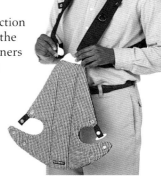

3 Close one side of the sling by feeding the toggle through the ring and snapping it securely closed.

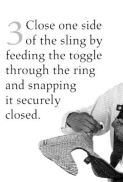

4 Hold your baby so that she faces you. If she is very young, support her head with your hand. Feed her leg through the hole on the fastened side of the sling. Keep your arm around her on the open side to ensure that she doesn't fall.

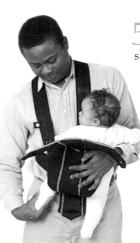

5 Support your baby in the seat of the sling with one hand while you fasten the toggle and snap under her arm with the other.

A padded back *supports your baby's head*

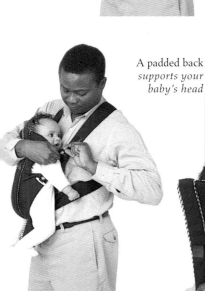

6 Close the top fasteners so that an arm hole is created on each side. The back flap supports a younger baby's head and neck.

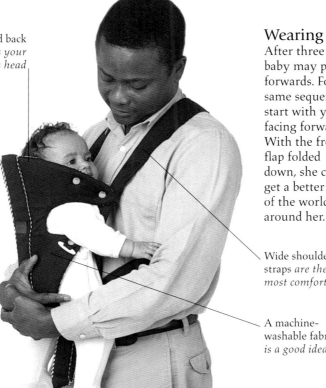

Wide shoulder straps *are the most comfortable*

A machine-washable fabric *is a good idea*

Wearing the sling

After three months, your baby may prefer to face forwards. Follow the same sequence, but start with your baby facing forwards. With the front flap folded down, she can get a better view of the world around her.

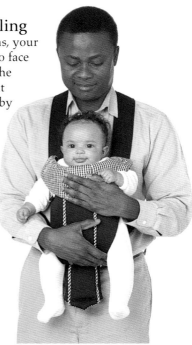

Handling and physical play

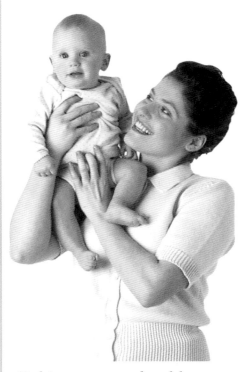

Sit him on your shoulder
Sit your six-month-old baby on your shoulder, so that he's taller than you are: he'll be exhilarated by this new perspective. Remember to hold him carefully.

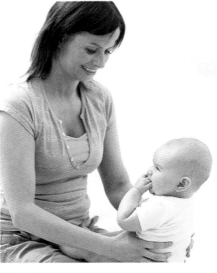

Play bouncing games on your lap
Your four-month-old baby will love the feeling of being jogged up and down by your knees, in time to a favourite rhyme. Hold your baby carefully, in case he jerks.

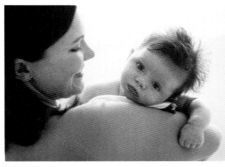

Let him see the world
Your baby will love to see the world. Hold him securely in your arms and perch his cheek gently on your shoulder. Twirl around slowly and let him enjoy the view.

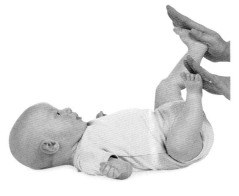

Let him kick
It's best not to let your baby become too dependent on being held. Let him spend some time kicking on the floor – you can get down to his level, too.

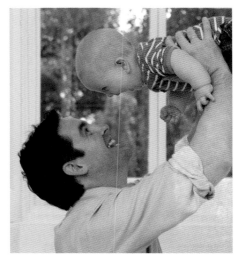

Eye-to-eye contact
Your baby will love you to swing him up high. Your face is always the best entertainment of all. You must be very careful not to jerk your baby's neck or head. Never throw him up in the air.

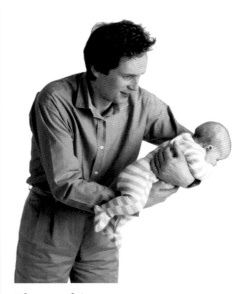

Play rocking games
Rock your baby to and fro, going higher if he likes the game. This type of rocking motion is a good way to soothe him, too. Make sure you hold your baby properly, so he doesn't slip from your hands.

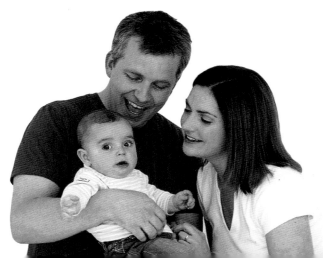

Winding down
However boisterously you play with your baby, have a few minutes of gentle cuddles afterwards. Always take your cue from your baby; forget rough-housing for today if he's not responding with his usual giggles.

Feeding your baby

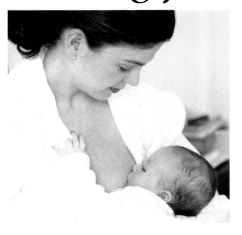

Breastfeeding is recommended for all infants with very few exceptions, because breastfed babies are generally healthier, with fewer ear, chest, gastrointestinal, and urine infections. They also suffer fewer allergies, and suffer less from asthma, eczema, diabetes, and obesity. Breastfeeding also has benefits for you. Nursing your baby immediately after delivery reduces the risk of excessive uterine bleeding, and continuing to breastfeed helps you return to your pre-pregnancy weight more quickly.

What mothers say about breastfeeding

Some women know early on in pregnancy that they want to breastfeed. Others are unsure. It is natural to have questions about which method might be the best option for you. Even if you have made your decision, it is best to learn about breastfeeding before your delivery. You can talk to other mothers who breastfed, your doctor, your community health nurse, lactation consultants, and your local breastfeeding support group. Breastfeeding clinics are also useful, if you have any particular concerns. You can call the National Breastfeeding Helpline at 0300-100-0212 as well.

"I knew that by breastfeeding I was giving my baby the best milk he could have. I could tell he was digesting it easily, and I knew it had exactly the right blend of nutrients."

Breast milk contains substances that help protect your baby from disease until his own immune system has matured. These also protect against allergies, which is important if there is an allergy in your family.

"I loved the convenience of breastfeeding my baby: the milk was always there, always sterile, always at the temperature he liked."

If you are out visiting friends, travelling, or just enjoying a day in the park, breast milk is the ultimate convenience food.

"The breast was always the best method of soothing my baby whenever he cried."

Breastfed babies are less fussy than bottle-fed babies. They have less constipation, less wind, and suffer fewer illnesses. Breastfeeding also allows you and your baby to come closer physically and emotionally, and this strengthens the bond between you.

"I was extremely worried that my breasts would become saggy with breastfeeding, but my obstetrician told me that if the breasts are going to go saggy, the changes already happen during pregnancy."

During the first few months, breasts will be fuller as feeding time nears. After that, you'll notice only occasional feelings of fullness, such as after your baby has had a longer sleep.

"I was tired and sore after my Caesarean section and the baby was nursing often. My mother and husband helped a lot, and it worked out very well."

All mothers need help in the weeks after delivery. They need the time to focus on the baby, and to get the hang of breastfeeding.

"I was convinced that I wouldn't be able to breastfeed – my bust was so small. But I had plenty of milk, and my baby certainly didn't mind my small breasts."

All mothers have enough milk for feeding their babies. If your baby is not gaining weight adequately, review your technique, feed more frequently, and discuss the issue with your healthcare providers.

"At first, I found it really hard nursing at night, but then the lactation consultant showed me how to nurse lying down. Now that he is in his sleeping box beside me, he nurses whenever he needs to."

Nursing lying down is a great way for you to rest. However, it is very dangerous for babies under six months of age to sleep with their parents, either sharing an adult bed or a sofa or an armchair, especially if either parent is a smoker, using sedating medication, alcohol, or recreational drugs. If you do let your baby sleep in your bed, consider a co-sleeping box, and perhaps keep a reassuring hand on your baby. See also the safety guidelines on page 126.

"My husband was a great help after the baby came, but said he felt left out when I was the breastfeeding. I told him how good he made me feel by all the things he was doing, and how much I loved him. It was a special moment for both of us."

Fathers and mothers are both important in their children's lives. The father's support is essential for the child's development and well-being.

Demand feeding

Feeding on demand simply means giving your baby a feed whenever he is hungry, without following a timetable. His digestive system is too immature to cope with large meals at infrequent intervals; little and often must be the rule at first. There is nothing to be gained by keeping your baby waiting for a feed once he has cried to be fed – he will only get so distressed that he will refuse to suck. In the early weeks, his hunger is the usual reason for waking and crying. As his digestive system matures and his stomach grows, he'll take more at each feed, and the intervals between feeds will become longer.

How often will he demand food?

Your baby will demand food whenever he needs it, and to begin with this will be often. Newborn babies will have no discernible pattern of feeding. By day three or four, feeds will be every two or three hours, and there may be eight or so feeds a day, with a lot of short feeds during the evening. At night you may be feeding your baby two or three times because few babies under the age of six weeks are able to sleep for more than five hours without waking with hunger. Breastfed babies need more frequent feeds than bottle-fed babies because breast milk is more easily and quickly digested than formula.

By three months, your baby may be settling into a regular feeding routine. Do bear in mind that babies don't grow at a regular rate, they have growth spurts, and their hunger fluctuates accordingly.

Special cases

Premature babies Your pre-term baby may have a small appetite, but he will need frequent feeds. Pre-term babies tend to sleep a lot, and may not wake and demand food even though they need it, so when applicable, wake your baby every three hours and offer a feed.

If you have managed to express milk for your baby while he's been in hospital, you will be able to breastfeed once you get him home. It isn't always easy for a baby to adapt to taking milk from a human nipple. To help him, express a little milk before a feed (see page 94) so that the nipple stands out, and rub breast milk over it to give him the taste.

Twins It is possible to breastfeed twins successfully. It's fine to feed them one at a time. When you have gained more confidence, you might find it possible to feed them both at the same time, their legs tucked under each arm, and their heads lying in your hands.

Wind and winding

Whether your baby is breast- or bottle-fed, give him chance to burp up swallowed air when he pauses for a rest; the wind may be making him feel full. If he doesn't burp after about half a minute, give up: he probably doesn't need to bring up any air.

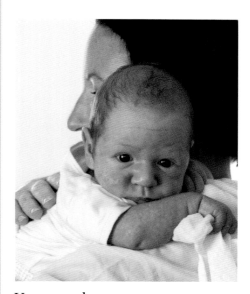

Your newborn
To help your baby bring up wind, put him against your shoulder and rub his back. Make sure his head is supported. He may bring some milk up too (known as possetting), so keep a clean cloth handy.

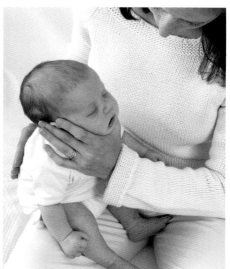

Your older baby
By three months, when your baby can sit up for short periods, jiggling him gently on your lap while you rub his back will help him burp up swallowed air. Make sure you still support his head.

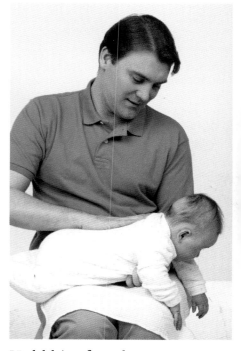

Hold him face down
At any age, holding your baby face down across your lap or in your arms may help him bring up wind. Rub or pat his back gently, but rhythmically, to help him to burp.

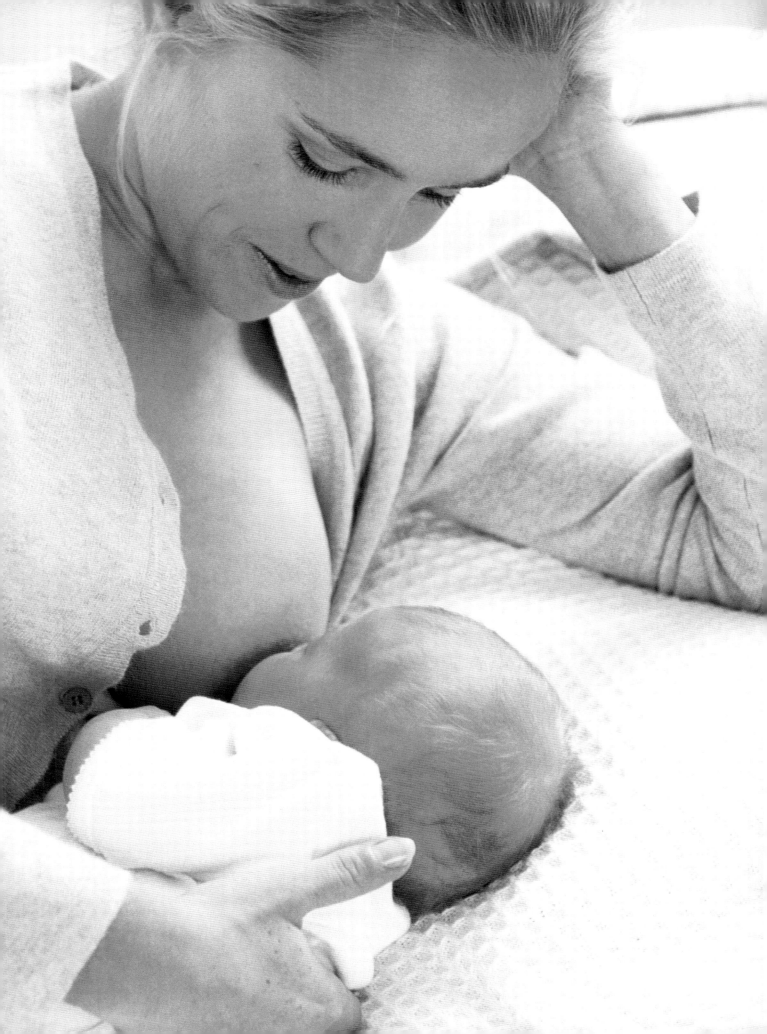

Breastfeeding your baby

Breastfeeding can be a very rewarding aspect of caring for your baby, and you'll be giving her the best nourishment – so don't be deterred if you encounter a few problems in the early days. You and your baby have to learn this new skill together, so if at first she doesn't seem to know how to suck, or doesn't suck for very long, be patient with her. She doesn't need a lot of food just after the birth. If breastfeeding seems difficult at first, your midwife or health visitor will be able to help you, and there will be plenty of friends and relatives to offer advice. Several breastfeeding associations also provide support. Once you're over the first few weeks, you can look forward to months of successful and satisfying feeding.

Getting comfortable

Settle yourself comfortably. The more relaxed you appear to your baby, the easier she will settle to feed. If you're in private, take your top off: with no clothes in the way, you will give her plenty of opportunity for skin contact, and might find it easier to get her "latched on" – that is, properly positioned on your breast and sucking efficiently.

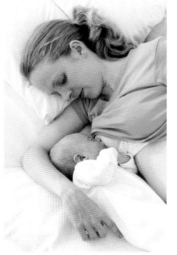

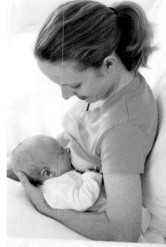

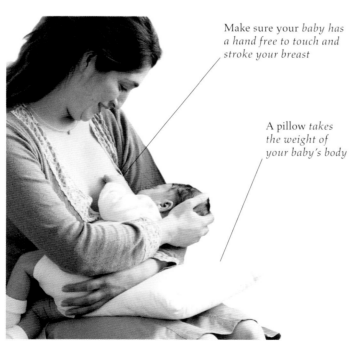

Make sure your *baby has a hand free to touch and stroke your breast*

A pillow *takes the weight of your baby's body*

Your young baby's early feeds
Sit comfortably in an upright position with your back supported. A low chair without arms is ideal, or sit up in bed with plenty of pillows propping your back. Your baby should be held close, chest to chest. Lift her up to your breast, rather than bending over her.

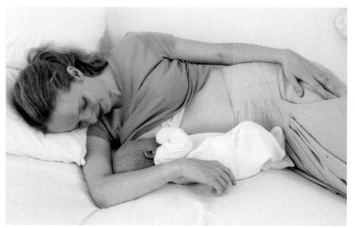

Your older baby's feeds
Once you are both adept at feeding, you will find you can nurse in almost any relaxed position. Sitting cross-legged on the bed or floor is excellent, especially if you can prop your back against pillows or furniture.

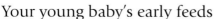

Your first breastfeeds
Finding the nipple

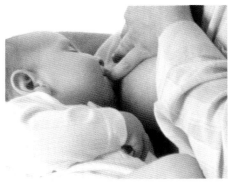 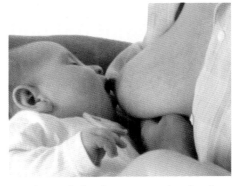 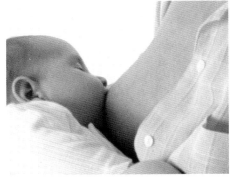

1 Your baby has an instinctive reflex that makes her search for your nipple to find food – this is called the "rooting" reflex. You can alert this reflex by stroking the cheek nearest you.

2 If your baby doesn't turn her head instinctively, try gently squeezing just behind your areola until a few drops form on your nipple. Touch her lips with this to encourage her to open her mouth.

3 Bring her head up close to your breast, so her chin is against it, and her tongue is underneath your nipple. Lift your baby to your breast, and let her latch on properly (see below).

Latching on

1 Once latched on, your baby doesn't just suck, she "milks" the breast with her jaws by pressing on the reservoirs of the milk at the base of the areola. If your baby just sucks on the nipple, you will get sore and she won't get any milk. If you feel a momentary piercing pain, breathe deeply to help you relax.

2 From your viewpoint, your well latched-on baby will have her jaws very wide and her mouth full of your breast. You can tell she is feeding properly when you see her temples and ears moving, showing that her jaw muscles are working hard.

The let-down reflex

Your baby's sucking action stimulates your breasts to release the milk they have stored. You may feel the warm rush of milk – the let-down reflex – as a tingling sensation soon after your baby has latched on. The stimulation sends a message to the pituitary gland to release oxytocin, which contracts the muscles around the mammary glands. Not everyone feels it though, so don't be surprised if you don't. If the reflex makes milk leak out of the other breast too, hold a breast pad over your nipple to catch drips, or use a breast shell (see page 96).

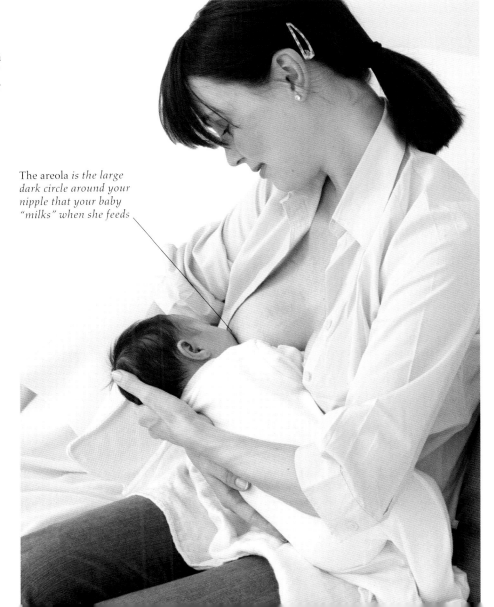

The areola *is the large dark circle around your nipple that your baby "milks" when she feeds*

Offering the other breast

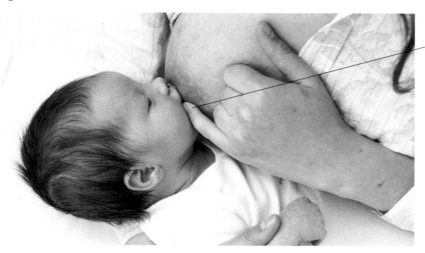

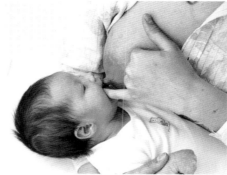

Use your clean *little finger to break your baby's suction*

1 Let your baby feed for as long as she wants to at the first breast, so she drains it – your breast will look smaller, and feel lighter when all the milk has gone. Your baby will often pause during her feed and just suck for a while. After a pause of several minutes when she is no longer taking in any milk, remove her from the breast, and wind her. Don't pull your nipple away – this will hurt. Slip a finger between her jaws to break the suction.

2 When your baby is off the nipple, slip a tissue or breast pad into your bra to catch any drips. Sit your baby up to wind her. Make a note to start her next feed on the other breast, so that they get equal stimulation.

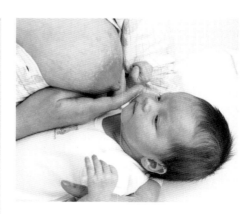

3 After a burp or two, and perhaps a short sleep, you can offer your baby the other breast. She may be hungry enough to drain this one, too, or she may just suck for comfort. She needs this as much as she needs the milk – so let her carry on.

4 When your baby's had enough to drink, she will fall fast asleep in your arms and let your nipple slip from her mouth. Don't worry if you think she has not taken a full feed; you can trust your baby to know how much she wants and needs at any time. If she feels hungry again, she will wake and let you know.

How your breasts produce milk

In the first few days after the birth, your breasts produce colostrum, a protein-rich food that supplies your baby with valuable antibodies against infection. Once you begin to produce milk on around the fourth day, your baby will naturally stimulate your body into producing a plentiful supply for her dietary needs.

The key to a good milk supply is feeding your baby when she wants to be fed – and in the early days that may mean at one- or two-hourly intervals. Breast milk production works on a demand and supply system: the more often your baby nurses, and the more she takes, the more your breasts will produce. Supplementary bottles of formula milk will undermine this system: if your baby's hunger is satisfied by a bottle, she won't be eager to suck and your breasts won't get the stimulation they need.

Breast milk isn't all the same. At the beginning of the feed, your baby takes foremilk, which is watery and thirst-quenching. Then she gets to the hindmilk, rich in calories and more satisfying. This is why it's important to let her suck for as long as she wants to at each feed: otherwise she will soon be hungry again.

What you need to do

All you need to do to produce enough milk is to eat a good, balanced diet with plenty of protein, to drink whenever you are thirsty – have a glass of juice or milk on hand while you feed – and to rest as much as you can. Your baby's natural appetite will do the rest.

You need a lot of energy to produce breast milk, so this is not the time to diet – you will feel run down and exhausted. Follow your appetite, and make sure you get the extra calories you need from fresh, vitamin-rich foods rather than "empty" carbohydrates. While you're breastfeeding you need to take a vitamin D supplement containing 10 micrograms (mcg). Everything else you should get by eating a varied and balanced diet.

When your milk comes in

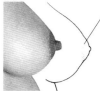

Normal breast **Engorged breast**

The areola is swollen and firm, so it may be hard for your baby to grasp; and the nipple is flattened

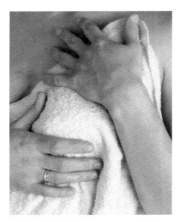

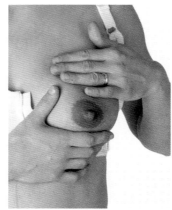

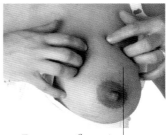

Draw your fingertips down towards the areola

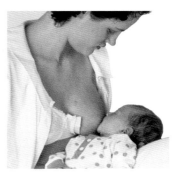

1 On about the fourth day of breastfeeding your breasts start to produce mature milk, as well as the colostrum that you've fed your baby up to now. You may wake up to find your breasts big, hard, and heavy and they can be quite uncomfortable. This is engorgement, and it may last for up to 48 hours. Your baby will find it hard to latch on because the nipple isn't sticking out, but is flattened by the swollen areola. The following tips should help her to feed, so clear the engorgement and ease your discomfort.

2 Before you try to breastfeed your baby, soften your breasts by laying warm flannels over them for several minutes. Or you may prefer to stand in the shower and splash warm water over your breasts.

3 Massage your breasts gently with your hands, and try to express some milk to relieve the swelling and help your baby get the nipple in her mouth (see page 94). Don't worry if you can't get the hang of expressing at this stage, you will soon.

4 When you put your baby to the breast, put your free hand on your ribcage under your breast and push gently upwards: this should help the nipple to protrude so your baby can get the areola in her mouth. Her sucking will quickly relieve the engorgement and discomfort.

"My baby son cries a great deal; could it be that he isn't getting enough milk from me to satisfy his hunger?"
When you are breastfeeding you can't actually see how much milk your baby is taking, so it's natural sometimes to worry that he is not getting enough. However, as long as you offer a feed whenever your baby cries, and he is gaining weight normally with occasional spurts, you have no need to worry that he will be undernourished. Remember that your baby will probably lose a little weight during the first days of life, and may not regain his birthweight immediately. It could also be that your baby is suffering from colic (see page 118).

"Will breastfeeding alter my figure for life?"
Your breasts may be slightly smaller after you have weaned your baby from the breast, because some of the fatty tissue in the breasts has been replaced by milk glands. Otherwise, you will probably regain your pre-pregnancy figure more quickly if you breastfeed. This is because the hormones released during breastfeeding encourage the uterus to shrink back to normal quickly, and the fat reserves that your body laid down during your pregnancy are used in the production of breast milk. Your waistline will also contract sooner than if you bottle-feed, and your pelvis returns to normal more quickly.

"When I am breastfeeding, do I have to be as careful as I was when I was pregnant about the drugs, medications I take, as well as my caffeine and alcohol intake?"

Q&A

What you eat and drink can be passed on to your baby through your milk, so it's still vital that you tell your chemist or doctor that you are breastfeeding before they prescribe any medicines for you. It's sensible to avoid stimulants such as alcohol and caffeine, too. If your baby won't sleep well, it may be worthwhile cutting coffee and tea out of your diet for a few weeks to see if the situation improves – the caffeine may be keeping him awake.

Expressing milk by hand

At some point, you might need to be separated from your baby, and will need to have breast milk available for him. By experimenting, you will find the best way for you to express milk – some mothers find manual expression works best, others like pumping, and some find both work well. It takes time and experience to learn how to stimulate the let-down reflex, so expressing only small amounts of milk does not mean that you don't have enough. Before you express by hand, sterilize the equipment, and wash your hands. Encourage the flow of milk by having a warm bath, or hold warm flannels over your breasts. Make yourself comfortable at a high surface, with the bowl in front of you.

Hand expressing

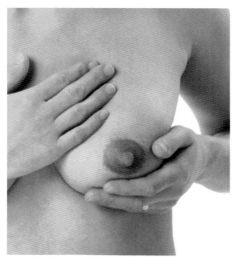

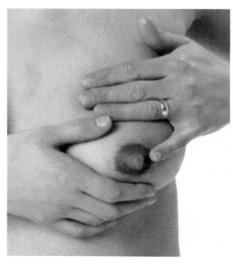

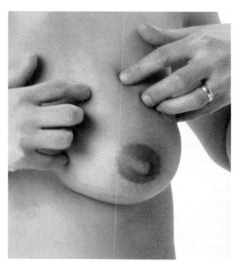

1 Support your breast in one hand and start to massage, working downwards from above the breast. Use your whole hand to massage the breast.

2 Work your way all around the breast, including the underside. Complete at least 10 circuits – this helps the flow of milk through the ducts.

3 Stroke downwards towards the areola with your fingernails several times. Use a rolling motion and avoid pressing on the breast tissue.

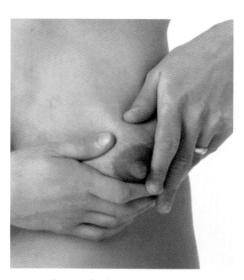

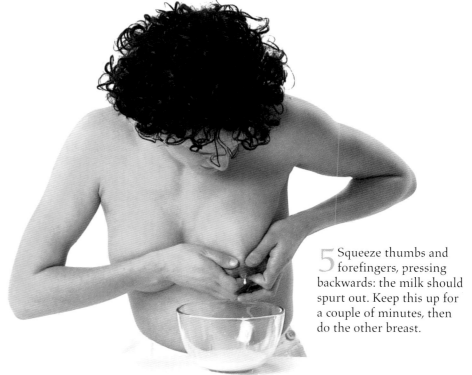

4 Apply gentle downward pressure on the area behind the areola with your thumbs and fingers, and rotate them gently to help access reservoirs.

5 Squeeze thumbs and forefingers, pressing backwards: the milk should spurt out. Keep this up for a couple of minutes, then do the other breast.

Expressing milk using a pump

Using a pump to express milk is often quicker and less tiring than expressing it by hand. Ease of use, durability, and suction adjustment are things to consider when choosing a breast pump. Ask your midwife or healthcare provider for advice. Your own personal circumstances are likely to dictate the pump you choose to some extent. For example, if you are frequently separated from your baby, or if you have twins, you might consider a double-sided electric pump, which will allow you to express milk in a shorter time. Or, if you plan to express milk only occasionally, a hand- or battery-operated pump may be the best option. In addition, the more expensive and powerful electric pumps can usually be hired. When pumping, it is important to make yourself as comfortable as possible in a chair with good back support. Relax as much as you can to ensure the best flow of milk.

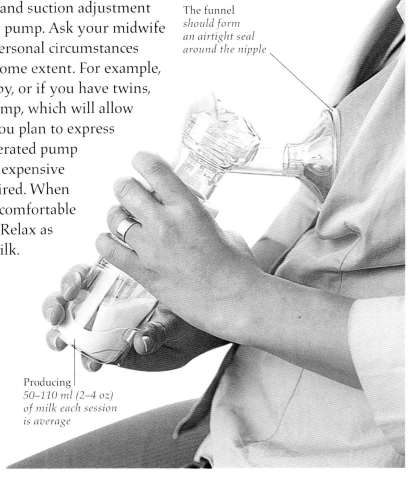

The funnel should form an airtight seal around the nipple

Producing 50–110 ml (2–4 oz) of milk each session is average

Preparing your pump

Pumps can vary, so read the instructions carefully. Stimulate your breasts beforehand, as described for expressing milk manually on the facing page. This is important for stimulating the let-down reflex, and pumping efficiently. Place the funnel of the pump over the areola to form an airtight seal. Your nipple should be positioned so that it is in the middle of the funnel. Once attached, start the pump. It is recommended that you don't go for longer than 20 minutes per breast. Ideally you should swap between your breasts as soon as milk flow from one begins to decrease.

Pumps

Manual pump

This type of pump has improved in recent years, and is now more effective and easier to use. A manual pump allows you to control the rate of pumping, but some women still find the device tiring.

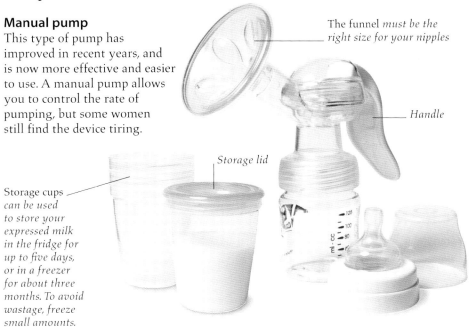

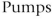
Storage cups can be used to store your expressed milk in the fridge for up to five days, or in a freezer for about three months. To avoid wastage, freeze small amounts.

Storage lid

The funnel must be the right size for your nipples

Handle

Battery pump

Battery-operated pumps take the work out of pumping, but the rate is not as easy to control as it is with manual pumps. Some battery pumps come with an adaptor so that they can also be operated by electricity mains if desired.

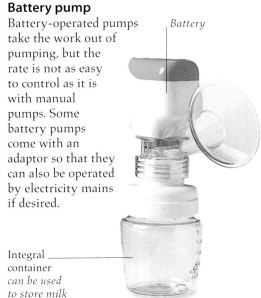

Battery

Integral container can be used to store milk

Breastfeeding problems

Get professional help quickly if you have any problems with breastfeeding: struggling on alone is discouraging, and something minor such as a blocked duct can lead to mastitis if it doesn't clear. Don't stop feeding if you encounter the problems below: you will only become engorged with milk, and make any problem worse. Take good care of your breasts.

Wear a comfortable nursing bra, both day and night for the early weeks: don't wear one that is too tight, as it may constrict the milk ducts. Be gentle when you massage your breasts. Let the air get to your nipples as often as possible, and wash them with water, not soap as it dries the skin. Dry thoroughly. You may even use a hair dryer on a low setting to do this.

Leaking breasts

Your breasts may leak copiously between feeds in the early weeks.
Treatment Breast pads inside your bra will absorb some drips, but change the pads frequently as wetness near your skin may make you sore. If you leak a lot, try using a plastic breast shell, and, in extreme cases, wear breast pads over it.
Prevention None, but leaking breasts are proof of a good milk supply, and help prevent engorgement. Don't be too concerned because the leaking will diminish as your milk supply matches the demands of your baby.

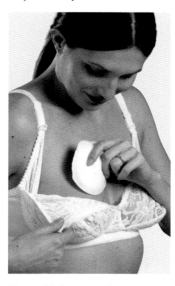

Disposable breast pad
A breast pad will absorb drips and small leaks and can help you stay dry and comfortable if you experience leaking. You can use disposable or washable breast pads.

Blocked ducts

A small, hard, tender, red lump in the breast usually means that one of the milk ducts has become blocked.
Treatment Bathe the breast in hot water and massage it gently, then put your baby to the breast. You might want to apply a heat pack on the affected side while you breastfeed. You may get a moment's intense pain when your baby latches on, but the duct should clear. If it doesn't clear, see your doctor that day.
Prevention Make sure your breastfeeding technique is sound and your baby is latching on properly.

Mastitis

A blocked milk duct may become infected, producing flu-like symptoms. Seek medical help urgently: if untreated, mastitis may lead to a breast abscess, which may need surgery.
Treatment Your doctor will prescribe antibiotics, and you must finish the course. Continue to feed your baby from both breasts as normal.
Prevention Regular feeding from both breasts will help prevent mastitis. Never let a tender lump in your breast go longer than a day without treatment.

Sore or cracked nipples

Prevention is always better than cure – sore nipples are nearly always caused because your baby is not correctly positioned at the breast and not latching on properly. Make sure she takes a large mouthful of breast and not just the nipple into her mouth. If your baby doesn't latch on properly don't pull your nipple out – that will hurt even more – but break the suction by putting your finger into the corner of her mouth, take her from the breast and start again. Sometimes the problem can be a badly fitting bra that puts pressure on your nipples, and breast pads and bra linings can make it worse by trapping moisture.
Treatment for sore nipples Try the following suggestions:
● Ask you health visitor to help you make sure your baby latches on properly.
● Try expressing a little colostrum or breast milk and then rubbing it gently onto your nipples – many people find that this works wonders.
● Dry your nipples after a feed using a hairdryer on a cool setting.
● Let the air get to your nipples for several hours a day. If you have a cracked nipple you will probably feel a sharp, shooting pain in your breast as your baby sucks. Rest the breast for a day by expressing milk. A crack will usually heal within a few days.
Prevention Make sure that your baby takes the areola into her mouth. Keep your nipples dry between feeds.

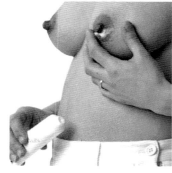

Cracked nipples
A purified lanolin cream formulated for breastfeeding may help the healing process.

Your emotions and let-downs

Your let-down reflex is strongly associated with your emotional state of being. When you are embarrassed, irritated, exhausted, or anxious, your breast milk doesn't always appear as readily as when you are relaxed. A few minutes of quiet cuddling with your baby in private should help relax both of you and make you and your baby ready to nurse.

Feeding the older child

Until the age of about six months, babies need only milk. After that, they are ready and able to start complementary foods. Milk will still be the most important food for the first year of life and remains an important food afterwards. Talk to your healthcare provider about how to introduce solids. Remember that you can easily and inexpensively make your own healthy foods for your baby. Start by offering your baby solids in small amounts, ideally at the same time as you have your own family meals if practical, so that her routine will coincide with that of the rest of the family. In the meantime, she will continue to nurse whenever she needs to, and for as long as she needs to.

How often will she nurse?

As your baby grows, her feedings will become more varied in duration and frequency. She'll nurse for hunger, thirst, when cold, tired, and when she just wants a cuddle. Remember that her varied nursing pattern does not mean that your milk is drying up. This is a perfectly normal pattern for a growing baby. There will be still more changes when you introduce her to solids.

How do I wean?

Gradually replace one breastfeeding at a time with milk by bottle or cup (depending on the age of your child). See page 106 for suggested guidelines when switching to bottle-feeding. If your baby is less than 12 months of age, replace breast milk with formula; otherwise, check with your doctor.

You may want to stop the night-time breastfeeding last, especially if this is a time for you and your baby to bond.

Going back to work

It is perfectly possible to return to work and continue breastfeeding, but it means planning ahead. While you are away, your baby will have to take milk from a bottle or, if she is over six months, from a trainer cup with a soft spout. So aim to get her used to it before you return to work.

If you want your baby to have breast milk only, you will need to express milk at work during the day to keep your milk supply stimulated. Or you may want her to have formula milk during the day but continue to breastfeed when you are at home. Your milk supply will respond to your baby's changing needs.

- Stock up on expressed milk in your freezer for a few weeks before you go back to work. Let it thaw naturally and warm it by putting the container in a bowl of warm water (not a microwave).
- At work you will need sterile equipment and a private place to express milk during the day, plus access to a fridge to store it. Transport the milk in an insulated cool box.
- If necessary, boost your milk supply by giving extra feeds during the evening and night.
- Ask your baby's carer to delay the late afternoon feed so your baby will be ready for a breastfeed when you get home.
- Leave formula ready to be made up in case your baby demands an extra feed while you are away.

How long should I nurse for?

No international group or organization has put a limit on the duration of breastfeeding and all encourage extended breastfeeding. The World Health Organization recommends two or more years, or as long as mutually desirable. When your baby is ready to stop, she will just nurse less and less.

Continuing breastfeeding
You can continue to nurse your baby for as long as you feel comfortable doing so. The more breast milk a baby gets, the healthier she will be.

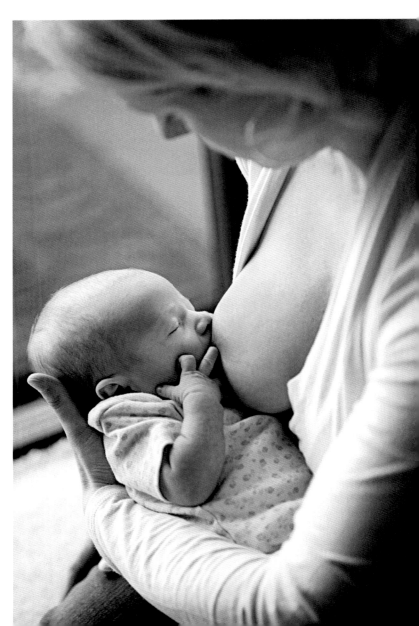

Bottle-feeding your baby

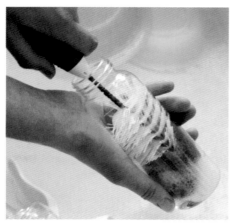

Bottle-feeding has two advantages – your partner can also do it, and you can see how much milk your baby is taking. Your health visitor will watch your bottle-fed baby's weight carefully in case he is putting on too much weight because you are overfeeding. It's important to sterilize bottles carefully, and to follow the manufacturer's instructions closely when making up a feed; formula that is too weak or too concentrated is harmful to your baby.

Equipment for bottle-feeding

For a baby who is fully bottle-fed, you will need at least eight full size (250ml/8oz) bottles. Buy extra teats, and keep them ready in a sterile jar in case one gives an inadequate flow of milk (see page 100).

Some bottles are supplied with discs that seal them, while the more modern, wide-necked bottles can be sealed with the protective cap. Disposable bottles are also available for travelling.

Bottles and other equipment

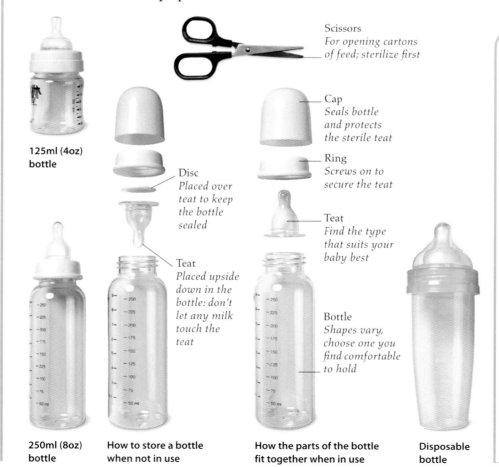

Scissors
For opening cartons of feed; sterilize first

Cap
Seals bottle and protects the sterile teat

Ring
Screws on to secure the teat

Teat
Find the type that suits your baby best

Bottle
Shapes vary, choose one you find comfortable to hold

125ml (4oz) bottle

Disc
Placed over teat to keep the bottle sealed

Teat
Placed upside down in the bottle: don't let any milk touch the teat

250ml (8oz) bottle

How to store a bottle when not in use

How the parts of the bottle fit together when in use

Disposable bottle

Bisphenol A (BPA)

Bisphenol is a chemical in the plastic used to make many babies' feeding bottles. In some circumstances – if the bottles are heated or scratched through repeated washing – the chemical can leak into the feed. Although the dose the baby receives is very small, there is some evidence that it may be harmful to the developing reproductive, neurological, and immune systems, and as a precaution some countries are withdrawing from sale all bottles containing the chemical. The bottles to avoid are the clear, shatter-proof polycarbonate plastic bottles, which often have the number "7" in the recycling triangle, or the letters "PC" near the recycling triangle. The safest bottles are made of glass or softer plastics, such as polyethylene, polypropylene, or polyamide. Sources of these can be found on the internet.

Teats

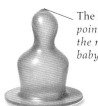

The holes *must point towards the roof of your baby's mouth*

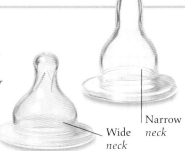

Wide neck

Narrow *neck*

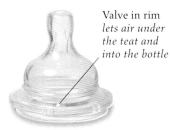

Valve in rim *lets air under the teat and into the bottle*

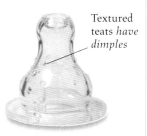

Textured teats *have dimples*

Orthodontic teat

The teat must go into your baby's mouth with the hole facing upward, so that the milk sprays over the roof of his mouth. An orthodontic teat is good for babies who are otherwise breastfed, as it mimics the shape of the mother's nipple more closely, and may be more acceptable. The shape also promotes correct development of the baby's mouth.

Standard neck teat

The standard shape of teat gives a sucking action that is not really like sucking from your breast, and babies who are otherwise breastfed may find them difficult to use. Teats are available with different rates of flow: slower flow rates are better for newborns and breastfed babies, while faster rates are more suitable for older bottle-fed babies.

Anti-colic teat

An anti-colic teat lets air into the bottle as your baby sucks the milk out. This stops the teat from collapsing, so enabling him to get a steady stream of milk, and perhaps lessening the likelihood of him developing colic from swallowing air. Like standard neck teats, anti-colic teats are available with different flow rates to suit your baby's needs.

Textured teat

These silicone teats are dimpled to make their texture more like that of an actual nipple. This type of teat is not interchangeable among different makes of bottle. As your baby sucks, his lips push against the squashy base, and the teat moves back and forth in his mouth. Fit the teat and ring together before assembling the bottle ready for filling.

"There are so many different types of formula – how do I know which one to buy?"
A cow's milk-based, iron-fortified formula remains the most acceptable alternative to breast milk. Some babies have problems digesting standard formula. If you think that your baby is having a problem with a milk-based formula, ask your doctor or health visitor for advice. If your healthcare provider identifies a problem, you may be advised to buy an alternative formula that is not milk-based, but do not do this without seeking professional advice first.

"Formula is expensive. When can I switch to regular milk?"
Cow's milk is very different in composition from breast milk, and a poor source of iron. It should only be introduced as a drink when your baby is eating a wide range of other foods, usually at about 12 months of age.

"The rest of my family uses low-fat milk products – when can my baby use these?"
Low-fat milk products (skimmed, 1 per cent fat, and 2 per cent fat) should not be used until your child is at least two years old. Low-fat milk products have excessive amounts of minerals and protein, are low in fat content, and lack essential fatty acids. Although popular with adults, they are not appropriate for very young children.

"How do I know when to wind my baby?"
If your baby is sucking happily, there is no need to stop feeding to wind him – wait until there is a natural break in the feed, and if he doesn't bring up any wind, carry on feeding as normal. If you're bottle-feeding, he'll swallow less air if you feed him in as upright a position as possible.

Q&A

Formula: what's in it?

Formula is sweeter than ordinary cow's milk, and as close in composition to breast milk as manufacturers can make it. Cow's milk is not well suited to your baby's needs – it doesn't contain all the nutrients essential for growth, and it can be difficult for him to digest. Most infant formulas are adapted from a cow's milk base, but are well supplemented with many other ingredients. Vegetable oils are added to replace cow's butter fat, and lactose is used to sweeten the mixture. Some formulas are fortified with iron, while others are derived entirely from soya. Use soya-based formulas only if your healthcare provider previously recommends them. If your baby vomits after a bottle; has diarrhoea, cramps, or excessive wind; wheezes; develops a rash; or is irritable, call your doctor immediately, and discuss the problem. Babies can dehydrate very quickly.

Washing your baby's feeding equipment

Your baby's teats, bottles, and other feeding equipment must be kept scrupulously clean. They can be cleaned either by hand, in hot, soapy water, or you can put them into your dishwasher to save time and energy. For babies under six months old, it will also be necessary to sterilize all equipment before use. Dummies and teething rings will also have to be thoroughly cleaned before use.

Using a dishwasher

An efficient way to wash your baby's feeding equipment is to put it in your dishwasher, making sure it goes through the hot drying cycle. The high heat is usually sufficient to kill any bacteria. Teats may have to be boiled separately because dishwashers can turn them into unusable sticky blobs.

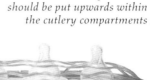
Dishwasher-proof teats should be put upwards within the cutlery compartments

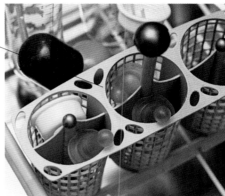

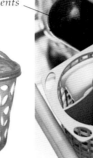

Dishwasher basket holds bottles, rings, and caps, and has grippers on top to keep teats in place

Hand-washing

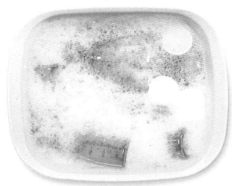

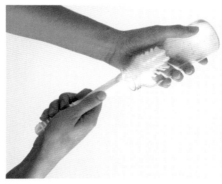

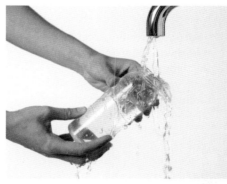

1 Put the rinsed-out bottles, teats, caps, rings, discs, jug, funnel, spoon, and knife into hot soapy water, and wash them thoroughly.

2 Scrub inside the bottles with the bottle brush to remove all traces of milk. Make sure you scrub carefully around the necks and the screw heads.

3 Make sure that you rinse the bottles, teats, and any other equipment thoroughly under running water. Use a pin to clear the holes in the teats.

Taking care of teats

Your baby can only feed happily if the nipple allows him to suck out formula at the right rate. When you tip the bottle up, you should see two to three drops a second: too small a hole will mean that your baby gets frustrated in his efforts to suck out enough formula; too large and the formula will gush out. Nipples do deteriorate, and the holes clog up. Have some spare sterile teats stored in a jar, so you can easily swap an imperfect teat for a fresh one. Throw away teats if the holes are too large; holes that are too small can be enlarged with a needle. Check the flow again afterwards.

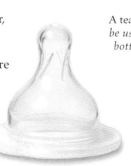
A teat brush should be used to clean the bottles thoroughly

Good hygiene and sterilizing

Formula, when warm or held for too long at room temperature, is a breeding ground for bacteria that cause vomiting or diarrhoea. These diseases, although not serious in an older child, can be life-threatening in a young baby. Before filling your baby's bottle make sure your hands are clean. Until your baby is six months old, sterilize the bottle and everything coming in contact with it either by boiling or using sterilizing tablets. You can also buy a steam sterilizer or microwave steam unit specially designed for sterilizing bottles. Never store bottles of made-up formula in the fridge. Always make a fresh feed.

Equipment for sterilizing

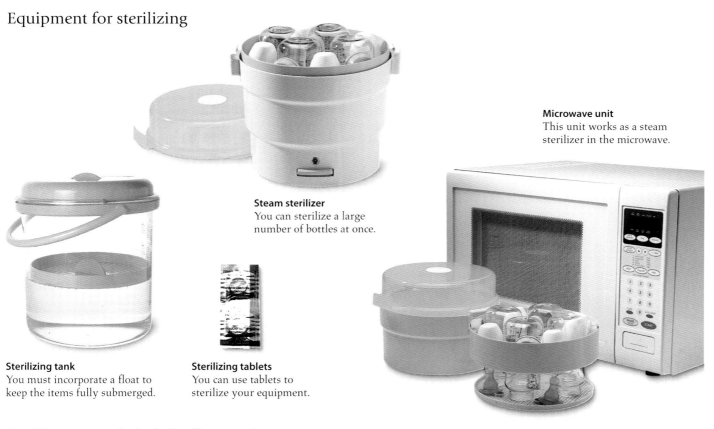

Microwave unit
This unit works as a steam sterilizer in the microwave.

Steam sterilizer
You can sterilize a large number of bottles at once.

Sterilizing tank
You must incorporate a float to keep the items fully submerged.

Sterilizing tablets
You can use tablets to sterilize your equipment.

Sterilizing your baby's feeding equipment

Sterilize all your baby's feeding equipment either by using a sterilizer or a steam sterilizer.

The occasional use of the boiling method will also sterilize, although repeated use will spoil the quality of the teats. If using the boiling method, wash the equipment and boil for five minutes. Use tongs to remove the hot bottles, and leave them until they are quite cold before filling.

If using tablets, fill the sterilizing tank with cold water, and add the tablets. When they have dissolved, put the equipment in, filling the bottles so they can't bob up. Leave for at least the minimum time, then take out items as needed and rinse in boiled water. Drain on kitchen paper.

All items must be fully submerged during the boiling period

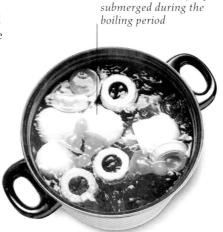

The boiling method

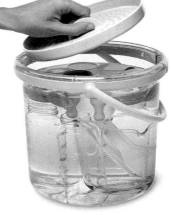

Sterilizing with tablets

Making up your baby's feed

It is important to make up a fresh bottle for your baby for each feed. Have a sterile empty bottle ready, and fill it with cooled boiled water whenever your baby requires a feed. Until your baby is at least one year old, give him an infant formula milk, which is modified cow's milk. Your health visitor will help you choose a brand. You can upset your baby by switching brands, so never do so without professional advice. Do not give cow's milk until your child is one year old.

Making up a powder formula

Infant formula is most commonly and inexpensively available as powder in tins, which you mix with cooled boiled water as needed. The instructions on the tins should tell you the correct number of level, loosely filled scoops to add to each measure of water. It is very important to maintain these proportions exactly. If you add too much formula, the feed will be dangerously concentrated: your baby may gain too much weight, and his kidneys may be damaged. If you consistently add too little powder, he may gain weight too slowly. Always use fresh, cold mains water to make your baby's feeds, and boil it once only. Some types of water should never be used:

● water that has been repeatedly boiled, or left standing in the kettle
● water from a tap with a domestic softener attached – the extra sodium (salt) can damage your baby's kidneys
● water from a tap with a domestic filter attached – filters can trap harmful bacteria
● mineral water – the sodium and mineral levels may be harmful.

The recommended method to make up your baby's feed is by mixing the formula directly in the bottle (see page 103).

Ready-mixed infant milk

Some brands of infant milk are also available ready-mixed in 250ml (8fl oz) sealed cartons. You need to add no water to the milk. If the brand of formula you are feeding your baby comes in this form, then you have a very convenient – but expensive – option.

The milk in the carton has been ultra-heat treated (UHT). Store unopened cartons in a cool place, and do not use after the "best before" date. Once opened, the milk can be stored in the fridge for up to 24 hours, either in a sterile, sealed bottle, or in the carton. However, unless you can be sure that you won't forget when you put the carton in the fridge, it's probably safer to pour all the milk out when your baby wants a feed, and throw away any he doesn't drink.

How much will my baby want?

On average, your baby needs 150ml of milk per kilogram (2½fl oz per 1lb) of body weight every 24 hours. You need to keep your baby on just formula milk even after you start weaning at six months. As a rough guide, a six-month-old baby will take a maximum 250ml (8fl oz) per feed, a five-month-old baby 200ml (7fl oz) per feed, a four-month-old baby 180ml (6fl oz) per feed, and so on. The risks of overfeeding are greater than underfeeding. Individual parents should consult their healthcare providers.

Should I give anything else?

While your baby is taking formula milk, extra supplements are not necessary. Vitamin supplements are advised from year one, when your child goes on to ordinary cow's milk. Never add anything to your baby's feed. Because formula is modified cow's milk, it can, in very rare cases, set off an allergy. Should this happen, go back to breastfeeding or see your doctor to discuss alternatives. Your doctor may suggest a specially prepared formula, which contains proteins that have been broken down so they do not cause an allergic response.

The right milk to give your baby

Type of milk		Birth	6m	9m	12m	18m
Infant formula	Cow's milk modified to resemble human breast milk. Supplements are not necessary.	→→→→→→→→→→→→→→→→→→→→→→→→→				
Follow-up formula	**Optional.** Modified cow's milk, intended for babies of six months to two years. Contains iron and vitamin D, so supplements are not needed.			→→→→→→→→→→→→→→→		
Full fat cow's milk	Introduce as main milk drink from 12 months; extra iron and vitamins A, C, and D may be needed. Can be given mixed with cereal from six months.					→→→→→

Making up powder formula in the bottle

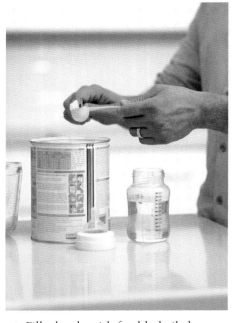

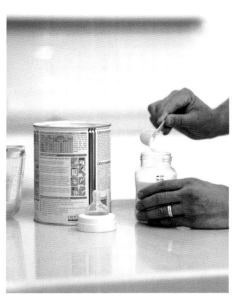

You will need

- Tin of powder formula
- Bottles and teats
- Kitchen paper

1 Fill a bottle with freshly boiled water. Open the tin of formula, and use the scoop inside to scoop up some powder. Level each scoop with the back of a sterilized knife: do not heap the scoop, nor pack the powder down inside it.

2 Drop each scoop of powder into the bottle. Add only the number of scoops recommended for that amount of water. The powder will dissolve quickly in hot water. Always add one scoop at a time; never add extra.

DHA and ARA supplemented formulas

DHA and ARA are fatty acids found naturally in breast milk and are added as supplements to some formula mixtures. There is some evidence that they may boost eyesight and language development in the first year, but by the age of three no difference has been found between babies fed this and those who were not given a supplemented formula. The supplemented milks are more expensive, and in a few babies may cause gas and bloating.

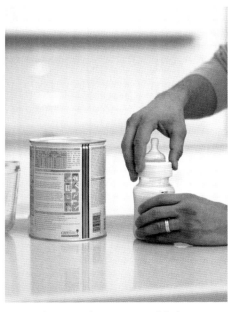

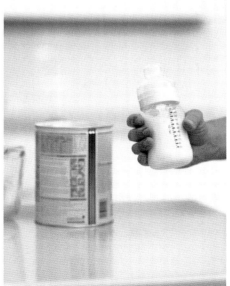

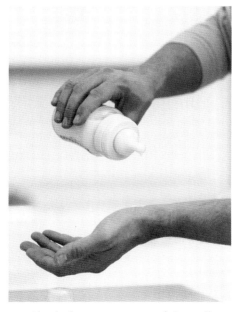

3 Make sure that you've added the right amount of formula. Put the disc, ring, and teat on the bottle. Screw on tightly. Put the lid on the top before shaking.

4 Shake the bottle to make sure the formula mixes thoroughly in the water. Cool the bottle in a bowl of cold water or under a cold running water tap.

5 Check the temperature of the milk before offering it to your baby by shaking a few drops on to your wrist. The milk should feel neither hot nor cold against your skin.

Using ready-mixed formula

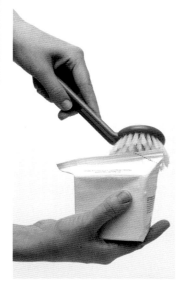

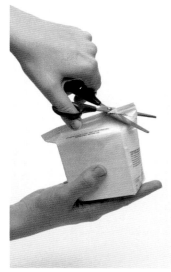

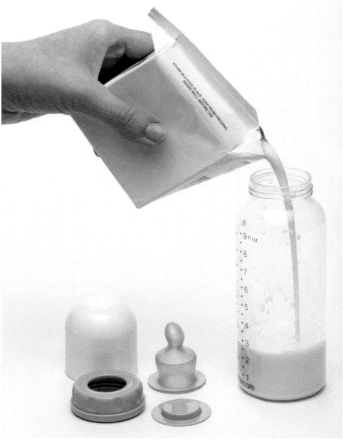

1 With a clean brush, scrub the top of the carton under running water. Also rinse a sterilized bottle with boiled water. Put to drain on kitchen paper.

2 Cut the top corner off. Make sure the pair of scissors you use is sterilized. Don't touch the raw edges of the carton – you may contaminate the milk.

You will need

- Carton of infant milk
- Feeding bottle
- Scrubbing brush
- Scissors

3 Empty the whole carton into the bottle (see page 102 for storage of this type of milk).

Protecting your baby from an upset stomach

If you take the precautions listed below, you should be able to protect your baby from the bacteria that cause stomach upsets (gastroenteritis).
- Sterilize all feeding equipment before you use it, even if it is brand new.
- If you do not have a fridge, make up each feed only when you need it.
- If your baby doesn't finish his bottle at a feed, throw the milk away as his saliva will have contaminated it.
- Throw away any milk warmed for your baby, even if he doesn't touch it; the process of warming the milk encourages bacteria to grow.

- Store opened cartons of ready-mixed formula in the main part of the fridge (not in the door). Don't keep the feed for longer than 24 hours.
- Leave the bottles in the sterilizing solution until you need them (it's effective for 24 hours) so that they can't be contaminated by bacteria in the air. Take the teats out after the minimum time, drain on kitchen paper, then store in a sterile jar.
- Don't drain sterilized equipment on your draining board or dry it on a tea towel. Drain only on kitchen paper.
- Wash your hands well with soap and water before touching the sterile feeding equipment.

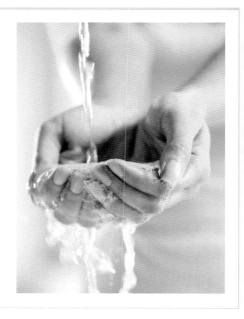

When away from home

If you're going out for more than a couple of hours, take cooled boiled water in a sterilized bottle and the measured formula powder in a dry container, and mix when your baby needs a feed. You can then take a flask filled with hot water, and warm your baby's bottle in this. Never carry a warm feed in a flask: bacteria will grow in the formula, and may cause a stomach upset. Cartons of made-up feed are even more convenient when you're away from home: the milk has been ultra-heat treated (UHT), so it needs only to be stored in a cool place to stay safe. Take sterile bottles and teats in a sterile container and pour out each feed as your baby needs it.

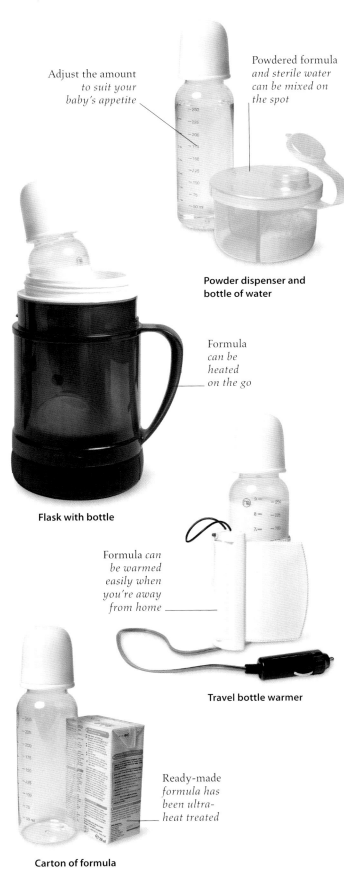

Adjust the amount *to suit your baby's appetite*

Powdered formula *and sterile water can be mixed on the spot*

Powder dispenser and bottle of water

Formula *can be heated on the go*

Flask with bottle

Formula *can be warmed easily when you're away from home*

Travel bottle warmer

Ready-made *formula has been ultra-heat treated*

Carton of formula

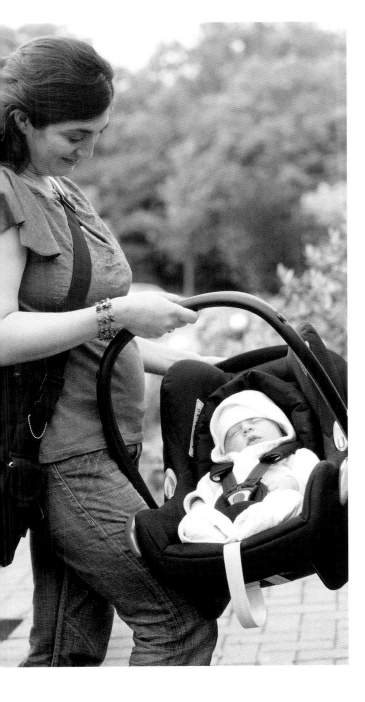

Giving your baby a bottle

Feeding your baby is the most important thing you can do for her – but don't make the mistake of thinking that the milk in the bottle is all she needs, or that "anyone" can feed her. Your love, your cuddling, and your attention are just as important to your baby as the milk itself. Always hold her close and cuddle her against you, smile and talk to her – just as you would if you were breastfeeding. Never, under any circumstances, leave your baby alone with her bottle: she may choke.

Right from the beginning, give your baby as much control over feeding as you can. Let her set the pace, pausing to look around, touch the bottle, or stroke your breast if she wants to – it may take as long as half an hour to empty the bottle if she's feeling playful. Above all, let her decide when she's had enough milk.

Make yourself comfortable, put a bib on her, and have a muslin cloth at hand for when you wind her in case she brings up any milk.

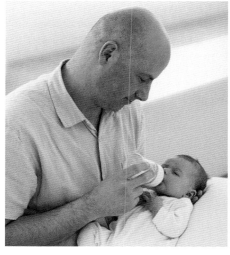

Bottle-feeding your baby
Your partner can now share in the joy and closeness of feeding your baby.

From breast- to bottle-feeding

If you have to change over to bottle-feeding from breastfeeding for any reason, remember that the transition needs a gradual approach and professional advice. Replacing one breastfeed with the bottle every third day is the best method – or you can go more slowly. You may start by replacing a lunchtime breastfeed with a bottle. If your baby won't take it, try again at the same feed the next day – you could offer a different type of teat (see page 99), or moisten the teat with a few drops of breast milk to encourage her. After three days with one bottle-feed, replace a second daytime feed with a bottle, and wait another three days before tackling a third feed. Carry on like this until eventually your baby has a bottle for her night-time feed.

Getting the bottle ready

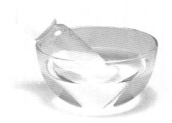

1 Always prepare a fresh feed. If the milk requires cooling, do so by keeping the bottle under a running cold water tap or standing it in a bowl of cold water.

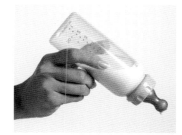

2 Check the flow of milk: it should be two to three drops a second. A small hole makes sucking hard; a large one lets the milk gush out. If the teat isn't right, get another sterile teat, and test the flow.

"My baby never seems to finish her bottle: is she getting enough?" **Q&A**

If your baby is feeding poorly, it could be a sign of illness, or of a serious underlying condition that needs medical attention. Check to see how much milk your baby should have for her weight (see page 102), and see if that matches what she actually takes. If you are at all concerned, talk to your health visitor about the problem, and make sure your baby is weighed regularly at the clinic, where her weight will be plotted on a growth chart (see pages 254–257). Poor feeding, if combined with inadequate weight gain, is always a cause for concern.

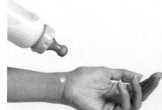

3 Test the temperature by tipping a few drops on to the inside of your wrist – it should feel tepid. Cold milk is safe, but your baby may prefer it warm.

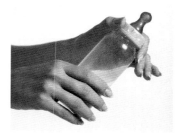

4 Unscrew the ring to let the air into the bottle. Then screw it back before giving to your baby as he sucks milk out. This will stop the teat from collapsing and halting the flow.

Giving your baby her bottle

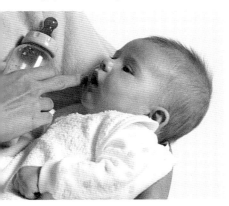

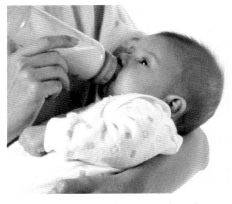

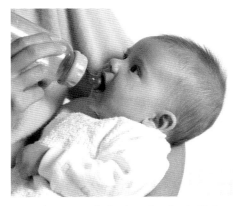

1 Stroke the cheek nearest you, she should turn and open her mouth. If she doesn't, or is older, let some drops of milk form on the teat, then touch her lips with it to give her the taste.

2 Hold the bottle firmly so that she can pull against it as she sucks, and tilt it so that the teat is full of milk, not air. If the teat collapses, move the bottle around in her mouth to let air back into the bottle.

3 When your baby has finished all the milk, pull the bottle firmly away. If she wants to continue sucking, offer her your clean little finger: she will soon let you know if she wants more milk.

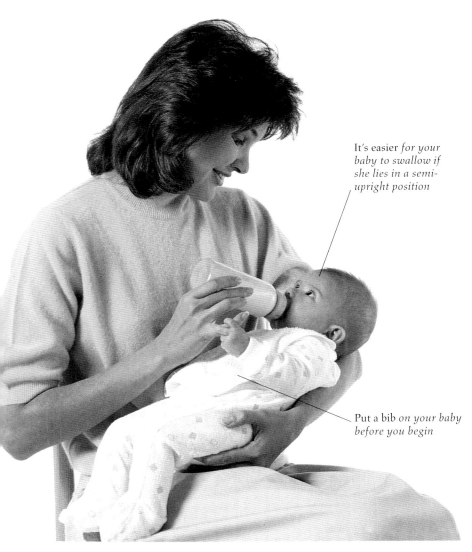

It's easier for your baby to swallow if she lies in a semi-upright position

Put a bib on your baby before you begin

If she won't let go

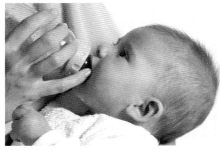

If your baby doesn't want to let go of the bottle even after a long suck, slide your little finger between her gums alongside the teat.

Sleeping during a feed

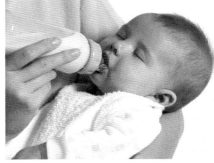

If she dozes off during her feed, she may have wind, which is making her feel full. Sit her up, and wind her for a couple of minutes, then offer her some more milk.

Introducing solid food

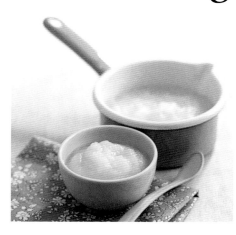

From the age of six months, your baby will be ready to try some solid food. Getting him used to unfamiliar tastes and textures may help him to avoid a "faddy" phase when he gets older. Let him eat as much as he reasonably wants – you want mealtimes to be enjoyable. Do not force him to eat foods that you think are good for him, but try to offer him choices. Including your baby in family mealtimes from an early age will help him learn essential social skills.

Equipment for first solids

The essential items you'll need for feeding your baby his first tastes include a clean plastic spoon, a bowl, and a bib to keep his clothes clean. Soon he will need beakers for drinks, and once he's sitting up steadily you will need a highchair. You don't need to sterilize equipment for solid food, just wash it well in very hot water, rinse, drain, and dry with kitchen paper.

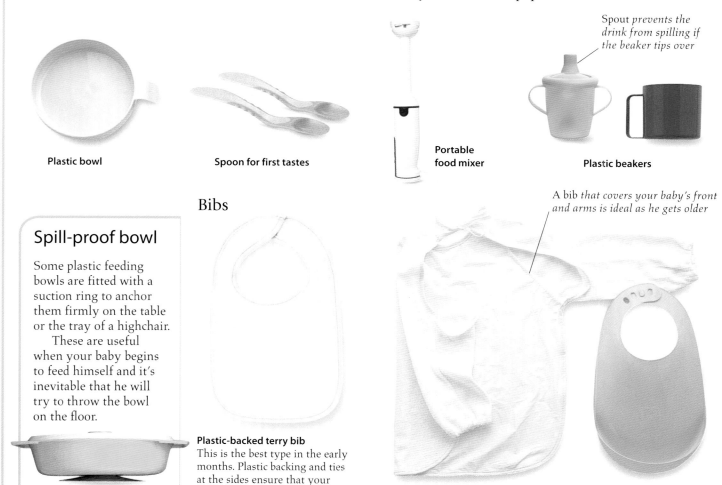

Plastic bowl

Spoon for first tastes

Portable food mixer

Spout *prevents the drink from spilling if the beaker tips over*

Plastic beakers

Spill-proof bowl

Some plastic feeding bowls are fitted with a suction ring to anchor them firmly on the table or the tray of a highchair.

These are useful when your baby begins to feed himself and it's inevitable that he will try to throw the bowl on the floor.

Bibs

A bib *that covers your baby's front and arms is ideal as he gets older*

Plastic-backed terry bib
This is the best type in the early months. Plastic backing and ties at the sides ensure that your child's clothes are protected.

Bib with sleeves

Plastic bib

Chairs

Highchair

Your baby needs a highchair from the age of about six months, or from when he can sit up steadily. Always strap him into the chair with a safety harness, and never leave him unsupervised. Put the chair on a plastic sheet to protect the floor, and involve your child in family meals by sitting him next to the table.

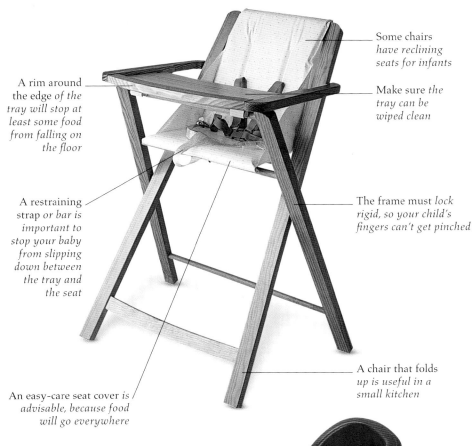

Some chairs have reclining seats for infants

Make sure the tray can be wiped clean

A rim around the edge *of the tray will stop at least some food from falling on the floor*

The frame must lock rigid, so your child's fingers can't get pinched

A restraining strap *or bar is important to stop your baby from slipping down between the tray and the seat*

An easy-care seat cover *is advisable, because food will go everywhere*

A chair that folds up is useful in a small kitchen

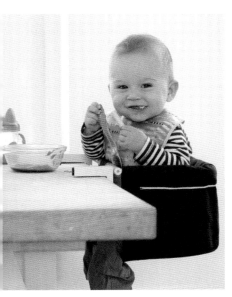

Clip-on chair

A seat that clamps onto a table is convenient when you're away from home – but follow the manufacturer's guidelines carefully, because there are several types of table on which this chair must not be used. Use a safety harness, and protect the floor underneath.

Booster seat

From the age of about 18 months, your child can reach the level of the table with a booster seat strapped securely to an ordinary chair. Adjust the height by turning the seat over. It's harder for a child to fall off a booster seat than just a cushion placed on the chair.

Why wait to feed your baby solids?

In the past, babies used to be fed puréed foods from a very early age. But we now know that the digestive system of a very young baby isn't ready for solid foods. His gut and kidneys can handle formula or breast milk, but not much else. Allergies, indigestion, constipation, diarrhoea, and obesity are less likely if you wait until your baby is at least six months old before starting to give solids. Very young babies cannot easily

move food from the front to the back of their mouth, and have such poor head control that it is difficult to hold them securely to feed them semi-solid foods. By six months, most can sit supported in a chair and swallow food from a spoon. They may have only one or two teeth, but their gums are hard, and they can chew. A seven-month-old baby will turn his head away to indicate he has had enough or wants to self-feed.

Food tastes and preferences

Food smells, tastes, and feels different from breast milk or formula, and it comes in mouthfuls, rather than a continuous stream. Don't worry if your baby refuses or spits out food at first. Let him play with his food, and as soon as he has teeth, give finger foods he can hold himself. All this will encourage your baby to experiment with this strange new way of feeding.

What to feed your baby

The best foods to give your baby are fresh foods that you prepare and cook yourself.

Texture Tailor the texture of the food to what she can happily cope with. As she gets older, it's normal to see occasional chunks of whole food on her nappy, but if they appear regularly, go back to mashing for a few weeks longer. Make her food wet and easy to swallow. Moisten puréed, mashed, or minced foods with boiled water, breast milk, formula, the cooking liquid (if unsalted), fruit juice, or yogurt.

Temperature Always let the food cool to lukewarm.

Introducing a new food If there is a family history of allergy, offer each new food on its own, and wait for at least 24 hours before giving it again to see how your child reacts. If diarrhoea, sickness, or a rash follows, don't offer it again for several months.

Seasoning Don't use salt. It can damage young kidneys, and your baby won't mind bland flavours.

What to avoid Until she is at least one, avoid nuts and any salty, processed, or fatty foods. Also avoid cow's milk, soft cheese, and honey. Use fresh eggs, and give yolks only once she is seven months old.

First foods (six months)

Texture Give your six-month-old baby semi-liquid purées, bland and smooth, and without any lumps.

Preparation
- peel carefully
- cook: steam or boil
- remove pips and strings
- purée or sieve

Other good foods

Peas, marrow, well-cooked green beans, cauliflower.

7–8 months

Texture Foods can be minced or mashed to the texture of cottage cheese, adding liquid or yogurt. Give plenty of finger foods that are easy for your baby to pick up so she feeds herself. For example, sticks of raw vegetables, bite-sized pieces of peeled fruit.

Preparation, fruit/vegetables
- peel carefully
- remove ends and strings
- purée or sieve.

Preparation, meat/fish
- trim fat and skin off
- cook: grill or poach
- remove all bones
- mince to fine consistency.

Other good foods

Wheat cereals, parsnip, tomato (remove skin first, and sieve), sweet corn, soaked and dried apricots, egg yolks (hard boiled).

Foods to avoid Biscuits, cake, ice cream, pastry, fried foods, citrus and berry fruits, peanut butter, low-fat dairy foods.

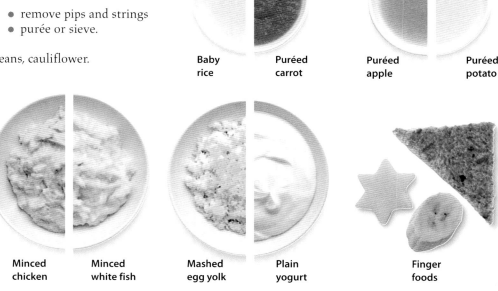

Baby rice   Puréed carrot   Puréed apple   Puréed potato

Minced chicken   Minced white fish   Mashed egg yolk   Plain yogurt   Finger foods

How to store your baby's food

Have nutritious, home-cooked food for your baby always on hand by making up batches of purées and freezing them. Purée fruits and vegetables separately, and cool them quickly by standing the bowl in cold water. Pour the purée into ice-cube trays, cover them well with plastic wrap, and then freeze. When frozen, empty the cubes out, and store in sealed freezer bags, one type of food per bag. Label with the name and date, and don't keep for longer than one month.

Half an hour before a mealtime, put some cubes in a bowl to thaw – one or two will be enough at first. Stand the bowl in hot water to heat the purée, then transfer it to your baby's bowl, ready to feed her. Stir to make sure it is warmed evenly.

You can keep prepared food for your baby in the fridge for up to 24 hours; always cover it first. After your baby has finished her meal, throw away any food that her spoon has been dipped into, including commercial baby foods if you have fed her straight from the jar. Never keep, as saliva may have contaminated the food.

8–9 months

Texture Introduce your child to chunkier textures now, so you can chop food rather than mashing it. Give plenty of finger foods to encourage feeding skills. Stay nearby when she is eating these in case she chokes.

Preparation, fruit/vegetables
● peel carefully
● remove pips and strings
● give in slices or sticks or grate, if raw
● chop or mash, if cooked: leave plenty of lumps.

Preparation, meat/fish
● trim fat and skin off
● cook: grill, stew, or poach
● mince into small lumps.

Other good foods
Toast, red meat, home-cooked dishes, such as lasagne, soup, or shepherd's pie (cooked without salt).

10–12 months

Texture Your child is eating almost everything the family eats, chopped into bite-sized pieces. Continue to avoid salt in your cooking; you can salt your own food at the table.

Preparation, fruit/vegetables
● peel carefully
● remove pips and strings
● if cooked, steam whenever possible.

Preparation, meat/fish
● trim fat and skin off
● cook: grill, stew, or poach
● chop into small pieces.

Other good foods
Pork (if thoroughly cooked), stronger-flavoured green vegetables, such as cabbage, green pepper, whole peeled tomato.

Foods to avoid Spicy, fatty, or salty foods, sugary foods, fruit squashes, cow's milk, soft unpasteurized cheeses, honey, raw strawberries, blueberries, and cranberries.

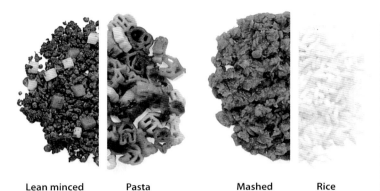

Lean minced beef or lamb   Pasta   Mashed lentils   Rice

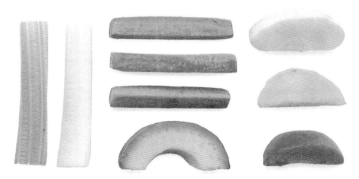

Finger foods

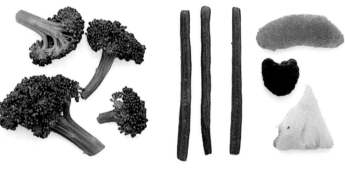

Steamed broccoli   Green beans   Fruits

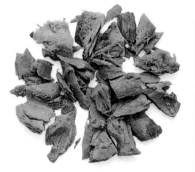

Tinned tuna

Develop a water habit

Many children never drink plain water, but have fruit juices or squashes instead. Some derive as much as a third of their daily calorie requirements from these drinks, which reduce their appetite and give no real nutrients. If they are sweetened, these drinks contribute to tooth decay, too. Offer water when your child is thirsty between meals, so she doesn't develop a "fruit juice habit". Colas and similar fizzy drinks aren't suitable for young children, and neither are "diet" soft drinks, which contain high levels of artificial sweeteners.

Iron and vitamins

The best way to make sure your baby gets the nourishment she needs is to offer her a wide range of foods. The store of iron she was born with will begin to run out when she is about six months old. Good sources of iron include: red meat, liver, dried fruit, breakfast cereals, lentils, egg yolk, and green vegetables, such as peas and spinach. Your baby will be able to absorb more iron if she eats foods containing vitamin C (found in fruit and vegetables) at the same time. Don't give her tea – it will reduce the amount of iron she absorbs from her food.

Warning

Never give a pre-school child peanuts. Apart from a risk of choking, it's easy for a small child to inhale a fragment accidentally, and if this happens, the oil the peanuts contain can cause severe irritation in the lungs.

Introducing first tastes

At around six months, your baby is probably ready to try small amounts of solid food although there is no rush if she seems happy and content on milk alone. Remember that for the first weeks you're simply introducing her to the idea of eating solid food from a spoon; breast milk or formula is still providing her with all the nourishment that she needs. Start at the breakfast or lunchtime feed, avoiding teatime because of the possibility of a food upsetting her and giving you both a disturbed night's sleep. Your baby will most likely be more co-operative if you let her partially satisfy her hunger first, so "sandwich" a teaspoon of baby rice or fruit purée between two halves of her normal breast- or bottle-feed. The whole process might take as long as an hour.

Give a feed first

Sit down comfortably with your baby's bowl of food within reach. Put a bib on her, then give her half her usual breast- or bottle-feed: let her empty one breast, or give her half her bottle. Help her bring up any wind. She will go on needing her milk feeds for several months to come. Your baby's digestive system is still developing, so it may be advisable to mix approximately one tablespoon of baby rice, for example, with enough breast milk or warm formula to give it a watery consistency. Babies over six months old are generally able to cope with thicker texture.

Commercial baby foods

Baby foods in jars, cans, or packets can be useful, especially when you're away from home or in a hurry. But your baby will be better off if you can keep them to a minimum in her diet. If you want to store some commercial food, avoid those with a list of ingredients that includes sugar, dextrose, sucrose, or salt, or that show water as the first item – this means that it's the largest ingredient, so the food may not be as nutritious as your home-made equivalent. Always check sell-by and packaging dates.

You will need

- Bib
- Small plastic bowl or egg cup
- Small plastic spoon
- About a dessertspoonful of fresh apple or pear purée, or baby rice
- Damp tissue or facecloth

Giving your baby her first tastes

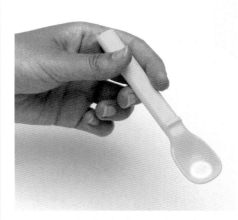

1 Scoop a little food on to her plastic spoon – enough to coat the tip. At first, she will probably eat only a teaspoonful or so. You can offer her more, but when she loses interest it is best to carry on with the rest of her milk feed.

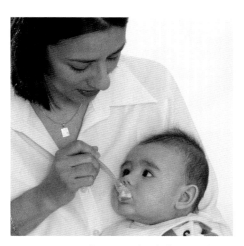

2 Try sitting her on a highchair at first, but if she resists, sit her on your lap. Put the spoon between your baby's lips, so she can suck the food off. Don't try to push the spoon in, she will gag if she feels food at the back of her tongue. She may be surprised at the taste and sensation at first, so be patient and talk to her encouragingly.

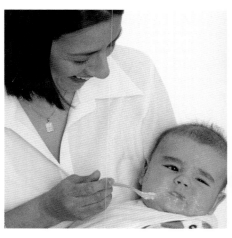

3 She may quickly discover that she enjoys this new experience. If she pushes the food out, scrape it up, and put the spoon between her lips again. When she's had about a teaspoonful of purée or baby rice, wipe her mouth and chin, and resume her milk feed.

Your baby's nutritional needs

How you balance breast- or bottle-feedings with solid foods will depend on your baby's temperament and your own lifestyle. The most important thing is not to rush her. The chart below is just one way you might approach feeding: it assumes you start at about six months. Discuss with your doctor the best time for your baby to start solid foods. If you are breast-feeding, your milk production system needs to wind down gradually – drop one feeding at a time, and leave at least three days before dropping another.

A stage-by-stage guide to infant feeding

Stage/age	What to do	Drinks	Early am	Breakfast	Lunch	Dinner	Bedtime
Weeks 1 and 2 Age 6 months (ages are guidelines only)	Give small tastes of baby cereal, or fruit or vegetable purée at lunchtime, halfway through the breast- or bottle-feeding. Give the same food for three days to accustom your baby to it.	If you are bottle-feeding, offer your baby occasional drinks of cooled boiled water.	■	■	■■■	■	■
Weeks 3 and 4 Age 6½ months	Introduce solid food at breakfast, halfway through the feeding: baby cereal or other single-grain cereal is ideal. Increase the amount of solid food at lunchtime to 3–4 teaspoonfuls.	Offer cooled boiled water in a bottle. Don't worry if she doesn't want any.	■	■■■	■■■	■	■
Weeks 5 and 6 Age 7 months	Introduce solid food at dinner, halfway through the feeding. A week later, offer two courses at lunch: follow a vegetable purée with a fruit one, giving 2–3 teaspoonfuls of each.	Introduce a trainer cup, but don't expect her to be able to drink from it yet – it's just a toy.		■■■	■■■■	■■■	■
Weeks 7 and 8 Age 7½ months	Offer solid food as the first part of lunch, then give breast or bottle to top up. She can have two courses at dinner now: some chicken, a vegetable, and a piece of banana, for example. At breakfast and dinner continue giving the milk feeding first. She may eat 5–6 teaspoonfuls of solid food at each meal now.	You can start to give your baby drinks in her cup, but hold it for her as she drinks from it.		■■■	■■■	■■■■	■
Weeks 9 and 10 Age 8 months	After lunch solids, offer a breastfeed or a drink of formula from a cup. After a few days with no lunchtime breast or bottle, offer solid food as the first part of dinner.	Offer formula or breast milk in a cup at each meal and water at other times.		■■■	■■	■■■	■
Weeks 11 and 12 Age 8½ months	Offer your baby breast milk or a drink of formula in a cup instead of a full feeding after her dinner. You may find she often refuses her breast- or bottle-feeding after her breakfast solids now.	As for weeks 9 and 10.		■■	■■	■■	■
Week 13 onwards Age 9 months	Offer a drink in a cup instead of the feeding before breakfast: now your baby is having solids at three meals a day. Breast milk or formula should be the main drink until one year. She can have cow's milk only from 12 months.	As before. Your baby may possibly be able to manage her own trainer cup now.		■■	■■	■■	■

Key
■ feeding   ▪ solid food

How your baby learns to feed herself

Your baby will be keen to try and feed herself long before she's able to do so efficiently. However messy an experience this is, be prepared for food to end up all over her face and clothes, in her hair (and yours!), and on the floor. Regardless of how drawn out it makes mealtimes, try to encourage her as much as you can – it is her first real step towards independence. Try to maintain a calm and relaxed attitude at mealtimes, and don't rush your baby: if she finds them interesting and enjoyable occasions, you are less likely to encounter problems over food and eating in the future.

At seven months

Your baby may be making determined efforts to feed herself by this age, but she won't be co-ordinated enough to get all the food she needs into her mouth. Feed her yourself, but don't stop her from playing with her food. Smearing it all over her face may be messy, but it's the first step in learning to feed herself; have a clean facecloth handy to wipe her with when she's finished. Give her plenty of different finger foods, too. They're easy to handle, so she will gain in confidence and dexterity.

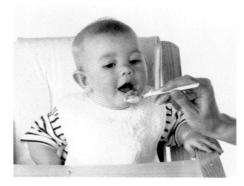

1 She will be hungry at the start of the meal. Keep the bowl out of her reach, and spoon-feed her.

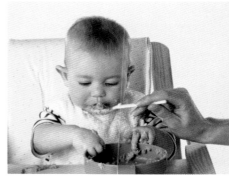

2 Once you've satisfied her initial hunger, let her join in, but continue feeding her yourself.

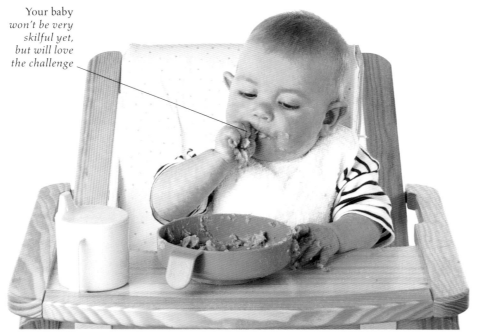

Your baby won't be very skilful yet, but will love the challenge

3 Your baby may get so absorbed in the pleasure of dabbling her fingers in her bowl and pushing the food into her mouth that she will lose interest in you feeding her with a spoon. If she's still hungry, she may cry and wriggle out of frustration because she can't get the food in quickly enough, so offer some more spoonfuls. Otherwise let her practise her feeding skills: feeling "I can do it myself" is important to her. The practice will also help her to develop a pincer grip. She knows when she's had enough.

Tips to help

● If she grabs your spoon, use two spoons at the same meal. Fill one and put it in her bowl, so she can pick it up. Keep your spoon ready. When her spoon turns over on the way to her mouth, pop your full spoon in, and fill hers, so she can try again.
● Have clean spoons ready for when she drops hers on the floor.

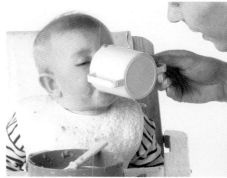

4 Solid food may make her thirsty, so offer formula, and tip the beaker for her – she won't be able to hold it herself yet. Introduce cow's milk from one year.

**"How much food should
I offer my baby?"**
Let your baby decide how much
food he wants at each meal. At six
months, start with no more than four
teaspoonful of food in his bowl,
and offer more if he eats it all. With
his pudding, start with about two
teaspoons. Some days he will eat
voraciously, others hardly anything. If
he is gaining weight normally, there's
no need to worry. Even if you think your
baby isn't taking enough food, he is.

**"My child will only eat cheese
and sandwiches. What can I do?"**
Food fads are extremely common in
young children, and thankfully usually
don't last for more than a couple of
weeks. Don't stop offering your child
other things at mealtimes, but don't
worry or get frustrated with him if he
won't eat them; he won't suffer unless
the fad goes on for several weeks. If
you are concerned that he is missing
vital nutrients, ask your health visitor
about vitamin drops.

**"Should I make him
eat things he doesn't
seem to like?"**
Respect your child's opinions. If he
doesn't like something, don't mix it
with something he likes: he will end
up disliking both. Try varying the form
in which you give a particular food. For
example, if he doesn't like vegetables,
he might eat them raw or liquidized
in soup; or egg custard might be a
good alternative to hard-boiled eggs,
if he always refuses to eat those.

Q&A

At 15 months
Your child will be making a good attempt
to feed himself with a spoon or fork with
rounded prongs, so cut his food into
bite-sized pieces. Give him his own
special bowl, spoon, and fork. He may
need your help on some days.

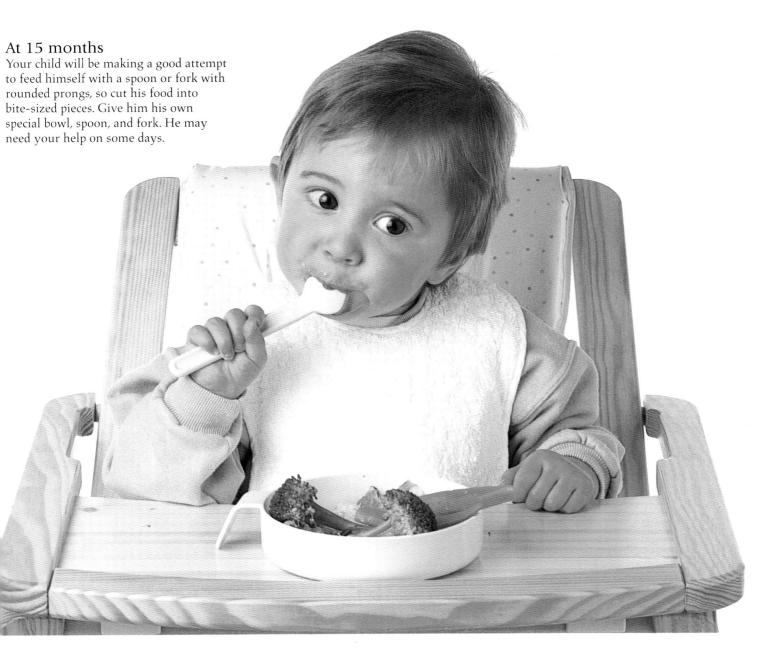

Eating and your older child

Around the age of two years, your child will probably be ready to graduate out of his highchair, and join the rest of the family at the meal table. Mealtimes are extremely important social occasions, and learning how to participate as a member of the family is a vital part of your child's continuing social development. What he eats is obviously important as well, but as long as you provide your child with enough nutritious food, you can leave it up to him to decide whether he eats it or not. Your child won't starve himself, and he knows best how much food he wants at any particular time.

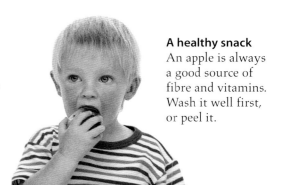

A healthy snack
An apple is always a good source of fibre and vitamins. Wash it well first, or peel it.

Avoiding mealtime problems

The secret of avoiding mealtime problems is to keep your own attitude relaxed and friendly. From the very beginning, make your child feel that eating is a pleasurable way to satisfy his hunger. It is always a mistake to turn eating into a battle of wills – you will end up upset, and he will refuse more strongly next time. Instead, keep the eating issue in perspective for both of you, for it should be an enjoyable experience:

● Give your toddler a varied diet, and give him some choice over what he eats. He will soon make his likes and dislikes clear to you.
● Don't punish him for not eating a particular food, and don't reward him for eating something either. "Eat up your carrots and you can play on your tricycle" will make any child think there must be something rather nasty about carrots if he has to be rewarded for eating them.
● Don't spend a great deal of time preparing food especially for him: you will only feel doubly resentful if he doesn't eat it.
● If he dawdles over his food, don't rush him to finish it. He's bound to be slower than you. If you would expect him to stay at the table while you finish your meal, then you must do the same, and wait for him to finish when he's being slow.
● Don't persuade him to eat more than he wants. Let him decide when he has had enough. He won't starve, and if he's growing normally, you know he's eating sufficient amounts to fulfil his dietary needs.

The right diet

Variety is the keynote of a good diet: if you offer different foods throughout the week, you can be sure that your child is getting the nutrients he needs. His diet will be unhealthy if for long periods he eats too much of some kinds of food, such as biscuits and cakes, or highly processed foods, such as sausages or hamburgers – to the exclusion of others.

Snacks and sweets

Your child will often need a snack to give him energy between meals. Rather than biscuits, offer him healthy, nutritious snacks, such as a piece of wholemeal bread, an apple, a carrot, or a banana. If he's not very hungry at the next meal, he won't have missed out nutritionally.

Sweets can be a battleground, but it's up to you to make the rules and stick to them. Certainly it's not fair or realistic to ban sweets altogether; he may learn to covet them even more. But sweets provide few nutrients and lots of empty calories, and they are also very destructive for your child's teeth.

Control your child's love of anything sweet by keeping sugary and sweetened foods to a minimum:

● Provide fruit or unsweetened yogurt for pudding at most meals. Cheese is excellent, too, because it neutralizes the acid that forms in the mouth and attacks tooth enamel.
● When you do let your child have sweets, offer them at the end of a meal, not between meals.
● Choose sweets that can be eaten quickly, rather than sucked or chewed for a long time.
● Give pure, diluted fruit juices rather than squashes, and give them only at meals; offer milk or water at other times.
● Don't use sweets as your main way of rewarding or punishing your child: they will become intensely valuable to him, so harder to control.
● Make brushing with fluoride toothpaste a routine at least after breakfast and before bed (see pages 144–5).

Ways to improve your family's diet

A healthy diet is one that includes a wide variety of foods. Although a low-fat diet is healthiest for adults, a child should be given full-fat foods until the age of five.
● Use fresh rather than processed foods – fresh foods will contain more nutrients, and less salt and sugar.
● Use vegetable margarine and oil instead of butter.
● Eat chicken or fish instead of red meat at least three times a week.
● Steam vegetables rather than boil them to preserve nutrients, or serve them raw.
● Buy wholemeal bread instead of white.
● Fruit has a lot of nutritional value. Feed your child a wide variety of fruit as it contains essential vitamins helpful in the growth of your child.

Crying and your baby

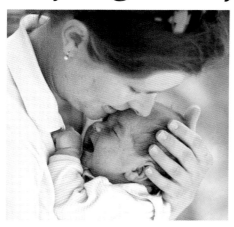

Until he is about three months old, and more aware of the world around him, your baby may seem to cry for much of the time he is awake. Your instinct will be to pick him up and cuddle him, and this is exactly what he needs – you need not worry that by doing so you are spoiling him or encouraging him to cry more. Your baby needs to know that he can rely on you. If he cries so much that you feel your patience running out, seek help from your health visitor.

Ways to soothe your newborn

The important thing when your baby cries is to respond quickly and calmly, without making a lot of anxious fuss: leaving him to cry will agitate him more. If your baby is crying for no obvious reason, try one of the methods below to soothe him. However, your baby should not become dependent on any of them. Never shake your baby, no matter how tired or angry you feel.

Seven ways to soothe your crying baby

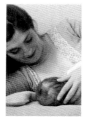

Offer a feed In the first few months, hunger is the most likely reason for your baby crying, and offering a feed is the most effective way to soothe him – even if that means frequent feeds throughout the day, and also at night. If your baby is bottle-fed, and sucks hungrily at his feeds with short gaps between bottles, try offering him cool boiled water in a sterile bottle – he may be thirsty.

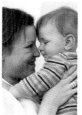

Cuddle him Very often this will be just the sort of loving contact your baby needs to calm down and stop crying. If he quietens when you hold him upright against your shoulder or face down in your arms (see page 83), it may have been wind that was making him cry. If he has been passed around for friends and relatives to hold, he may have become overstimulated, and just wants a few quiet moments being cuddled by you or your partner.

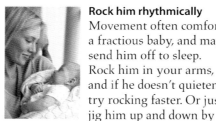

Rock him rhythmically Movement often comforts a fractious baby, and may send him off to sleep. Rock him in your arms, and if he doesn't quieten, try rocking faster. Or just jig him up and down by shifting from foot to foot, perhaps with your baby in a sling on your tummy (see below). Or put him in his carrycot or a rocking chair and push him to and fro. Alternatively you could even take him around the block in his pushchair.

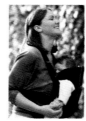

Carry him Often you will be able to soothe your baby simply by putting him in the front pack and carrying him around with you. This leaves your hands free, and your baby will be soothed both by the close physical contact and the motion as you move around. If your baby is crying because of something you've had to do to him – changing his nappy, bathing, or dressing him, for example – this may be the best way to calm him, and will probably even send him off to sleep.

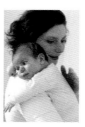

Pat him Rhythmically patting and rubbing his back or tummy will often calm him down, and may help him to bring up wind. It may comfort him when you first put him down to change his nappy, too.

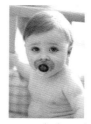

Give him something to suck Almost all babies are soothed by sucking. Your clean little finger will probably work like magic. He may well suck his own fist from an early age. You could even use a natural-shaped dummy (see page 124), but remember to sterilize it before every use.

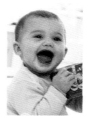

Distract your baby Something to look at may make your baby forget why he was crying. Bright, colourful patterns may fascinate him: he will often gaze intently at postcards, wallpaper, or your clothes. Faces and mirrors are also excellent distractions.

Seven reasons your baby might be crying

Often you won't really know why your young baby is crying or why he stopped. If you've tried the simple remedies, such as feeding and a cuddle, and you've tried the soothing tactics that have worked in the past (see previous page), all without success, then there may be another reason. Listed below are some other possible causes of his crying.

Illness may be making your baby cry, particularly if his crying sounds different from normal. Always call your doctor if your baby shows any symptoms that are unusual for him. A blocked nose from a cold may stop him feeding or sucking his thumb, so he can't comfort himself in the way he's used to, even though he may not be very ill. Your doctor can prescribe nose drops to help him breathe easily (see pages 180–1).

Nappy rash or a sore bottom may make your baby cry. Take his nappy off, clean him thoroughly, and leave him without a nappy for the rest of the day: just lay him on a towel or terry nappy. Take steps to stop the rash worsening (see page 150).

Colic, often called three-month or evening colic, is characterized by a pattern of regular, intense, inconsolable screaming at a certain time each day, usually the late afternoon or evening.

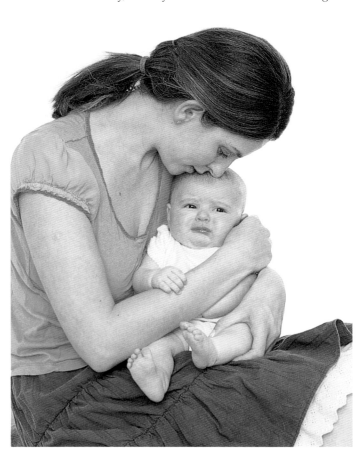

Soothing your baby
Bounce your baby gently in your arms and talk or sing to him – most babies are soothed by both sound and movement (see previous page).

The pattern appears at about three weeks, and continues until 12 or 14 weeks. The crying spell may last as long as three hours. Always ask for medical advice the first time your baby screams inconsolably. Colic isn't harmful, but you might misdiagnose it and miss other serious symptoms.

His surroundings may make your baby cry. He might be too cold: your baby's room temperature should be about 16–20°C (61–68°F), a temperature comfortable for lightly clothed adults. Avoid overheating – don't pile on too many bedclothes. If the back of your baby's neck feels hot and damp, he's probably too hot; remove some bedclothes, and undo some clothes to help him cool off. If he is sweating, a towel under the crib sheet may make him more comfortable. Bright lights can make him cry too, so make sure neither an overhead lamp above his changing mat, nor the sun, are shining in his eyes.

Activities he hates can't always be avoided, however loudly he voices his dislike. Dressing and undressing, bathing, having eye or nose drops are all activities a new baby commonly dislikes, but all you can do is get them over with as quickly as possible, then give your baby a cuddle to calm him down.

Your own mood may be a reason for your baby's distress. Perhaps it's evening and you're feeling tired; perhaps your baby's tetchiness is making you irritable. Knowing that your baby is often just reacting to your own emotions may help you to be calmer with him.

Too much fussing can sometimes make an upset baby cry all the more. Passing him between you, changing a nappy unnecessarily, offering a feed again and again, discussing his crying in anxious voices, may all make him more agitated. If there's no obvious reason for his crying, don't keep trying to find one: he probably just wants a calming cuddle.

Coping with colic

All you can do if your baby has evening colic is learn to live with it, in the certain knowledge that he isn't ill and that the colic will eventually pass. If none of the methods listed on the previous page help, the following may work:
● Gripe water is harmless and comforts some babies. Don't resort to any other medication. Remember colic can't be cured.
● If you are breastfeeding, try excluding dairy products from your diet, and avoid caffeine.
● If you are bottle-feeding, anti-colic bottles are very effective.
● Rarely, colic may be due to a milk allergy, so ask your health visitor's advice about changing to a hypoallergenic formula.
● Try to have an evening out. Leave your partner or a relative in charge, and enjoy some time to yourself.

Your crying older baby

From about three months of age, you may notice a real change in your baby. Now he's much more aware of what goes on around him, he's responsive and interested in everything; he's much more of a person altogether. He'll still cry a lot, and will continue to do so for many months to come, but by now you'll have a better idea of why he is crying.

Six reasons why your older baby might be crying

Hunger is still an obvious reason for your baby to cry. As his first year progresses, and he becomes mobile and moves on to solid food, he will often get tired and fractious between meals – his life is a busy one, as he is led by his own curiosity. A snack and a drink may restore his energy, and cheer him up.

Anxiety will be a new reason for crying from the age of seven or eight months, because by then your baby will have discovered his unshakable attachment to you. You are his "safe base"; he'll be happy to explore the world, provided he can keep you in sight. He may cry if you leave him, or if he loses sight of you. Be patient with him, and gently encourage him to get used to new people and situations.

Pain, from bumps as he becomes mobile, will be a frequent cause of tears. Often it will be the shock that makes him cry, rather than any injury, so a sympathetic cuddle and a distracting toy will usually help him forget it quickly.

Wanting to get his own way will often be a cause of friction and tears, particularly from the age of two. It's worth asking yourself if you're frustrating him unnecessarily, or perhaps trying to assert your own will; but sometimes he will need to be checked for his safety. If he gets so angry that he throws a tantrum, don't shout at or try reasoning with him, or punish him afterwards. It's best to ignore the tantrum completely. Wait until the fit of temper has passed, then continue with whatever you were going to do (see also page 176).

Frustration will become an increasingly common reason for your baby crying, as he tries to do things currently beyond his capabilities. You can't avoid this, although you can make life easier for him by, for example, putting his things where he can reach them. Distraction is the best cure: introduce a new game or toy, and his tears may soon be forgotten. Or help him, if he's struggling, but don't take over completely.

Overtiredness will show itself in whining, irritability, and finally tears. By the end of his first year, your child's life is so full of new experiences that he can run out of energy before he's run out of enthusiasm. He needs you to help him relax enough to get the sleep he needs. A quiet time sitting on your lap listening to a story may work, and a calming, enjoyable bedtime routine (see pages 124–5) that you stick to every evening will help, too.

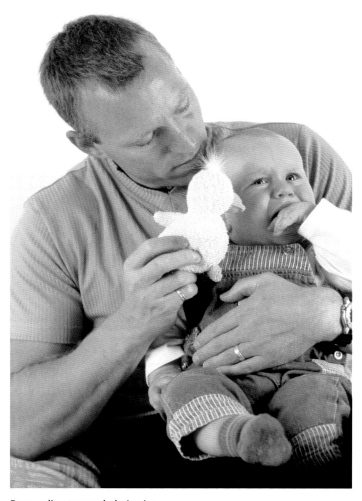

Responding to your baby's cries
All babies thrive on the company of their parents. When he's upset, put your baby on your lap and distract him with his favourite toy.

"Every new tooth my toddler cuts is preceded by days of crying. What can I do to help him?" Q&A

The first teeth shouldn't cause your baby any trouble, but the back teeth, which are usually cut during the second year, can be painful. Your child will probably dribble a lot, and have a red cheek for a couple of days. There are ways you can help him cope with the discomfort:
● Rub his gums with your little finger.
● Give him something firm to chew on: a carrot is ideal, chill it in the fridge first. Make sure that he does not bite off a piece and choke on it.
● If you use a water-filled teething ring, put it in the fridge, not the freezer: frozen rings can cause frostbite.
● Avoid giving repeated doses of medicines or teething gels.

Sleep and your baby

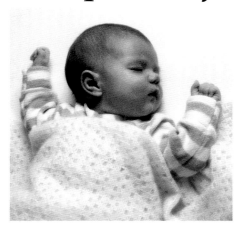

Lack of sleep for you will be a fact of life for many weeks before your baby settles into a routine that coincides more closely with yours. Until your baby is about three months old, she may not sleep longer than three or four hours at a stretch. She will need daytime naps as well until she is at least two-and-a-half years. From about six weeks, try to establish a consistent bedtime and nap routine, and try your best to stick to it. It's best to put her down while she is still awake, so she learns to fall asleep by herself.

Equipment for sleep

It doesn't matter what kind of mattress you buy for your baby to sleep on as long as it's firm. Foam mattresses are fine, provided they are at least 8–10cm (3–4in) thick. Ventilation holes are unnecessary. Until your baby is a year old, tuck the bottom of the top sheet and blankets well under the end of the mattress, so that the top ends come only half way up the cot. Put her to sleep so that she is lying half way down the cot, with her feet near the end of the cot, to prevent her from slipping beneath the covers.

What to sleep in

Moses basket A newborn baby may feel more secure in a Moses basket than in a larger cot. A Moses basket is also easily portable, and can be taken with you from room to room. However, it can only be used for the first few months, until your baby outgrows it.

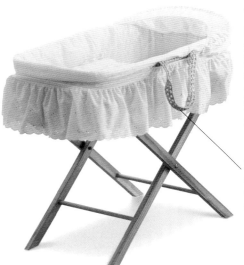

Handles *enable you to transport your baby easily while asleep*

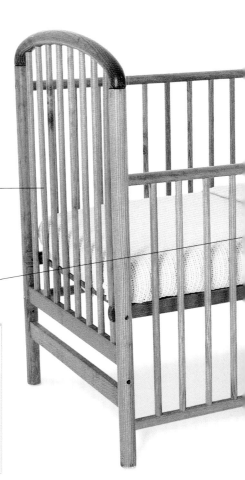

The spaces *between the bars should not be less than 2.5cm (1in), and not more than 6cm (2½in)*

A fitted sheet *made of 100% cotton is easy to put on, and is comfortable for your baby*

Motion-sensor

The newer motion-sensor baby monitors come with a pad that you place under the crib mattress. A baby is never completely still, even when she is asleep. The motion-sensors pick up your baby's slightest movements, and should your baby remain absolutely still for a specified period of time, an alarm will sound. The device is worth considering, especially if you're concerned about Sudden Infant Death Syndrome (SIDS) (see page 123). Make sure the device conforms to European safety standards.

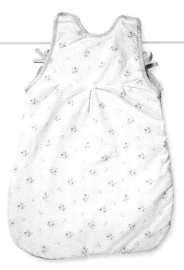

Your baby's bedding

Sheets and blankets

Cotton sheets and cotton cellular blankets are the best options for your baby's bedding. Cotton is a naturally breathable fabric, which helps to ensure that your baby does not get too hot. This is especially important when she is too small to throw off her covers herself.

Quilt

Quilts and comforters, while attractive, should only be used for babies over the age of one year. This is because older babies can easily kick them off, if they become too hot in the night.

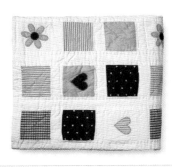

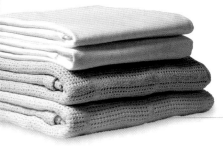

Baby sleeping bag

Sleeping bags are worn over a sleepsuit, and must only be used without any other covering (see page 125).

Toys for the cot

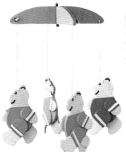

Mobile

Hang just out of reach above your baby's cot; a colourful mobile will amuse her.

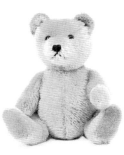

Teddy bear

Keep soft toys out of the cot for the first 12 months.

Your baby's room

- Keep the room warm, but not hot: 16–20°C (61–68°F) is ideal. At this temperature, a sheet plus one or two layers of cellular blankets is enough.
- Install a dimmer switch or nightlight, so you can check on your baby while she's asleep without disturbing her.
- You will need a baby alarm installed in your baby's room, unless you live in a small flat. The type that can be plugged in wherever you are is the most flexible (see below).

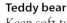

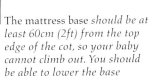

The mattress base should be at least 60cm (2ft) from the top edge of the cot, so your baby cannot climb out. You should be able to lower the base

Follow exactly the instructions on what size mattress to buy. It must fit snugly all round, so your baby can't get her face or head trapped

Your baby will be sleeping in a cot from around three months to around three years, so it's worth investing in a sturdy, well-made one. Safety is paramount; choose a cot that conforms to European Safety Standards

Baby monitors

Baby monitors have two separate units – one part is left close to the baby, and the other goes with whoever is listening. A microphone means you can sit anywhere in the house, and know your baby isn't crying. Ranges can vary from around 75m (68ft) up to 300m (275ft), and many monitors come with additional features such as an integrated nightlight

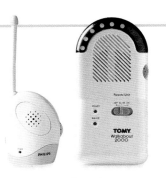

and remote digital room temperature display. As with any baby equipment, look for European safety marks to show that goods are safety approved.

Day- and night-time sleep

Your newborn baby will sleep as much as she needs to; the only trouble is she may not take her sleep when you would like her to. In the early days, she will sleep in short bursts randomly throughout the day and night. The chart below shows how her sleep pattern might develop. As the months pass, her longest period of sleep aligns itself with the hours of night, and her wakeful times become longer. However, babies vary. Don't worry if yours takes longer than you expected to sleep through the night.

Emphasizing day and night

Right from the newborn stage, make a clear distinction between how you treat day- and night-time sleep to help your baby learn which time is for play and which for sleep. During the day, put her to sleep in a carrycot, pram, or Moses basket; if you're using a cot already, save it for night-time only. A carrycot or pram can go outside, in a shady spot, always covered with an insect net, and with the brakes on. When indoors, make sure pets can't get into the room where your baby is, but there is no need to keep the house especially quiet for her. When your baby cries, pick her up, and make the most of her waking time: help her to associate the daylight hours with play and wakefulness.

At night, put your baby in a baby sleeping bag, so her jerking limbs won't wake her, and put her to sleep in her cot, if you're already using one. Keep the room dark. When she wakes and cries for a feed, pick her up and feed her quietly, talking as little as possible, and changing her nappy only if she's very wet or dirty. She will gradually learn that night-time feeds are business only, not social times, and her sleep pattern will become more like yours as the weeks go by.

Your toddler's naps

From the age of about six months, bedtime becomes a more and more important ritual in your baby's day, and she needs to be tired and ready for bed if she is to sleep through the night. She needs some daytime sleep to give her energy for her active life, and will go on needing it throughout toddlerhood, but don't let her nap for too long. Give her two hours for each nap (she may wake earlier), then wake her. She may be grumpy and confused if she was deeply asleep, so give her plenty of time before introducing the next activity.

Q&A

"My 13-month-old baby wakes up at 6am, and won't go to sleep again. Is there anything we can do?"

Early-morning waking probably just means your baby has had enough sleep. Leave a few toys in her cot each night to occupy her when she wakes, and a drink in a non-spill beaker in case she's thirsty. When she calls out for you, changing her nappy and offering some new toys in her cot may gain you an extra hour's sleep.

If early waking is a regular pattern, adjust the baby's sleep times through the day so she has a later bedtime. You could try putting thick curtains up in her bedroom, so the sun won't wake her up too early in the morning.

How much will my baby sleep?

Age of baby	Night-time							Day-time													Night-time			Key
	1	2	3	4	5	6	7	8	9	10	11	12	1	2	3	4	5	6	7	8	9	10	11	12	
4 weeks																									
3 months																									Night-time sleep
6 months																									
12 months																									
18 months																									
2 years																									Day-time sleep
3 years																									

Getting the temperature right

The risk of cot death is increased when a baby is overwrapped or overheated, especially if she is feverish or unwell. And yet it is important not to let your baby become chilled. The ideal room temperature should be between 16 and 20°C (61–68°F) – a comfortable temperature for a lightly clothed adult. If the room is at this temperature, a baby who is wearing a sleepsuit and a vest should not need more than one or two lightweight blankets to cover her. To prevent restricted chest expansion, wrap your baby from the waist down. Wrapping a baby snugly in a blanket stops her limbs jerking, and often helps her settle more easily. Whatever method you use, make sure your baby doesn't get too hot or cold. Don't add extra bedding if your baby is unwell, and don't expose her to direct heat from a hot water bottle, electric blanket, or heater.

Sleeptime safety

- Never let your baby sleep with a duvet or a pillow until she is at least two years old.
- Put your baby to sleep on her back. Doctors now know this is the safest position. Babies who sleep on their front run an increased risk of cot death.
- Use a firm mattress with a fitted sheet.
- Don't let your baby get too hot or too cold.
- Don't smoke; and keep your baby in a smoke-free atmosphere.
- Place your baby in the feet-to-foot position, so she can't slip down beneath the covers (see below).
- Never hang toys over the cot within easy reach of your baby.

Cot death Each year, a few babies die unexpectedly in their cots. There is no explanation for cot death, or Sudden Infant Death Syndrome (SIDS), but doctors have suggested some safety precautions (see left) that can help to minimize the risk of cot death occurring. If you always put your baby to sleep on her back, make sure that she is not exposed to cigarette smoke, and be careful to see that she does not become overheated – you can greatly reduce the risk of cot death.

If you think your baby is unwell, consult your doctor straightaway.

Putting your baby in the "feet-to-foot" position

Place your baby's feet at the foot of the cot, so that she cannot wriggle her way under the covers, and tuck in the covers securely so they reach no higher than her shoulders and cannot ride up and cover her head. Babies whose heads are accidentally covered with bedding get too hot and run a greater risk of cot death.

Lay your baby *with her feet at the foot of the cot*

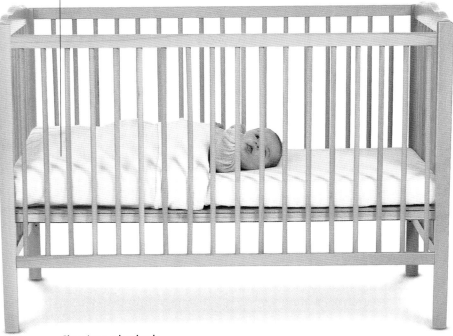

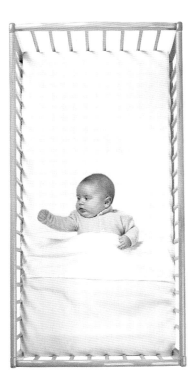

Sleeping on her back
Doctors believe that the safest sleeping position for your baby is lying on her back – there is no evidence to suggest that babies tend to vomit and then choke in this position.

Temperature regulation
Babies regulate their body temperature by losing heat from their face and head. If a baby slips beneath the bedclothes so that her face and head are covered, heat can't be lost as easily. Make sure the bedding is arranged so that this can't happen. Unless the room is very cold, babies should not wear hats indoors for sleeping.

Settling for sleep

There will be times when your baby won't settle down to sleep after a feed. Gentle rocking or a quiet period in your arms may help to relax him and send him off to sleep. Make sure you keep the following soothing methods for times when he is really fretful, so he does not develop incorrect sleep associations and become too dependent on them.

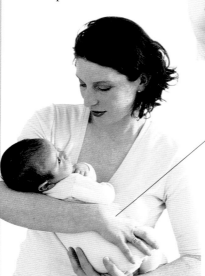

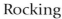
Gentle rocking soothes your baby

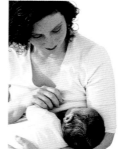

Sucking
Your baby will be soothed by sucking, either at the breast or on your clean little finger. He may suck his own fist. If you don't mind him having a dummy, use a natural-shaped one; you can limit its use to the first three months if you wish – he won't miss it at that age.

Soothing contact
Rubbing your baby's back rhythmically may soothe him enough to send him to sleep. Don't alter the rhythm or you will disturb him, and don't stop until his eyelids have closed.

A sling
If your baby wakes every time you put him down, try carrying him around in a sling: the motion of your body will keep him asleep (see page 85).

Rocking
Rock your baby to and fro in your arms to lull him to sleep. You may have to keep it up for some time, and he may wake every time you stop to put him in his cot, but it's still a tried and tested way to send him to sleep.

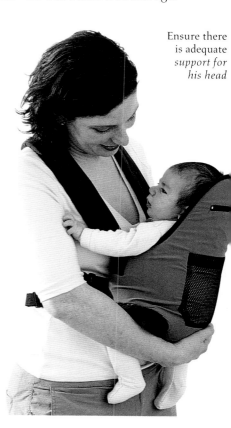
Ensure there is adequate support for his head

Your older baby's bedtime routine

From about six months, your baby will settle down to sleep more happily if the whole process of going to bed takes place in exactly the same way every day – babies love routine and rituals. From now on, he won't be quite so ready to go to sleep in strange surroundings, and his sleep patterns will be easily upset by a change in daily life, so try to impose the normal routine even if you're away from home.

What time is bedtime?
It's up to you and your partner to choose a time that fits in with your own routine, and one that you can stick to more or less every day. Make sure it's late enough that you're both home, and not so late that the routine takes up all your evening. Any time between 6pm and 8pm is perhaps the most suitable.

The bedtime routine
1 Start the routine in the same way every evening. A bath is ideal, because it's both fun and relaxing. If he doesn't like being bathed, 20 minutes spent playing a gentle game together might help him unwind.

2 If your baby still has a bedtime feeding, give it to him in his room, so he understands this to be a friendly, familiar place, not somewhere he is banished to at night while family life continues elsewhere.

3 Put your baby into his cot. If he is over one year old, you can give him a favourite teddy or a soft toy.

4 Now perhaps your partner could take over, so that you're both involved in the bedtime routine. This last half hour or so should always be the same, to mark it as the end of the day. You may want to sing a lullaby to help your baby drop off.

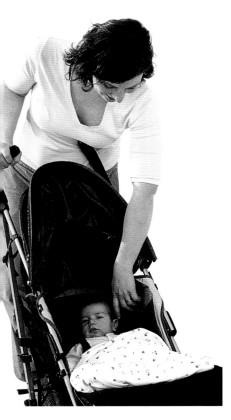

A car ride

If you get desperate, you can always try putting your baby in his car seat and going for a short drive round the block: the motion will probably put him to sleep automatically. When you return home again, leave him undisturbed in his car seat, and carry both indoors. Cover him with a blanket to keep him warm. Many parents find that this is an effective way to soothe an irritable but otherwise tired baby.

Other methods

Lullabies are an age-old method of soothing your baby to sleep. Your baby won't mind if you can't sing in tune, as long as you rock him to and fro. Playing music softly in his room may also help your baby to drop off to sleep. For difficult sleepers, a **soother CD** of the rhythmic swishing sounds he would have heard in the womb may work.

Rhythmic movements

Pushing your baby to and fro in his pram or pushchair will often soothe him to sleep, although he may keep trying to look at you. If this doesn't work, you can try taking your baby out in his pram for a walk in the open air. Make sure he is adequately dressed and covered for the weather. Use this soothing method only when your baby is particularly unsettled.

Sleeping bag

A sleeping bag will keep your baby comfortably warm all night. It is more practical than a blanket or quilt, and can make your night easier, too. Sleep sacks also reduce the risk of SIDS (see page 123) and suffocation. Your baby will soon learn to associate sleep with being put in his bag. Choose one without a hood, and make sure it is the right size around the neck so your baby won't slip down inside it. A 2.5 tog bag will be suitable for most of the year – you can adjust the amount of clothing your baby wears underneath as the weather gets warmer. A low tog (0.5 or 1 tog) bag is better for warm summer nights.

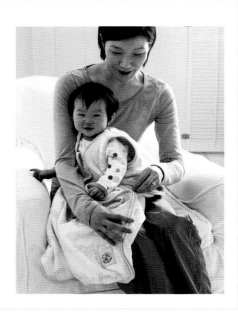

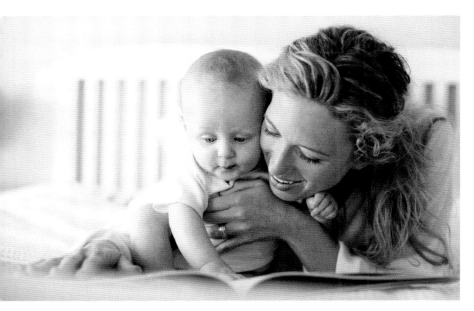

5 Read a story with your baby to relax him and help him wind down. Don't give up if you think he isn't paying attention: he will be tired, and won't respond to the pictures with his usual lively interest, but that doesn't mean he isn't listening or learning for that matter.

6 Tuck your baby up, making sure that his feet are at the foot of the cot if he is under one year old. Turn the light down, or switch a nightlight on. Spend a moment or two pottering around in the room before you go, so that he is still aware of your presence, as he drops off to sleep.

Sharing a bed with your baby

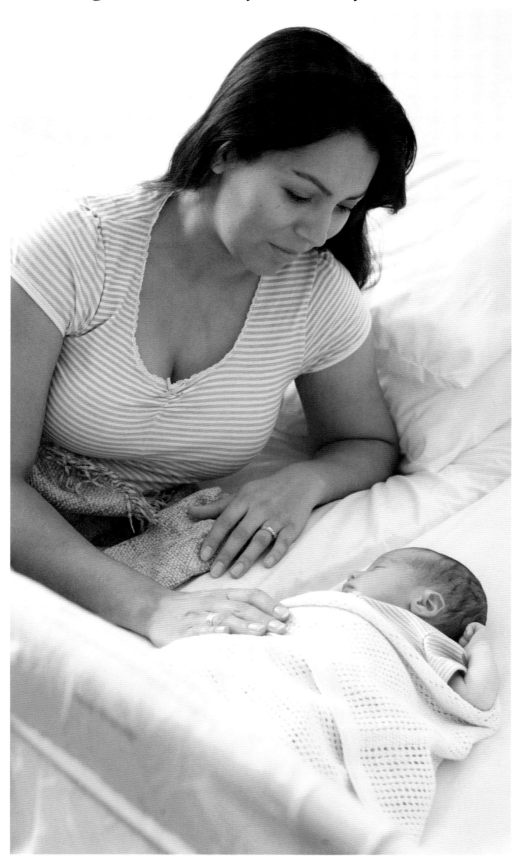

For the first six months, the safest place for your baby to sleep – night and day – is in a crib or cot in a room with you. But if your baby won't settle, it is very tempting to bring him to your bed. Snuggled close to you, he will fall asleep more easily. However, it may become a habit, which is hard to break – your baby may be very resistant to sleeping in his own cot when you decide it's time for him to do so. More importantly, co-sleeping can increase the risk of cot death, unless you take proper safety precautions. See the safety guidelines in the box given below if you decide to bring your baby into your bed.

Co-sleeping safely

● Don't sleep with your baby if you or your partner smoke, drink, or take drugs or medication that make you drowsy.
● Don't place your bed directly against furniture or a wall. Your baby could become trapped between the bed and the wall.
● Be careful your baby doesn't get too hot. Your own body heat will keep him warm, so he will only need light coverings.
● Don't let siblings share a bed with a baby younger than one year old.
● Consider buying a snuggle nest.

Overcoming sleeping problems

Establishing a routine

By three or four months, most babies start to sleep 15 hours a day (10 hours at night, and the remainder divided among three daytime naps). You may still be getting up once or twice a night for feeds at the beginning of this stage, but by the time your baby is six months old, she'll be physically capable of sleeping through the night. Whether she actually will depends on whether she's learning sleep habits and patterns that will encourage this. She will still need about 14 hours of sleep a day, and may sleep for as long as seven hours at a stretch, with two one-and-a-half to two hour naps a day. She no longer needs a feed during the night. By nine months to a year, your baby will probably be sleeping for about 10–12 hours at night, and napping twice a day for an hour and a half to two hours at a time.

You can prevent a lot of future sleeping problems if you try to establish a consistent bedtime routine as early as possible (see page 124–5). From the time your baby is three months old try to:
● keep bedtime and nap times as regular as you can
● put her down to sleep at night before she nods off, so that she doesn't become dependent on you to fall asleep
● help her to learn how to settle and soothe herself – by sucking her thumb, or cuddling a favourite blanket or small cuddly toy, which is always put in her cot with her. Most babies discover such a "comfort object" for themselves, and it works wonders, but once the favourite is established, make sure that you always have a duplicate handy for the inevitable night when it can't be found at bedtime
● give her a massage between bath and bedtime. This should make her feel relaxed and prepare her for sleep.

Night waking

Lots of babies, especially newborns, are night owls. During the day, they sleep, wake to feed, then after a little while, go happily back to sleep. At night, however, they seem much more unsettled, stay awake for longer, and often cry much more. Things usually get better when your baby is a few weeks old, but if they don't you can try to reset her biological clock by helping her differentiate the night from the day.
● Try to wake her at the same time each morning, however tempting it is to let her sleep longer, so you get some rest for a few more minutes.
● Try waking her when she has slept for about four hours during the day, and even if she doesn't seem to want to feed, play with her and talk to her. When she wakes at night, keep the lights dim and be as quiet and soothing as possible.
● Don't panic and change her bedtime routine. Night waking is usually a temporary issue, and resolves itself in most cases.

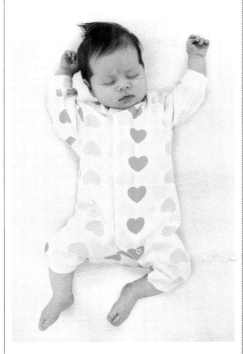

Daytime sleep
During the day, don't close her curtains when you put her to sleep and don't try to keep the house unnaturally quiet.

Unsettled babies

How do you deal with a baby who either refuses to go to sleep, or who wakes and won't settle easily during the night? This depends on the baby's age. A newborn needs cuddling, while a toddler needs routine. If by the time your baby is six months she is still waking frequently, or refusing to settle to sleep, there are two approaches you can use (see below) – try them both, and see which works best for you and your baby. If all else fails, and you resort (as many parents do) to bringing your baby into bed with you, remember that this does raise the risk of cot death (see page 123). A "snuggle nest"– a box that protects your baby – is the safest way to do this.

1. The checking routine
If your child is crying, go back into her room. Pat her on the back, and tell her that everything is OK, but that it is time to go to sleep. Don't pick her up or cuddle her; be gentle but firm. Leave. Wait about five minutes, then check again. Do this repeatedly until she falls asleep, extending the time between each visit, but never leave her crying for more than 15 minutes without going back in to reassure her.

2. The flexible routine
Don't let your baby cry it out. Instead, try to see if there's any obvious cause. Comfort her to sleep; rock her or lie down with her until she drops off. You can buy CDs of special sleep-inducing baby music, or choose special songs that you sing to her as part of her bedtime ritual.

By six months, she may be starting to suffer from separation anxiety, she misses you, and needs to know you are still around. Giving her more daytime contact with you may help – for example, by breastfeeding, playing with her, carrying her in a sling. Or, as she becomes more physically active, she may simply be overtired. Try putting her to bed half an hour or so earlier than her usual bedtime.

Clothes and dressing

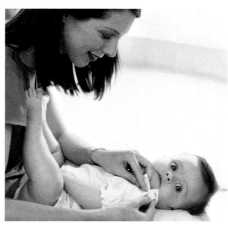

In the early weeks, your baby may need clean clothes as often as she needs a clean nappy. But once she turns into an active toddler, she will need far fewer items of clothing – she will outgrow them long before they are outworn. Choose clothes that are machine-washable, comfortable and unrestricting, with easy-to-manage fastenings and elasticated waistbands to help her learn to dress and undress herself. She shouldn't have to worry about her clothes, and nor should you.

Buying clothes for your baby

Clothes for a young baby should be easy to put on, and if possible made from natural fibres, which allow your baby to regulate her own temperature as well as she can. Don't use any biological powders or fabric conditioners to wash your baby's clothes, as they may irritate her skin. The basic item of clothing now and throughout the first six months is the all-in-one stretchsuit.

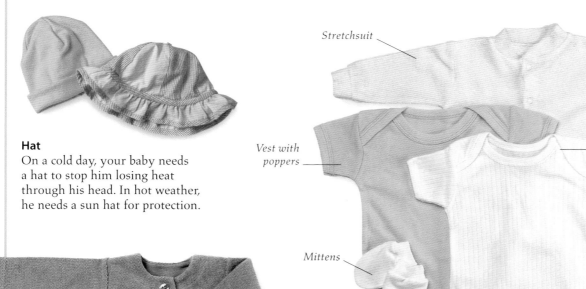

Stretchsuit

Vest with poppers

Envelope neck

Vest

Mittens

Hat
On a cold day, your baby needs a hat to stop him losing heat through his head. In hot weather, he needs a sun hat for protection.

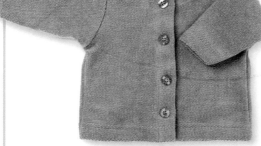

Cardigan
Avoid mohair or fluffy wool and any knit with large holes that could catch fingers.

Clothes with poppers
Look for clothes with poppers up the front and around the crotch – these will be easy to put on over nappies, which can be bulky. Envelope necks make it easy to put clothes over your baby's head.

Socks
These should be soft and roomy, so that toes are not restricted.

Clothing basics

For babies of any age, clothing should be easy to put on and take off and should allow plenty of scope for movement. Practical, easy-to-wash fabrics are essential as clothes will become dirty quickly.

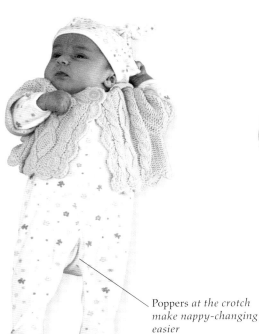

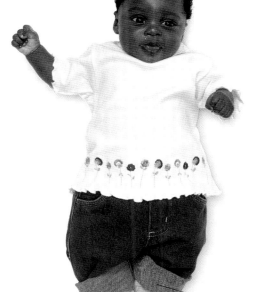

Denim jeans *look good and are hardwearing*

Rolled-up trousers

Larger trousers can be rolled up when your baby is small and rolled down as she grows.

Poppers *at the crotch make nappy-changing easier*

Stretchsuits

This perennially popular style is practical and hardwearing for when your baby starts to crawl.

Cotton *is breathable*

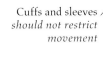

Dresses

Most dresses for baby girls come with matching pants to go underneath. Tights keep a baby's legs warm.

Easy-care fabric *is important*

Elasticated fabric bootees

These are useful in cold weather before she is walking; they must be very roomy inside.

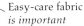

Cuffs and sleeves *should not restrict movement*

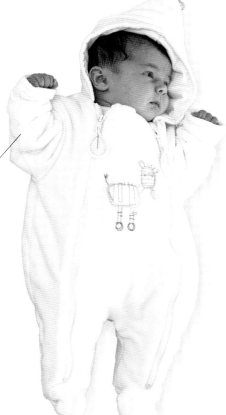

Outdoor clothes

Your baby should be adequately dressed in colder weather as she loses heat easily.

> ## Basic items for your new baby
>
> Start with the following in size 60cm, then add extra items as needed. Buy too much rather than too little, or you will be washing all the time. You need:
>
> - eight stretchsuits, minimum
> - six vests
> - two cardigans
> - two nighties
> - two pairs of socks
> - fabric bootees
> - tie-on mittens
> - sun hat or woolly hat
> - outdoor clothes (winter).

How to dress your baby

Dressing and undressing your baby is a lovely opportunity to let him learn about his own body as you stroke and caress his soft skin. He may hate being dressed, but you can make it pleasurable with lots of nuzzling, cuddles, kisses, and chat; be especially gentle, too. Gather up the clothes you need, and undo all the poppers. Lay your baby on his changing mat.

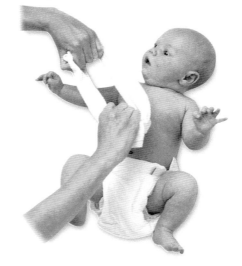

Putting on a vest

1 Hold the vest with the front facing you, and gather it into your hands. Put the back edge at your baby's crown.

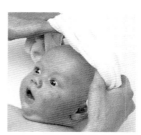

Position the back edge at the top of his head

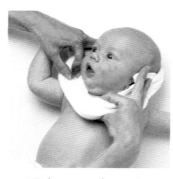

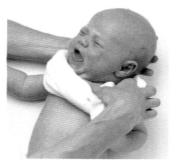

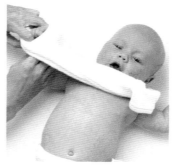

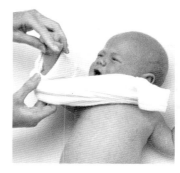

2 With one swift, gentle movement, bring the front edge of the vest down to your baby's chin. Hold all the fabric gathered up together, and stretch it as wide as you can, so that none of it drags on his face and upsets him.

3 Gently lift your baby's head and upper body, and pull the back of the vest down so it is round his neck and lying behind his shoulders. Lower him to the mat without jolting or letting his head flop.

4 If your baby's vest has sleeves, put the fingers of one hand down through the first sleeve, and stretch it wide, then with the other hand, guide his fist into your fingers.

5 Hold your baby's hand with your first hand, and ease the sleeve over his arm with the other. Pull the vest down below his arm. Do the same with the other sleeve, pulling the vest, not your baby.

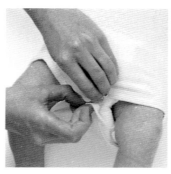

6 Pull the shirt over his stomach. Lift his lower body by his ankles, and pull the back down. Do up the poppers at the crotch.

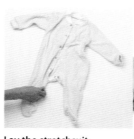

Lay the stretchsuit out flat

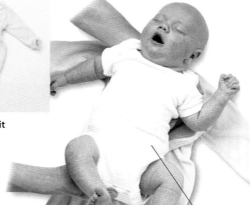

Putting on a stretchsuit

1 Pick your baby up while you lay the clean stretchsuit out flat on the changing mat, the front upward, and all the poppers undone. Lay your baby on top, his neck in line with the stretchsuit's neck opening.

A vest *underneath the stretchsuit is usually necessary in anything but the hottest weather*

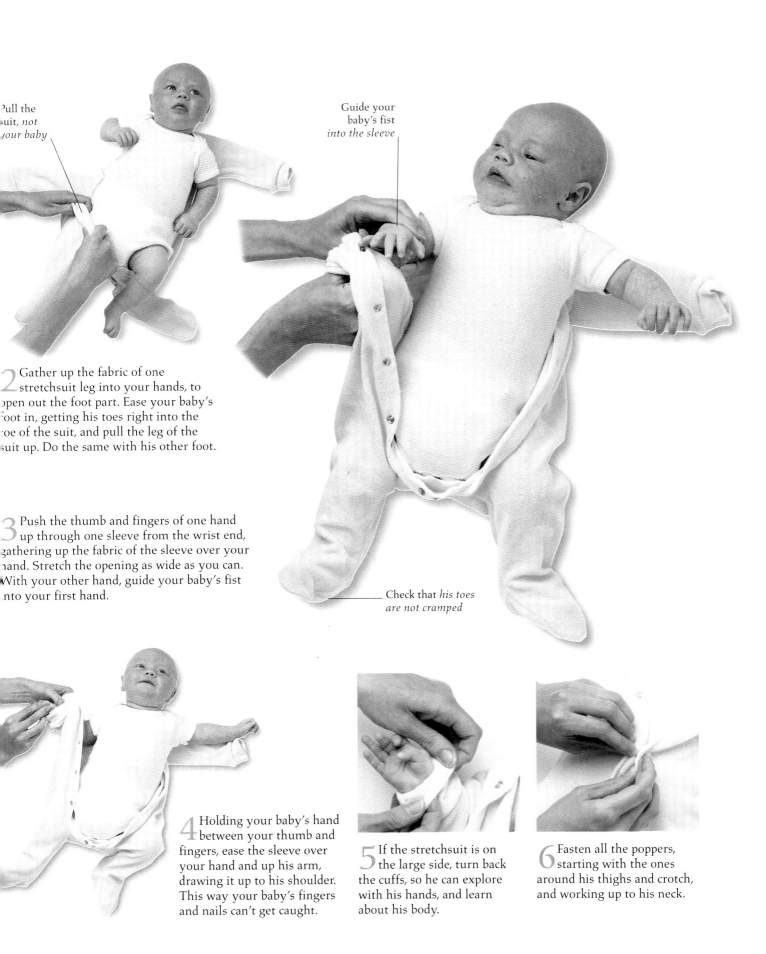

Pull the suit, *not* your baby

2 Gather up the fabric of one stretchsuit leg into your hands, to open out the foot part. Ease your baby's foot in, getting his toes right into the toe of the suit, and pull the leg of the suit up. Do the same with his other foot.

3 Push the thumb and fingers of one hand up through one sleeve from the wrist end, gathering up the fabric of the sleeve over your hand. Stretch the opening as wide as you can. With your other hand, guide your baby's fist into your first hand.

Guide your baby's fist *into the sleeve*

Check that *his toes are not cramped*

4 Holding your baby's hand between your thumb and fingers, ease the sleeve over your hand and up his arm, drawing it up to his shoulder. This way your baby's fingers and nails can't get caught.

5 If the stretchsuit is on the large side, turn back the cuffs, so he can explore with his hands, and learn about his body.

6 Fasten all the poppers, starting with the ones around his thighs and crotch, and working up to his neck.

Undressing your baby

Lay your baby on his changing mat. Your baby may be unnerved by the feel of cold air against his skin as you undress him, so nuzzle his bare stomach, and make the most of this opportunity for skin-to-skin contact. Have a towel on hand to wrap your baby in when you've undressed him, or dress him again quickly.

Taking off a stretchsuit

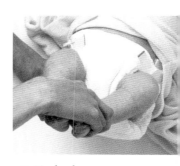

1 Undo the stretchsuit poppers. Hold one ankle inside the suit, and pull the suit leg off. Do the same with the other.

Hold his ankle *while you pull the leg of the suit off*

2 Undo the poppers on his vest, then lift his lower body by his ankles, and slide the vest and stretchsuit up underneath him as far as you can.

Be gentle *as you undress your baby*

Support *your baby's head*

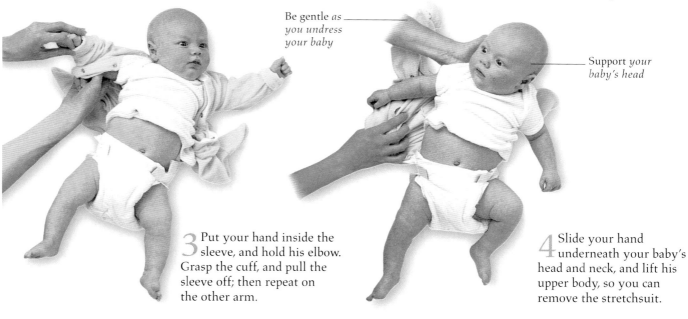

3 Put your hand inside the sleeve, and hold his elbow. Grasp the cuff, and pull the sleeve off; then repeat on the other arm.

4 Slide your hand underneath your baby's head and neck, and lift his upper body, so you can remove the stretchsuit.

Taking off a vest

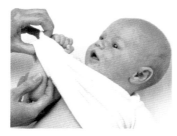
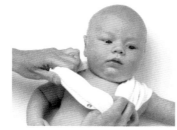
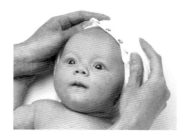
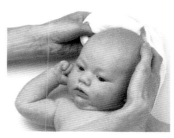

1 Hold his elbow inside the vest with one hand, bunch up the vest, and ease all the fabric over his fist. Do the same on the other side.

2 Gather up all the vest in your hands, so there is no spare fabric that might drag over your baby's face as you take it off.

3 Stretch the opening as wide as you can, then with one swift movement take it up and over your baby's face to his crown.

4 Slide your hand underneath your baby's head and neck, and lift his upper body, so you can slide out the vest.

How your child learns to dress himself

By about two years of age, your child will probably manage to pull off his own socks or T-shirt, and the majority of children will begin to dress themselves by the age of about three. You can encourage this new independence by buying clothes that are easy for your child to manage, and by letting him dress and undress himself as much as he can.

Ways to help

- Allow plenty of time – if you're not in a rush, you won't get too irritated by his slowness.
- Lay out his clothes in the order he needs to put them on.
- Buy trousers or skirts with elasticated waistbands. Always avoid zip flies for a pre-school boy in case he gets any part of his penis caught.
- Look for clothes with large buttons, toggles, or Velcro fastenings.
- Teach him to start doing buttons up from the bottom upward.
- Let him choose his "favourite" foot, then mark his shoe, so he can get it on the correct foot.
- Avoid anoraks with slot-in zippers.
- When you have to help, make a game of getting dressed, playing "peek-a-boo" as you pop garments over his head.
- Once he's dressed, let him stay dressed, even if he gets grubby.

Choosing shoes

Bare feet are best for babies who are learning to walk. They make it easier to balance, and walking barefoot makes for healthy feet. Once your child is ready to walk outdoors, he will need shoes, but even then let him go barefoot as much as possible. Shoes are necessary only to protect feet, not to "support" them – the muscles give all the support the foot needs. Buy shoes from a specialist children's fitter, who will measure the length and the width of the foot. Have the fit checked every three months. Buy new socks at the same time as new shoes: too small socks can be just as deforming as too small shoes.

What sort of shoes should I buy?

Any leather or canvas shoe is suitable, provided your child's feet have been properly measured so that the shoes fit in length and width. In practice, you may find that cheaper shoes, such as canvas sneakers, aren't available in half sizes and different width fittings. Wellington boots aren't usually available in half sizes, but they're still essential for wet weather walks. Buy them on the large side, and fit an insole.

Avoid all plastic shoes: plastic doesn't mould itself to the shape of your child's foot like leather. Never give your child hand-down shoes unless they fit well, or shoes he has to "grow into".

What to look for in your child's shoes

The space between *your child's big toe and the end of the shoe should be 0.5–1.25cm (¼–½in), no more and no less*

The fastening *should hold your child's foot snugly: buckles or Velcro are easiest for your child to manage*

Wide toes *are important to give your child's toes room to splay out inside*

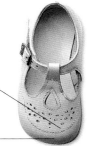
T-bar with buckle

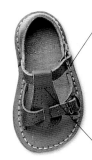
Open-toed sandal

The seams *must be smoothly finished, so nothing can rub your child's skin*

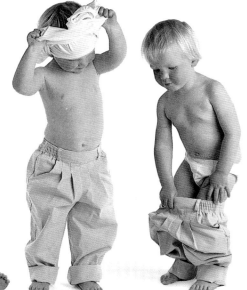

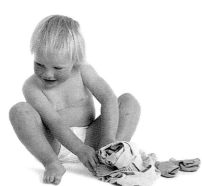

Undressing himself
Your two year old will enjoy the challenge of undressing himself, given lots of time.

Bathing and washing your baby

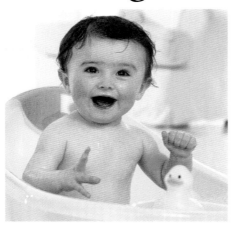

A large part of taking care of your new baby day-to-day will be keeping her clean. A newborn baby's skin is delicate and easily irritated by sweating, urinating, or dribbling. As your baby grows and starts to feed herself and explore the world around her, she will generally get more grubby, too. Topping and tailing or sponge bathing is quite enough to keep her clean, but most babies love being bathed, and bathtime will quickly become an important part of your daily routine together.

Equipment for bathing and washing

There are plenty of products available designed to make bathtime easier for you, but make sure that you only buy products intended for use on babies.

Adult shampoos, soaps, lotions, and creams contain too many additives and chemicals to be safe for your baby's delicate skin.

Equipment for bathing

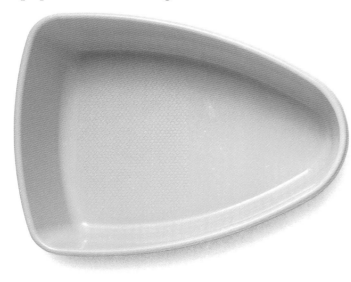

Baby bath
Until your baby is ready to go into an adult bath (between three and six months), a proper baby bath will make bathtime easy for you. Place it at a convenient height on a worktop, or put it on the floor. If you buy a special bath stand, make sure it puts the bath at the right height for you.

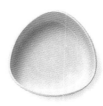

Small bowl of cooled boiled water   **Cotton wool**
You will need cooled boiled water and plenty of cotton balls to wash your baby's eyes, ears, and face.

Waterproof apron
A cotton fabric with waterproof backing will feel softer to your baby than PVC.

A rubber bath mat stops your baby from slipping down

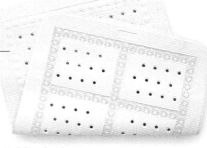

Rubber bath mat
Once your baby moves into the big bath, a suctioned rubber bath mat is essential to stop her from sliding on the bottom of the tub.

Baby toiletries

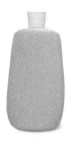

Bath liquid

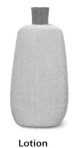

Lotion

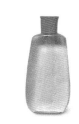

Oil

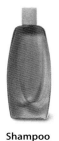

Moisturizer

Shampoo

Soap

Cotton swabs

Baby bath liquid makes an excellent alternative to both soap and shampoo. **Baby lotion** is useful for cleaning your baby's nappy area if his skin is very dry. **Baby oil** moisturizes your baby's skin when it is dry or scaly. **Baby moisturizer** can be used instead of baby oil. **Baby shampoo** may be needed once a week. **Baby soap** need only be used if you don't use bath liquid.

With a young baby, place her on your lap, and soap her all over, then rinse the soap off in the baby bath. Remember to hold her firmly. Use soap sparingly and rinse it off thoroughly – for the first few weeks water alone is quite enough to keep your baby clean. **Cotton wool buds** are useful for cleaning between your baby's fingers and toes and behind his ears, but never push them into his ears, nose, eyes, or bottom.

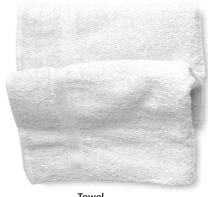

Towel

Keep a large, very soft towel for your baby's use only. Warm it on a radiator before you begin. Some towels have a corner piece that makes a hood.

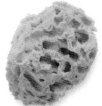

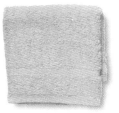

Flannel

Natural sponge

Keep a new flannel or sponge for your baby's use only, and wash the flannel regularly. Don't let an older baby put the sponge into her mouth.

Hair and nails

Hairbrush This should have soft bristles, and be small enough for your child to brush his own hair from about 18 months.

Baby nail scissors These have rounded ends and short blades, so there's no danger of hurting your baby by accidentally jabbing her.

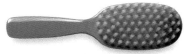

Baby hairbrush

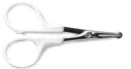

Nail scissors

Tips for washing your young baby

● Until your baby is six months old, always use cooled boiled water to wash her eyes, ears, mouth, and face. Boiling kills off any bacteria that may be present in the water.
● Only clean the parts you can see; do not try to clean right inside your baby's nose or ears, just wipe away any visible mucus or wax with damp cotton wool, otherwise you may push the dirt back up into the nose or ear.
● With a baby girl, never try to separate her vaginal lips to clean inside them. You will hinder the natural flow of mucus that washes bacteria out. Be very gentle.

● With a baby boy, never try to push back his foreskin to clean under it: you may hurt him, or tear or damage the foreskin.
● Always wipe from front to back when you are cleaning a baby girl's nappy area. This prevents germs from spreading from the anus into the vagina and causing infection.
● When wiping your baby's eyes and ears, use a fresh piece of cotton wool for each one, or you may spread infections.
● Always leave cleaning your baby's bottom until last, and use a fresh piece of cotton wool for each wipe. Dip the cotton wool in warm tap water.

Topping and tailing

Topping and tailing simply means cleaning only the parts of your baby that really need cleaning – her hands, face, neck, and nappy area – without undressing her completely. Top and tail your baby as part of your morning or bedtime routine – it's an effective alternative to a bath, particularly during the first six weeks when your baby will not feel very comfortable about bathing in the baby bath. Make sure the room in which you are topping and tailing her is warm. Boil some water for washing your baby's face and pour it into a small bowl to cool. Wash your hands. Lay your baby on her changing mat and undress her down to her vest.

You will need

- Small bowl of cooled boiled water for your baby's face
- Bowl of warm tap water
- Pieces of cotton wool
- Tissues
- Warm towel
- Nappy-changing equipment
- Clean clothes

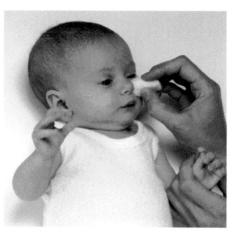

1 Wipe each eye from the nose outwards with cotton wool dipped in the boiled water. Use a fresh piece for each wipe, and for each eye. Dry gently with a tissue.

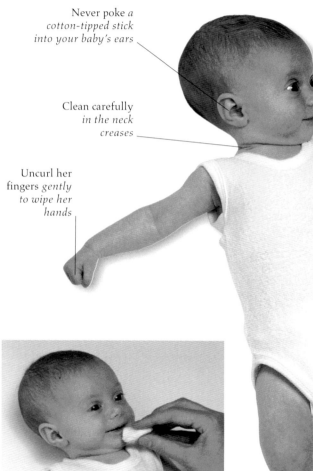

Never poke *a cotton-tipped stick into your baby's ears*

Clean carefully *in the neck creases*

Uncurl her fingers *gently to wipe her hands*

Wipe each eye *with fresh cotton wool*

Remove all traces *of milk and dribble*

Pull up her vest *to clean her tummy and nappy area*

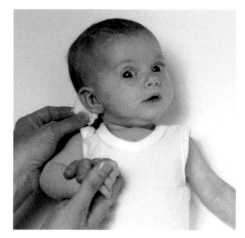

2 With fresh moist cotton wool, wipe each ear. Don't try to wipe inside: just wipe over and behind it. Use a fresh piece for each ear, and dry with the towel. Wipe away dirt behind her ears.

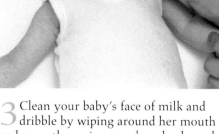

3 Clean your baby's face of milk and dribble by wiping around her mouth and nose, then wipe over her cheeks and forehead. Dry with the towel.

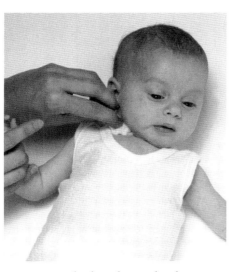

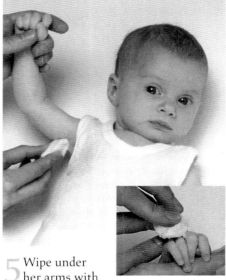

4 Wipe under her chin and in her neck creases with fresh moist cotton wool, as sweat here can irritate her skin. Dry well.

5 Wipe under her arms with fresh moist cotton wool, gently pulling her arms up to flatten out the creases. Clean between her fingers. Dry well.

Cleaning your baby's cord stump

The shrivelled-up stump of your baby's umbilical cord will probably have dropped off by the time she is just over a week old. Careful cleaning makes sure infection cannot set in, and helps the cord separate.

Once the stump of cord has dropped off, you will need to clean the navel daily until it is fully healed.

Consult your doctor or health visitor as soon as possible if the navel looks red, swollen, inflamed, or pus starts to weep at the base of the stump. A small amount of bleeding is normal, and usually nothing to worry about.

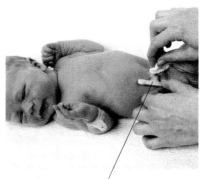

Clean the *stump with a cotton swab*

It is essential to wash your hands before you start. Gently clean the cord stump with cotton wool balls and clean water. If it is soiled use soapy water. Dry thoroughly and leave it exposed to the air as much as possible. Fold the front of your baby's nappy down so it is clear of the cord and avoid getting any urine on it.

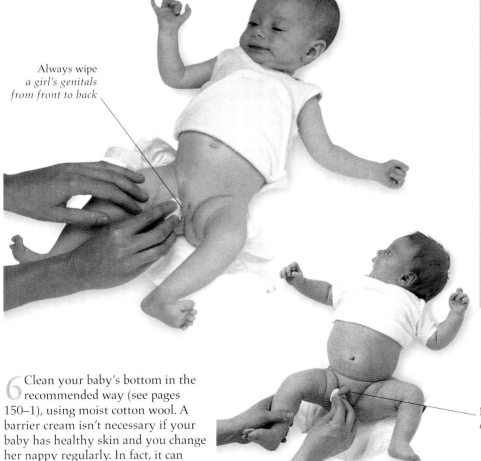

Always wipe a girl's genitals from front to back

6 Clean your baby's bottom in the recommended way (see pages 150–1), using moist cotton wool. A barrier cream isn't necessary if your baby has healthy skin and you change her nappy regularly. In fact, it can make her nappy less absorbent.

Never pull back *a boy's foreskin*

Bathing your young baby

Most babies come to love the sensation of being bathed, but a new baby often dislikes the feeling of being "unwrapped", and you may feel nervous of holding your baby's small, slippery body. In the first weeks, you can simply top and tail your baby to keep her clean, but practise with a full bath once a week, and a hair wash every two weeks. Make sure the room is warm. You can kneel, sit, or stand to bathe her, but make sure your back doesn't start to ache.

You will need

- Baby bath
- Changing mat
- Your baby's bath towel
- Hairwashing towel
- Waterproof apron
- Bowl of cooled boiled water to wash her face
- Pieces of cotton wool
- Baby bath liquid (optional)
- Nappy-changing equipment
- Baby oil
- Clean clothes

Getting ready for the bath

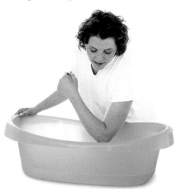

1 Test the water temperature with your elbow: it should feel just warm, and be 10cm (4in) deep. Add bath liquid, if used.

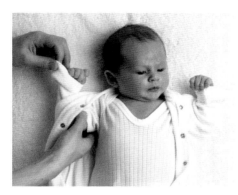

2 Lay the bath towel on the changing mat, place your baby on it, and undress her down to her nappy.

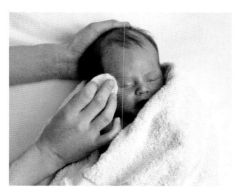

3 Wrap her up snugly in a towel and wipe her eyes and face with cotton wool dipped in boiled water.

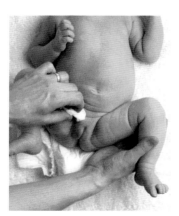

Cleaning her bottom

Lay her on her mat. Take off her nappy, and clean her bottom, wiping from front to back to prevent germs from the anus entering the vagina (see pages 150–1).

"My four-week-old baby has crusty patches on his scalp. What can I do about them?" Q&A

This is a harmless form of dandruff known as cradle cap. Rub your baby's scalp with aqueous cream, and leave overnight. Then wash the crusts off, and gently brush the scalp with a soft brush. If the cradle cap doesn't improve, ask your doctor or health visitor for advice.

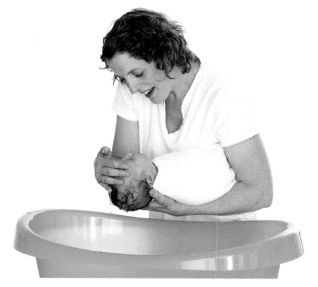

Washing your young baby's hair

Cradle her head in one hand, her back along your forearm, and tuck her legs under your elbow. Gently pour water from the bath over her head with a cupped hand. With most brands of bath liquid, you don't need to rinse her hair in fresh water. Bring your baby on to your lap to pat her head dry with a second towel.

Putting your baby in the bath

1 Unwrap the towel while she is on your lap. Support her head and neck on your forearm, your hand holding her firmly round her far shoulder and upper arm. Put your other hand under her bottom and thighs and lower her in.

One wrist supports her head, the other her thigh

2 Smile and talk to your baby all the time as you use your free hand to splash water gently over her body. Take it very slowly if she doesn't seem relaxed.

Hold her far shoulder all the time

Lifting her out and drying her

1 Two or three minutes in the water is enough for a very young baby. Lift her out of the water by sliding your free hand under her bottom: she will be slippery, so hold her firmly.

Support her head so it can't flop

2 Wrap her in the towel on your lap, and cuddle her dry. Put her on her mat, and dry all her skin creases. Put on a clean nappy.

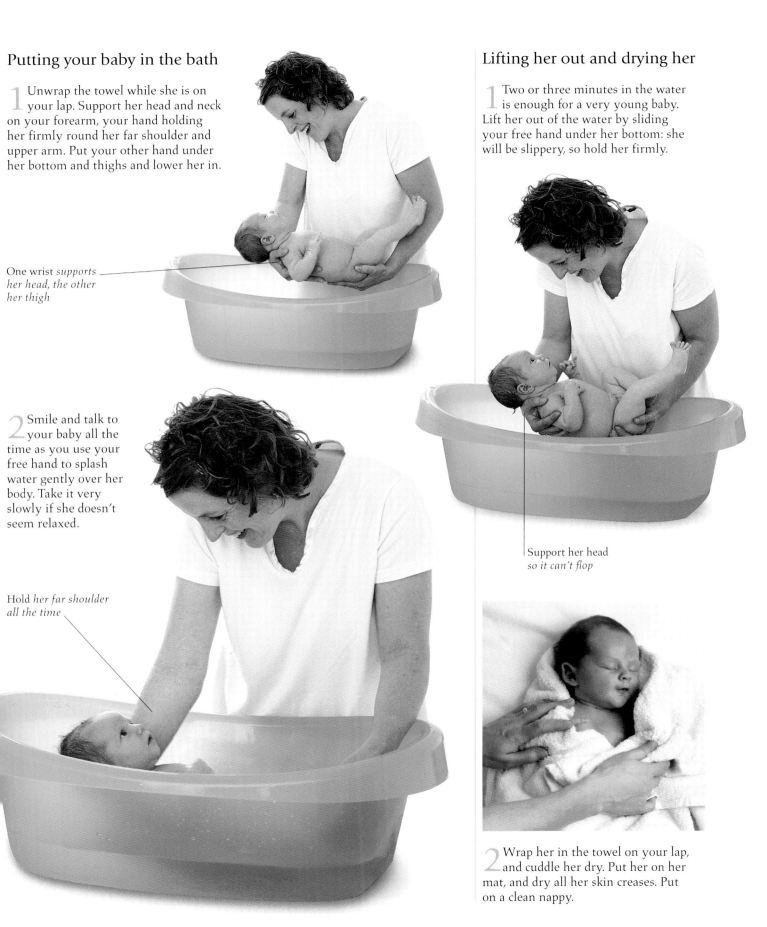

Bathing in the big bath

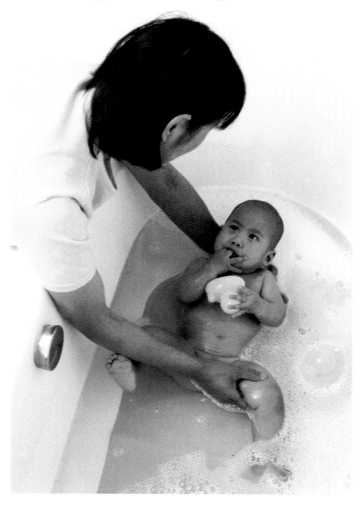

Your baby will probably be ready for the big bath at the age of six to seven months – and some babies are ready for the experience even earlier. If your baby hasn't yet learnt to enjoy bathtime, give him a few more weeks of being bathed in his baby bath, until he really is too big for it or is more confident. To bathe your six-month-old baby, arrange everything you will need beside the bath. Make sure the room is warm. Put your baby on his changing mat to wash his face, eyes, and ears, using cooled boiled water. Then undress him carefully, and clean his bottom thoroughly before placing him gently in the bath.

Washing your baby

1 Put the rubber mat on the floor of the bath and run in cold water, then hot, so that the water is just warm. Lay your baby on the rubber mat. Keep his head and shoulders supported on your arm, his ears clear of the water.

2 If you are using soap, roll the bar in your free hand then run your hand over his body. If you've put bath liquid in the water, just splash the water over him.

3 Rinse the soap off by splashing water gently over him. It may not be necessary to rinse off the bath liquid. Make sure to support his head when you lift him out. Take care, he will be slippery.

You will need

- Rubber bath mat
- Waterproof apron
- Baby bath liquid, or baby soap, and baby shampoo (shampoo not needed every time)
- Large soft towel
- Baby's own sponge or facecloth
- Cotton wool or a soft flannel for washing your baby's face
- Nappy-changing equipment
- Pouring and other toys for an older baby
- Toothbrush for an older child
- Clean clothes

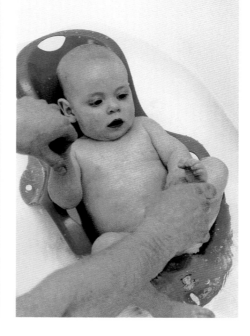

Bath seat

Once your baby can sit up by himself, you can put a bathtub seat or bath ring into the bath to make him more stable and leave your hands free. Choose one with strong suction cups to help keep the seat in place, and put it well out of reach of the taps. Remember though that this doesn't mean that you can leave him alone in the tub even for a second. He can still wriggle himself off the seat and slide into the water.

Drying him

Wrap him in his towel and cuddle him dry. Make sure that you dry him thoroughly, especially in the creases under his armpits, at the top of his thighs, and around the neck region. The area between the fingers and toes also need careful attention.

Making bathtime fun

Once your baby can sit steadily, bathtime becomes a wonderful playtime – not just a way of getting him clean. Search out some bath toys: things that pour, such as plastic beakers and funnels, sandcastle buckets with holes in, even plastic colanders, will fascinate him, and floating toys, such as boats or ducks, are ideal, too. About once a week, use a pouring toy to wash your baby's hair, but don't let water run over his face – he will probably hate it.

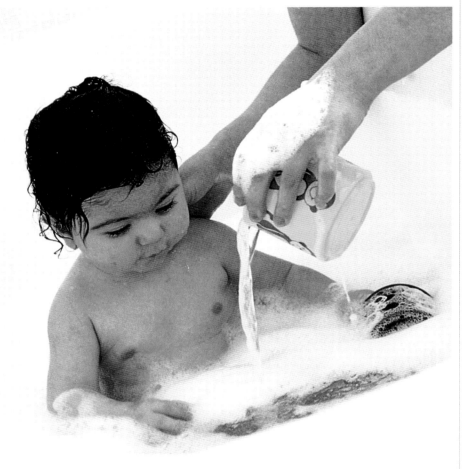

Washing your baby's hair

It is only necessary to wash your baby's hair about once a week. Wet the hair first. If using a baby shampoo, slide your supporting hand forwards and pour a small amount into the palm.

Support your baby's head with your free hand. Rub shampoo gently over his hair. Be careful not to get shampoo in his eyes. If you have bath liquid in the water, just wash the water over his hair.

Swap hands again and rinse the shampoo off with a wet, well-squeezed-out sponge or washcloth. You may want to turn this into a game to make it more enjoyable for him.

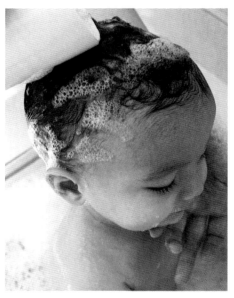

Applying shampoo
Use the tiniest drop of baby shampoo – apply it to your baby's wet hair and lather gently.

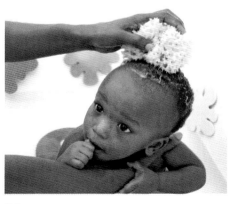

Using a sponge
Rinsing with a sponge or flannel can prevent shampoo and water from running down his face.

Bathtime safety

Always follow these few rules:
● Never leave a baby or small child alone in the bath or move out of easy reach, even for a second. It takes no time for a child to slip and drown, even in very shallow water.
● Even when your baby can sit steadily, keep a hand ready to support him if he slips.
● Never top up with hot water while your child is in the bath. If any topping up is necessary, mix hot and cold water in a jug so it's just warm, then pour it in.

● A rubber mat in the bottom of the bath is essential.
● Never let your child pull himself to standing in the bath even when he can stand steadily, and even though you have a rubber mat in the bath.
● Make sure the thermostat on your water heater is not too high.
● If the tap gets hot, tie a facecloth around it so your child can't burn himself on it.
● If you bathe with your baby, have the water cooler than you would usually have it.

Babies who hate water and washing

Bathing

Some babies are frightened by bathtime – and often a baby or toddler may suddenly take a dislike to bathing. If this happens, give up baths altogether for a short time: daily topping and tailing will keep a small baby clean, although a mobile baby will need an all-over sponge bath on your lap (see below). After two or three weeks, try having a bath with your baby to help him overcome his fear of the water. If your baby is particularly anxious, being held close to you will be comforting for him. Introduce some toys to make the experience fun for your baby. You can also buy special beakers with a rubber lip to pour water over him, which stops water going into his eyes.

Hairwashing

Babies and young children often particularly dislike having their hair washed, even if they love bathtime. If your child doesn't like having his hair washed, abandon it for a couple of weeks. Respect his dislike, but help him to be more reasonable about it: for example, go out together in the rain and show him how pleasurable raindrops feel on his face.

Reintroduce hairwashing at bathtime gradually. It may help to give him a facecloth to hold over his eyes and face: often it's the feel of water on their faces that children dislike most. If your child will wear one, you could try putting a plastic "halo" round his hairline to keep the water off his face.

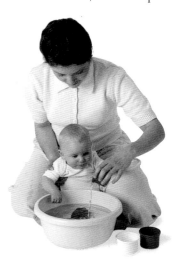

Handwashing

Even if your child dislikes having his hands washed, it's very important to do this before and after every meal. Make the experience more fun by washing his hands between your own wet and soapy ones.

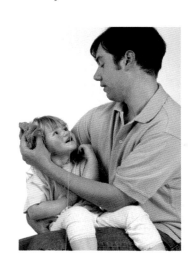

Playing with water

Sit your baby beside a bowl of water on the kitchen floor and let him splash and play. Pouring beakers and floating toys can often persuade a child that water can be fun.

Sponging her hair

You can keep your child's hair clean by sponging out any bits of food and dirt that she may have in her hair with a damp facecloth or a sponge.

Giving your baby a sponge bath

If your baby doesn't like water, there is no need to bathe him: once he can hold his head up, a daily sponge bath on your lap is enough. First, lay him on his mat and wipe his eyes, face, and ears with clean pieces of cotton wool. Sit him on your lap and keep everything you need within reach.

You will need

- Large bowl of warm water, with a little baby bath liquid added
- Small bowl of cooled boiled water and cotton wool for your baby's face
- Waterproof apron
- Your baby's own sponge or facecloth
- Warm towel
- Nappy-changing equipment

Top half

1 Take off the top half of your baby's clothing. Wet the sponge, squeeze it out well, and wash his neck. Dry well with the towel. Remember to dry thoroughly in all the creases, because leaving excessive moisture in them can lead to skin irritation.

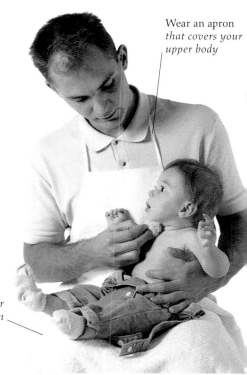

Wear an apron *that covers your upper body*

Put the towel *over your lap before you begin*

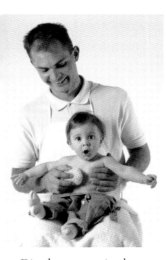

2 Dip the sponge in the water again, squeeze it out so it doesn't dribble, then wash all over his chest and tummy. Dry him well with the towel.

3 Hold your baby's arms up to wash and dry his underarms where sweat and fluff can accumulate. Wash and dry his forearms, then let him dip his hands in the bowl of water if he wants to. Make sure you dry them well with the towel.

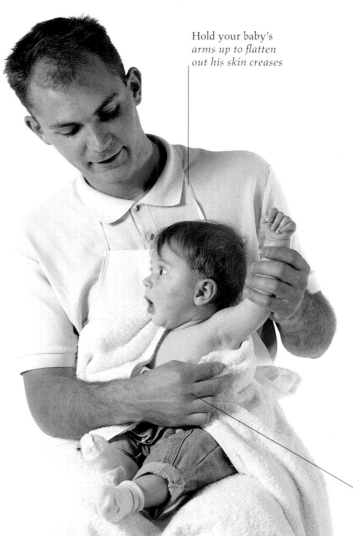

Hold your baby's *arms up to flatten out his skin creases*

Hold your baby *firmly all the time: he will wriggle*

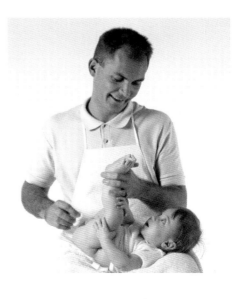

4 Lean him forwards over your arm to wash and dry his back and shoulders. He won't like water trickling down his back, so squeeze the sponge out.

Lower half

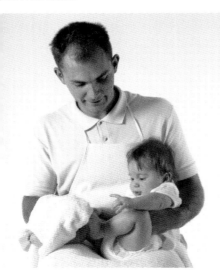

1 Put a clean vest on your baby, and take off his trousers and socks. Wash his feet and legs next. Gently pat him dry, particularly between his toes.

2 Finally, take off your baby's nappy and clean his tummy, genitals, and bottom in your usual way (see pages 150–1). Lay him on your lap if you feel confident, or put him on his mat. Put on a clean nappy and dress him in his nightclothes.

Caring for your child's teeth

It's never too early to start looking after your child's teeth. It is recommended that you use a toothbrush as soon as a tooth appears. However, if you are nervous about using a brush, you can wipe his teeth and gums with a wet handkerchief. As soon as you feel comfortable, introduce him to a baby-size toothbrush: clean his teeth for him (see below) after breakfast and at bedtime. Taking care of the first, or "milk",

teeth helps to ensure that the permanent teeth coming through at around six years are correctly positioned and in healthy gums – and you will be establishing good, lifelong habits in your child.

The more teeth cleaning seems like a game, the more your child will co-operate. Playing dentist, cleaning your own teeth with him, and spitting out messily into the washbasin will all help.

Cleaning your baby's teeth

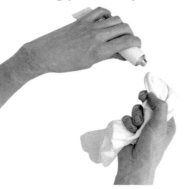

1 Wet a clean handkerchief. Sit your baby on your lap. Wrap the handkerchief round your finger and smear on a pea-sized helping of fluoride toothpaste. There's no need to use toothpaste if your child objects, or wants to eat it, but if you do use it, choose a brand suitable for young children.

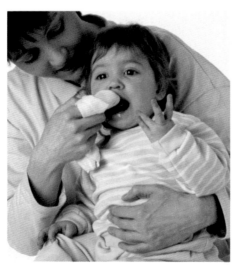

2 Rub your finger over your child's gums and teeth. Let her spit into the washbasin if she wants to copy you.

Why do teeth decay?

Teeth decay because bacteria in the mouth react with sugar to form acid, which eats through the hard enamel covering the teeth. Sweets and sugary foods and drinks increase the risk of tooth decay, particularly if they're eaten between meals because the teeth are bathed in sugar most of the time. Give your child healthy snacks, such as sticks of cheese and carrots or dried fruit. Give sweets infrequently as a treat, and brush your child's teeth afterwards.

Fluoride

Fluoride is a chemical that hardens tooth enamel, and even heals small breaches in it. Brushing twice daily with a fluoride toothpaste will help protect your child's teeth from decay. Fluoride may also be present in some water supplies. If you are unsure about using fluoride toothpaste check with your dentist.

Too much fluoride?

You needn't worry if your child swallows a little toothpaste as you brush his teeth, but he might love the taste so much that he wants to eat it from the tube. Don't let him. Even if this isn't the case, research has shown that young children don't have complete control of their swallowing reflex, and typically swallow toothpaste when brushing. This is why it is recommended that you give your child only a pea-sized amount. All children up to three years old should use a toothpaste with fluoride level of at least 1,000ppm (parts per million). After three years old, they should use a toothpaste with a fluoride level of 1,350ppm–1,500ppm. If he's getting fluoride from water, the extra in the toothpaste might be excessive.

Visiting the dentist

It's sensible to get your child used to seeing the dentist before he is likely to need any treatment. He can go to the dentist even before he has a full set of teeth. This will allow him to get used to the noises, smells, and surroundings, and prepare him for future visits. If he seems frightened, sit him on your lap in the chair and show him what the equipment does. By the time he is about two and a half he should have dental check-ups every six months. Your dentist will advise you on helping your child to care for his teeth – so see him even if you are sure your child's teeth are healthy. If there are cavities, it's vital that they are spotted in good time.

How the teeth come in

Your baby might cut his first tooth at any time during the first year, and he will be teething into his third year. Babies' teeth usually appear in the same order.

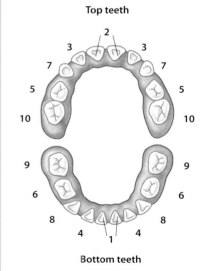

Top teeth

Bottom teeth

Teaching your child how to clean his teeth

As soon as the teeth come through, start cleaning your child's teeth for him with a wet toothbrush and a pea-sized helping of fluoride toothpaste. Brush them for him for as long as he will let you; he will probably want to brush his teeth himself from about the age of two. Always supervise your child – he needs to brush his teeth correctly. Teach him by standing behind him in front of a mirror, and, holding his hand, showing him the correct movements.

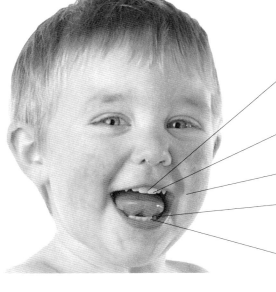

Top teeth: *brush downwards, away from the gums*

All biting surfaces: *brush to and fro along the flat tops of the teeth all around the mouth*

Get the brush *right to the back of your child's mouth*

Brush the gums *with a circular motion, both on the outside and inside by the tongue*

Bottom teeth: *brush upwards, away from the gums*

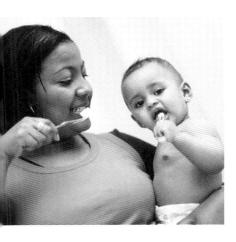

Making a game of teeth cleaning

Play games at bathtime to encourage your child to copy you; clean his teeth properly afterwards.

Cleaning your child's teeth

Stand your child on a step at the washbasin, with you behind her and to one side. Hold her head back so you can see into her mouth as you brush. Let her rinse and spit out – that's most of the fun.

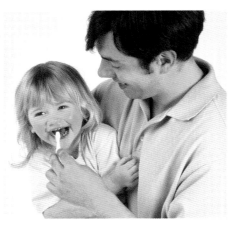

Cutting nails

Your newborn baby

Keep your newborn baby's fingernails short so that there's no chance of him injuring himself by scratching his skin.

A young baby's nails are so soft that the easiest way to trim them may be to peel the ends off with your fingers or teeth. Or you can buy a pair of baby scissors or nail clippers with specially rounded ends. Hold his hand firmly, and press the finger pad away from the nail to avoid nicking the skin as you cut or clip.

Make sure that you always cut the fingernails straight across, otherwise the side edges might grow into the skin. Check for any sharp points when you finish.

If your baby wriggles while you are trying to cut his fingernails, don't try to fight him. Instead, trim them while he is sleeping peacefully.

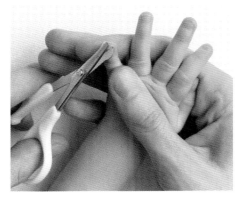

Your older baby

Sit your baby on your lap, with him facing forwards. Hold one finger at a time and cut his nails with special baby scissors. It is best to follow the shape of his fingertips.

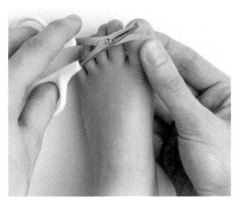

Cutting toenails

Lay a young baby on his mat; sit an older baby on your lap. Hold his foot firmly as he may try to kick you. Most children dislike having their toenails cut, so it might be a good idea to do it while your child is asleep.

Nappies and nappy care

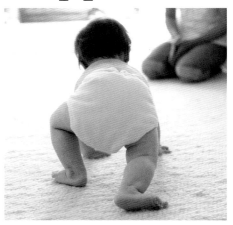

Leaving your baby in a wet or dirty nappy may cause nappy rash. Because your baby's bladder is small, she wets frequently, so, for the first few weeks, you will seem to be constantly nappy-changing. But as the months go by, her nappy will need changing less frequently. By the age of around two (although boys may take a little longer), she will start to recognize the feeling of a full bladder, and will soon be ready to give up nappies altogether.

The contents of your baby's nappy

One way of knowing that your baby is feeding well is by checking the contents of her nappy. Listed below are the common sights on a baby's nappy during the first few weeks of his life:

● **greenish-black, sticky tar (first two or three days only):** this is meconium, which fills the bowels before birth, and passes out in the first two or three days

● **greenish-brown or bright green semi-fluid stools, full of curds (first week only):** "changing stools" show that your baby is adapting to feeding through her digestive system

● **orange-yellow, mustard-like stools, watery with bits of milk curd in them, often very copious:** the settled stools of a breastfed baby

● **pale brown, solid, formed, and smelly stools:** the settled stools of a bottle-fed baby

● **green, or green-streaked, stools:** quite normal, but small green stools over several days may be a sign of under-feeding.

Consult your doctor if:

● your baby's stools are very watery and smelly, and your baby is vomiting and off food: diarrhoea is life-threatening in a young baby (see page 223)
● you see blood on the nappy
● anything at all worries you.

Types of nappy

Your baby won't much mind whether you use disposable or fabric nappies, provided the nappy fits snugly, and she's not left in a wet or dirty one. Disposables give your baby a neat, slim-line appearance. Cloth nappies are bulkier, and so the clothes you buy your baby may need to be a few centimetres larger to accommodate the nappy. But they also support your baby's hips, an advantage if your doctor suspects a loose hip joint. Reusable nappies have developed a lot since the time terry nappies were the only choice available. Because they are much easier to use, they are becoming more and more popular among parents. They are cheaper than disposables, and can be environmentally friendly, too. See pages 148–9 for more on types of nappies.

All-in-one disposable nappy

Padded *in the middle*

Velcro fasteners

Cotton pre-fold nappy

Changing your baby's nappy

Make sure you have everything you are going to need and choose a warm place to change your baby's nappy. Since you will be changing her nappy frequently, make your changing area a pleasant place for both of you – a mobile above your baby's head, a teddy nearby, transfer motifs stuck to the walls or furniture will all amuse your baby and encourage her to lie still for you. A changing mat is cheap and convenient, and your baby will be safe if you put the mat on a clean and dry floor. A specially designed changing table may be useful for storing clean nappies and toiletries, but your baby can fall off a table. If you do put the mat on a raised surface, never turn your back on your baby even for a second.

Changing time
Changing your baby's nappy is the perfect opportunity for you or your partner to talk to and play with her: incorporate lots of games and tickles, to make changing time fun.

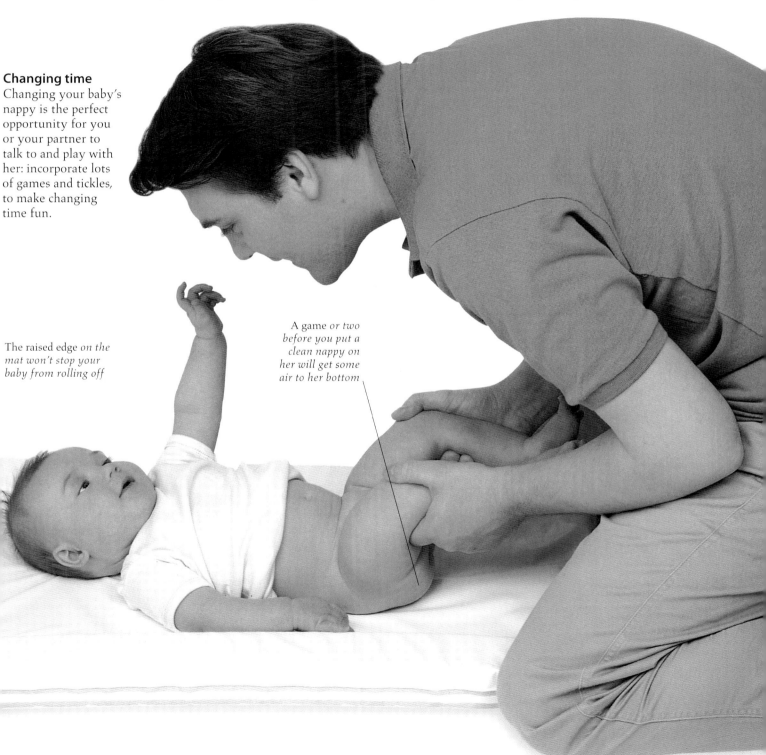

The raised edge *on the mat won't stop your baby from rolling off*

A game or two before you put a clean nappy on her will get some air to her bottom

Equipment for changing your baby's nappy

Although it may seem to be a daunting array of equipment at first, keeping a full set of everything you will need together in one place will make nappy-changing seem that much easier. You can flush used tissues and nappy liners down the lavatory, but put cotton wool, wipes, and disposable nappies, folded up and sealed, in a bin lined with a plastic bag. Drop reusable nappies into the appropriate bucket, before washing and rinsing them thoroughly (see page 153).

Equipment for cleaning your baby's bottom

Changing mat
A padded, wipe-clean mat with raised edges is invaluable. In warm weather, put a fabric nappy under your baby's head: the plastic may make her sweaty.

Clean the mat with a baby wipe

Baby wipes
These are useful for cleaning your baby's bottom, but if used regularly they may contribute to nappy rash.

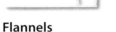

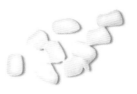

Flannels
Use some wet flannels, then some dry ones, to clean her bottom.

Tissues
These are needed to wipe away faeces and to dry your baby's bottom.

Cotton wool
Buy in a roll or pleats, and break off several pieces before you start the nappy change so you don't have to put a dirty hand into the bag.

Barrier cream
Use barrier cream sparingly, and only if your baby's bottom is sore. Be careful not to get any cream on disposable nappies as the tapes will not stick.

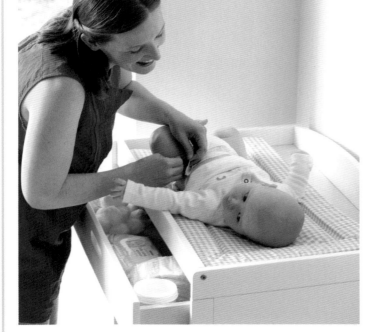

Changing your baby's nappy
Keep everything you need to change your baby's nappy nearby, in a place where you won't need to turn your back to her.

Baby bath liquid and lotion
A few drops of baby bath liquid added to the bowl of warm water is a good alternative to water alone for cleaning your baby's bottom. A little baby lotion on cotton wool is also effective.

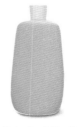
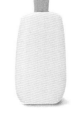

Baby bath liquid   **Baby lotion**

What kind of nappies should you use?

In a few months' time you will have gained enough experience to change a nappy in a matter of minutes, and almost in your sleep, but to begin with nappies and nappy-changing may seem to take up a disproportionate amount of your day. When you are deciding whether to use reusable or disposable nappies, you will be thinking about cost, convenience, and comfort for your baby. Reusable nappies, as well as being cheaper than disposables, are now so easy to use and wash that they will probably be your first choice for regular use. Most are shaped like a disposable nappy and fasten with Velcro, poppers, or plastic clips. Some local councils offer a nappy laundering service. Disposable biodegradable liners, which catch the faeces but allow moisture to seep through, make dealing with a dirty nappy easier – the liner is simply flushed away. You can also choose from a wide variety of shapes and sizes to suit your baby. You will need about 15–20 nappies.

Disposable nappies are more expensive, and in the first few weeks you may find yourself changing your baby 10 times a day, and have 70 non-biodegradable nappies to dispose of each week. However, there are times when you are travelling or on holiday, for example, when you will really need the convenience of disposables. In this case, think about choosing the more environmentally friendly biodegradable nappies, which can be composted. Many are also made from recycled materials that are free from chemicals and are unbleached (so they may have a beige tinge to them).

Reusable nappies
All-in-one reusable nappy

All-in-one reusable nappies offer the convenience and all the features of a disposable nappy. They combine an absorbent nappy and nappy liner and an outer waterproof shell that prevents leakage. They fasten around the baby's hips with Velcro tabs and look similar to disposable nappies. They are less difficult to use than conventional fabric nappies and avoid the need for nappy pins, but are harder to wash and dry because the integral waterproof shell usually can't be put in the tumble drier.

Terries

The traditional terry-towelling squares are the cheapest and most basic reusable nappies available. These must be folded into a triangular shape, fastened with a nappy clip and used with a waterproof outer wrap – you can use plastic pants with popper fasteners to give a good fit. They dry quickly, but aren't as absorbent as some of the modern reusable nappies.

Pre-fold

These are basic cotton non-terry nappies that are folded into a rectangular shape

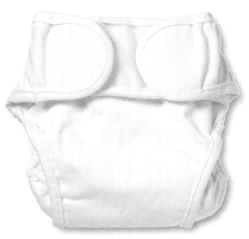

All-in-one reusable nappy

with a padded bit in the middle, and a waterproof outer nappy wrap, all secured with poppers or Velcro. These take less time to dry but may not be as absorbent as shaped nappies.

Shaped nappies

A shaped nappy is a cloth nappy shaped like a disposable nappy, which you use with a waterproof outer wrap. They fasten either with Velcro tabs or poppers.

Disposable nappies

Disposable nappies are sized according to your baby's weight. When you are happy with a brand, buy in bulk. "Ultra" or "High Performance" nappies are very absorbent, and will effectively keep the wetness away from your baby's skin. Some disposables have an outer cover that is breathable, allowing air to circulate next to the skin. "Standard" nappies are cheaper and bulkier, and you will have to change your baby more often. Nappies for boys have more padding at the front, while those for girls have more padding underneath.

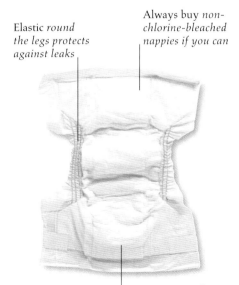

Elastic *round the legs protects against leaks*

Always buy *non-chlorine-bleached nappies if you can*

Disposable nappy

Experiment until *you find a brand with reliable adhesive tapes and good absorbency*

Cleaning a girl

Clean your baby girl's bottom thoroughly at every nappy change, otherwise she will soon get red and sore. Put your baby on her mat and undo her clothing and nappy. If she's wearing a fabric nappy, use a clean corner to wipe off the faeces. With a disposable nappy, open it out: wipe off the faeces with tissues and drop them into the nappy. Then lift your baby's legs and fold the nappy.

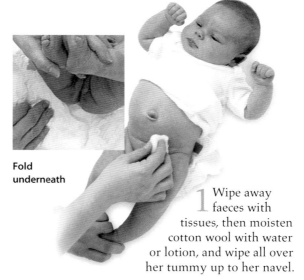

Fold underneath

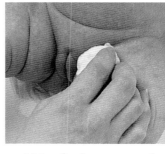

1 Wipe away faeces with tissues, then moisten cotton wool with water or lotion, and wipe all over her tummy up to her navel.

2 Using fresh cotton wool, clean inside all the creases at the top of your baby's legs, wiping downwards towards her bottom.

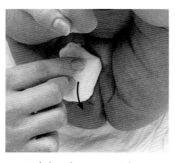

3 Lift her legs up with a finger between her ankles, and clean her genitals next. Always wipe from front to back to prevent germs from the anus entering the vagina. Do not try to clean inside the vaginal lips.

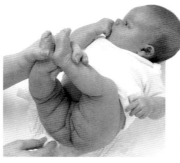

4 With fresh cotton wool, clean her anus, then her buttocks and thighs, working inwards towards the anus. When she's clean, remove the disposable nappy, seal the tapes over the front, and drop it in the bin.

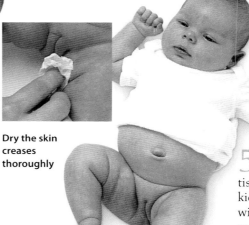

Dry the skin creases thoroughly

5 Dry her nappy area with tissues, then let her kick for a while without a nappy, so that her bottom is open to the air.

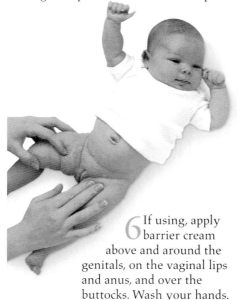

6 If using, apply barrier cream above and around the genitals, on the vaginal lips and anus, and over the buttocks. Wash your hands.

Nappy rash

All babies get a red or sore bottom from time to time. Consult your doctor if the rash won't clear up.

To avoid nappy rash:
- change your baby's nappy frequently
- clean and dry her bottom and skin creases thoroughly, using warm water and tissues
- avoid baby wipes
- leave your baby without a nappy as often as possible
- if using fabric nappies, buy tie-on or popper plastic pants, as these allow air to circulate
- wash and rinse all fabric nappies thoroughly.

At the first signs of redness:
- change nappies more frequently
- use a healing nappy rash cream
- leave your baby without a nappy on for as much of the day as possible
- if using fabric nappies, try a more absorbent type of liner
- stop using plastic pants: they make nappy rash worse because they help keep urine close to the skin. If you don't like the leaks, switch to disposables for a while.

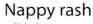

Cleaning a boy

Your baby boy's urine will go everywhere so you need to clean his bottom very thoroughly at every nappy change to guard against a sore bottom. Put your baby on his mat, and undo his clothing and his nappy. If he's wearing a fabric nappy, wipe off the worst of any faeces with a clean corner. With a disposable, undo the tapes, then pause (see right).

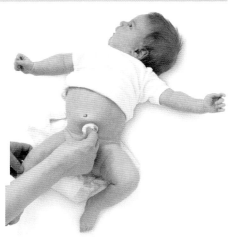
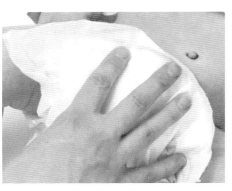

1 Your baby boy will often urinate just as you take his nappy off, so wait a couple of seconds with the nappy held over his penis to avoid urine going everywhere.

2 Open the nappy out. Wipe off the faeces with tissues, and drop them into the nappy, then fold it down under him. Start by wiping his tummy up to his navel with moist cotton wool.

Clean carefully under his testicles

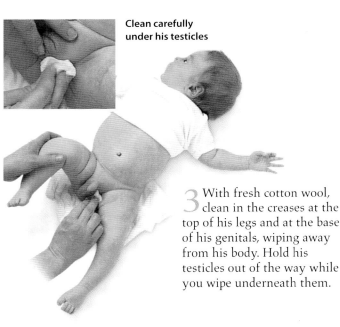
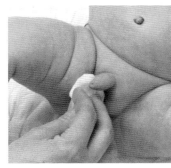
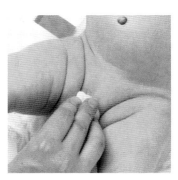

3 With fresh cotton wool, clean in the creases at the top of his legs and at the base of his genitals, wiping away from his body. Hold his testicles out of the way while you wipe underneath them.

4 With fresh cotton wool, wipe all over your baby's testicles, including under his penis, as there may be traces of urine or faeces here. Hold his penis out of the way, but take care not to drag the skin.

5 Clean his penis, wiping away from the body: do not pull the foreskin back to clean underneath, this will keep itself clean.

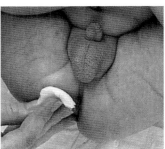
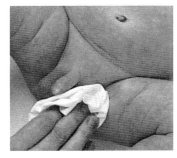
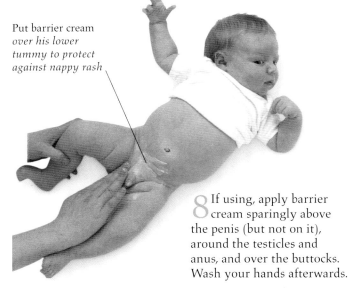

6 Lift your baby's legs to clean his anus and buttocks, keeping a finger between his ankles. Wipe over the back of his thighs, too. When he is clean, remove the nappy.

7 Wipe your hands clean, and then dry his nappy area with tissues. Let him kick for a while if he has a sore bottom. Always keep tissues at hand, just in case he urinates.

Put barrier cream *over his lower tummy to protect against nappy rash*

8 If using, apply barrier cream sparingly above the penis (but not on it), around the testicles and anus, and over the buttocks. Wash your hands afterwards.

Putting on a disposable nappy

Before you put on a new nappy, make sure that you clean your baby's bottom thoroughly and, if using, apply a barrier cream to help prevent nappy rash. Wipe your hands well on a tissue, as the nappy's adhesive tapes won't stick very well if you get grease on them or on the front of the nappy.

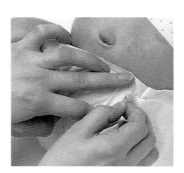

1 Open up the nappy with the tapes at the top. Lift your baby by her ankles with one finger between them, and slide the nappy under her, until the top edge lines up with her waist.

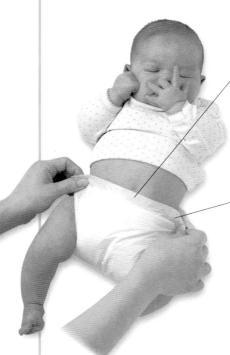

Bring the nappy *straight up: don't twist it to one side*

Spread the nappy *taut over your baby's tummy*

2 Bring the front up, pointing the boy's penis toward his feet (or he may urinate into the waistband).

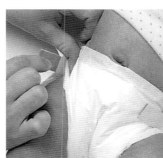

3 Hold one corner in position and, with the other hand, peel the tape, and pull it forwards to stick to the front, parallel with the top edge of the nappy.

4 Do the same with the other side, making sure the nappy is snug round your baby's legs, and not twisted round to one side.

Nappy bin

These are useful for discarding disposable nappies. The dirty nappies are put into the top of the bin, and the lid is closed and then rotated, sealing the nappy into a plastic wrapper. The bin only needs to be emptied once all the wrappers are used. This type of bin controls odours better than traditional nappy buckets, and makes it easier to dispose the contents quickly and hygienically.

Plastic wrappers *effectively seal in germs and odours*

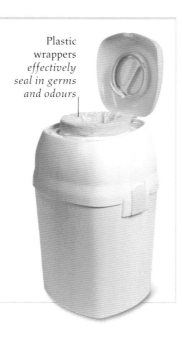

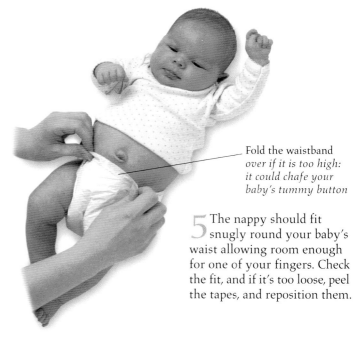

Fold the waistband *over if it is too high: it could chafe your baby's tummy button*

5 The nappy should fit snugly round your baby's waist allowing room enough for one of your fingers. Check the fit, and if it's too loose, peel the tapes, and reposition them.

Putting on a reusable nappy

Shaped nappies

These reusable nappies come in two parts: an absorbent inner nappy, sometimes used with a liner, and an outer wrapper. The inner nappy square is folded and placed inside the outer wrapper (as shown here), or sometimes a shaped or ready-folded inner nappy is used inside the wrapper. The inner nappy catches faeces and absorbs urine, while the wrapper holds everything in place, and prevents wetness from leaking through to the baby's clothes. If you use squares, it is a good idea to have them folded ready for use. Like a disposable, a reusable nappy should be changed when your baby soils it.

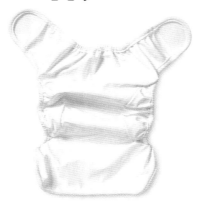

1 Lay the outer wrapper out flat, with the inside facing you and the tabs at the top.

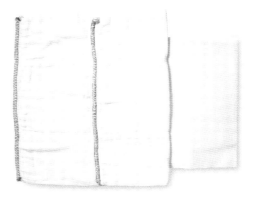

2 Take one of the absorbent nappies and fold it into thirds along its length, forming a long rectangle.

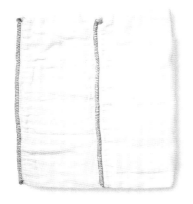

3 Fold the liner over the nappy, and then fold the nappy and liner again to form a long rectangle.

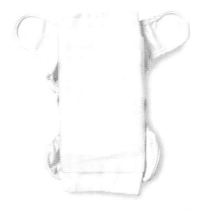

4 Place the absorbent nappy (with the liner on top) down the centre of the outer wrapper.

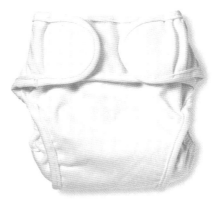

5 Put the baby down on the nappy, bringing the front up and fastening the tabs snugly around her hips.

Washing reusable nappies

There is no need to soak and sterilize nappies before washing them. Just put used nappies in a dry bucket until enough have accumulated for a washing machine load. If there are traces of dried faeces on the nappies you can do one of two things: you can either use the pre-wash cycle first to loosen the faeces, or you can be environmentally friendly and use a little squirt spray gun to get rid of most of the dried faeces into the toilet first. Machine wash at 60°C, which is hot enough to kill any bacteria. Use a non-biological washing powder. Do not add any fabric softener, as this reduces the absorbency of the nappies. Some manufacturers recommend an extra rinse cycle to make sure that all traces of detergent are removed. Try to dry outside on a line, if you can. Although the reusable nappies can be tumble-dried, constant tumble-drying may eventually affect their absorbency, and reduce the amount of use you get out of them. In addition, tumble-drying uses up a lot of energy, and will negate the environmental benefit of using reusable nappies.

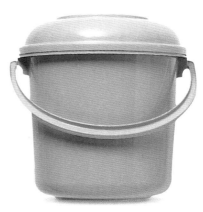

Maintaining hygiene
Choose buckets with different colours or lids: one for wet nappies, one for dirty.

Giving up nappies

Usually around the age of two, your child will start to recognize the feeling of a full rectum and a full bladder. The next step is knowing that a movement is on its way, and once your child grasps this she will train herself to get to the potty in time if it is easily accessible to her. Progress might be uneven: she may gain control over her bowels before her bladder, or vice-versa, so be patient with her.

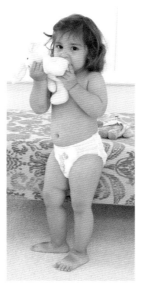

Tips to help
● Choose a time for potty-training when your child's life is relatively free of new situations and when you can approach it with a relaxed attitude.
● Set the situation up so she is more likely to succeed than fail in getting her functions in the potty – if she thinks she always fails, she will stop trying.
● When she's successful, show that you're pleased with her.
● When she has an accident, be sympathetic about it.
● Allow her to learn at her own pace.

Trainer pants
Towelling and a waterproof backing make these more absorbent than ordinary pants. Disposable trainer pants are also available.

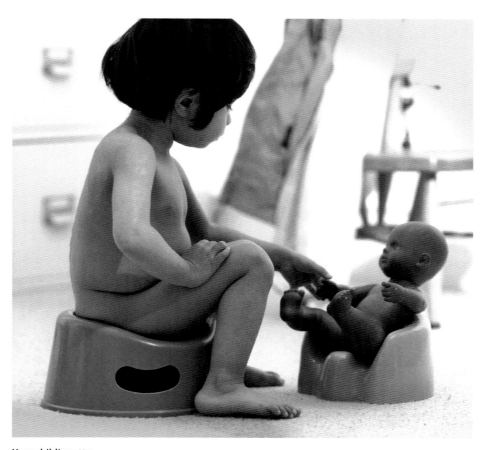

Your child's potty
Your child will soon understand what it's for, and will be proud of herself for learning a new skill. Always be encouraging and complimentary.

Achieving daytime control

1

Wait until your child is ready
Your child is ready to learn to use the potty if she:
● is aged two to two and a half
● recognizes that she's done something in her nappy, perhaps by pointing and shouting
● is often dry after a nap.

2

Introduce the potty
Show her a potty and tell her what it's for. Put it in the bathroom for a few days before doing anything further, so she gets used to it. Show her how to sit on it, but with her nappy on for now.

3

Set aside a suitable time
Set aside two weeks during the summer for potty training, when you can stay at home most of the time with your child playing outside in the garden, or when you're free for two weeks, during which time you can concentrate your efforts on potty training, and a few accidents won't disrupt the household. *Don't* start when your routines are already upset: a holiday away from home, for example, is not a good time.

4

Put her in pants, and remind her often to use the potty
For these two weeks, let your child wear pants or trainer pants, which will absorb at least a little of the urine. Have the potty nearby, and suggest she sits on it after a meal, a drink, a snack, or a nap, or whenever she shows any signs of needing it.

Achieving night-time control

5 · Help her to use the potty
Encourage her to sit on the potty, but do not pressure her. Pull down her pants and help her to sit down on it (tuck a boy's penis in). If she's managed to tell you she needs it, thank her.

If your child jumps up too soon
Suggest she sits there a little longer – about five minutes – and distract her with a toy or a book. If nothing happens, let her get up and carry on playing.

When she does go in the potty
When she does use the potty, always praise her. Wipe and clean her quickly, from front to back. Hold the potty steady as she stands up, and pull up her pants for her. Don't show disgust at the contents of the potty, just flush them down the lavatory, wipe the potty clean, then rinse it with disinfectant. Wash your hands.

6 · When your child has an accident, don't scold her
You can't expect her to remember to use the potty at this stage. If she wets or dirties her pants, don't scold her – it's really your fault for not reminding her to sit on the potty often enough. Clean her bottom with a sympathetic air and put fresh pants on her. If after two weeks your child shows no signs of understanding, and is not telling you she needs the potty on at least some occasions, she's not ready to give up nappies yet. Put her back in them for a few more weeks, then try again – you may have several two-week training stints before she gets herself to the potty on most occasions when she needs to.

7 · Leave a nappy off during naps
Once your child is using the potty fairly reliably during the daytime, and her nappy has been dry after a nap for about a week, you can leave her nappy off. Suggest she sits on the potty after she wakes from her nap. Napping without nappies will help her towards staying dry at night.

8 · When you go out
Until your child is fairly reliable, put a nappy on her when you go out, but try to make sure, without forcing her, that she uses her potty beforehand. If you're going on a car journey, put her in a nappy. Take a potty, spare clothes, and an old towel, in case of accidents.

9 · Suggest using the toilet
After a few weeks of using the potty during the day, suggest that she try being like you and use the lavatory. Help her pull her pants down and sit her on the seat for the first few times, until she gets the hang of it. For a boy, lift the seat and lid, and show him how to aim his penis, otherwise help him pull his pants down and climb up to sit on the seat. You can use a clip-on lavatory seat to make the hole smaller and less daunting for her. Stay nearby until she's finished, wipe her bottom, and help her down; she won't be able to wipe her own bottom until she is at least four. Wash her hands and yours.

Achieving night-time control

1 · Wait until she is dry at night
If you have taken a dry nappy off your child in the morning for about a week, you can start leaving her nappy off at night.

2 · Let her sleep without anything on her bottom at all
For the first week, put her to bed without a nappy or pants; protect the mattress with a waterproof sheet if you want to. Make sure she uses the lavatory before bedtime. She should sleep through without any problems. If she doesn't, and she wets the bed, she's simply not ready to give up night-time nappies yet.

3 · If she lapses into bedwetting
If your child starts to wet her bed after being dry at night for weeks or months, it's probably because she has suffered some sort of upheaval in her life. Never scold or punish her for bedwetting. If she wakes up wet in the night, be sympathetic and quickly dry her, and put her in clean pyjamas with a clean sheet on the bed. If it happens more than once, put her back in nappies until she's more settled and you have taken off a dry one for seven consecutive mornings. She may not be dry at night until she is five or six, but this is not unusual. Withholding a bedtime drink won't help her.

Reaching the toilet
Put a step out so your child can climb up. She will probably want to flush the lavatory when she finishes – that's part of the fun.

Getting out and about

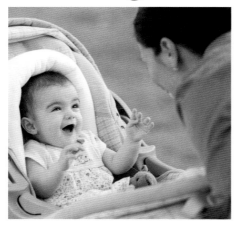

As she grows older your baby will love going out and about. She'll find everything fascinating and new – dogs, people, even supermarket shelves. To facilitate this, some form of pram or pushchair and a car seat are essential items. Other useful items are a sling for a young baby, or a backpack carrier if your baby is older. You will need a sun-blind to fix to the window on the sunny side of the car. A changing bag with a detachable changing mat is convenient for outings.

Methods of transport

Choosing a method of transporting your baby can be bewildering. In a nutshell, an ideal and practical choice is a carrycot on a chassis that can be converted to a pushchair. Your newborn needs protection from draughts and fumes, and a pushchair can't provide this. Once she is older, a sturdy, rigid-backed pushchair is a good choice.

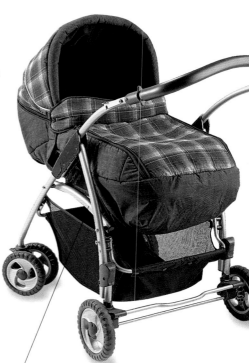

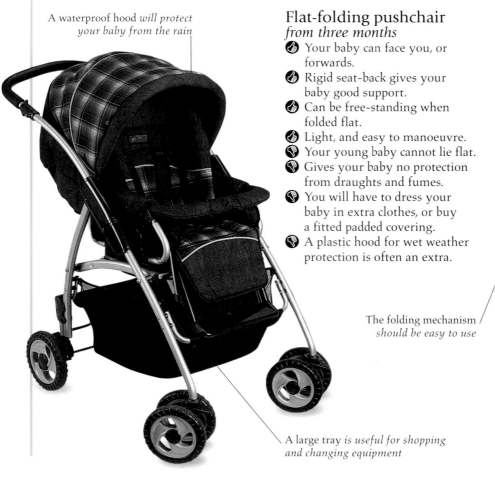

A waterproof hood *will protect your baby from the rain*

Flat-folding pushchair
from three months
- 👍 Your baby can face you, or forwards.
- 👍 Rigid seat-back gives your baby good support.
- 👍 Can be free-standing when folded flat.
- 👍 Light, and easy to manoeuvre.
- 👎 Your young baby cannot lie flat.
- 👎 Gives your baby no protection from draughts and fumes.
- 👎 You will have to dress your baby in extra clothes, or buy a fitted padded covering.
- 👎 A plastic hood for wet weather protection is often an extra.

The folding mechanism *should be easy to use*

Carrycot on a chassis
from birth
- 👍 Gives your young baby good protection from draughts and fumes.
- 👍 Your young baby can sleep in it day and night.
- 👍 Your baby can be snug under a weatherproof cover for outdoor use.
- 👍 Some types convert to take a pushchair seat.
- 👍 Chassis folds flat.
- 👎 Can be awkward to take on public transport.
- 👎 Some types are too wide to fit through a small door.

A large tray *is useful for shopping and changing equipment*

Pram on a pushchair
from birth
- 👍 Gives your young baby good protection from draughts and fumes.
- 👍 Gives your baby a comfortable ride.
- 👍 Can be used up to about one year.
- 👎 Hard to use on public transport.
- 👎 You need ample storage.

The car seat fixes easily onto the chassis

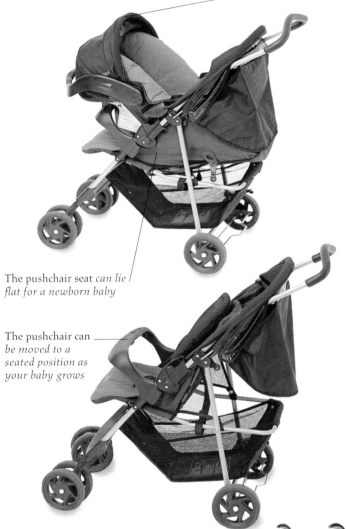

The pushchair seat can lie flat for a newborn baby

The pushchair can be moved to a seated position as your baby grows

Umbrella-folding pushchair
from about six months
- 👍 Folds up neatly, so it is good on public transport, and also when storage space is limited.
- 👍 The cheapest option; also the lightest.
- 👎 Soft seat-back gives poor support, so not suitable for babies under six months.
- 👎 Often no shopping tray.

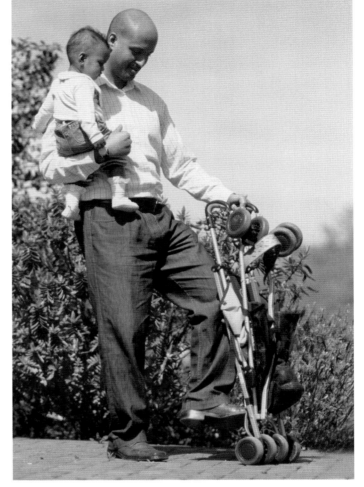

When your child is walking
Once she is up and about, she will be keen to explore her surroundings. This enthusiasm may tire her out at times, so be ready to pick her up, or take a pushchair with you. If you are worried about her safety when you take her outside, reins are the ideal way to keep your child from wandering off, while giving her more freedom than holding your hand. They also provide additional stability when she starts to walk..

Pram and pushchair safety
- Check that the pushchair is firmly locked into position before you put your baby in.
- In a pushchair, fit and **always** use a harness.
- In a pram, fit and **always** use a harness when your baby starts to sit up.
- Put the brake on as soon as you stop.
- Never let your child pull herself up or try to stand.
- Never hang bags on the handles: you may tip it up.
- Never let your child play with a folded pushchair.
- Make sure the pram or pushchair you buy conforms to the European safety standards.

Car travel

You must take steps to protect your child from injury by always restraining her on car journeys as described below. Currently, the law states that all children under the age of 12 must use some form of child car seat, unless they are taller than 135cm (4ft 5in). The law also stipulates that it is illegal to use a rear-facing baby seat in a front seat that is protected by an active frontal airbag. If it is at all possible, you should try to bolster these safety measures to make sure that in the event of a collision, your child is as protected as she can be.

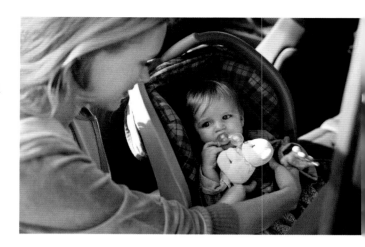

Being extra safe

Traditionally, only infants are put in rear-facing car seats. However, it is recommended that you put small children into these seats, too (provided the seat is big enough), since they have weak, underdeveloped neck muscles that are vulnerable in a front-end collision. In such an instance, if a child is in a rear-facing seat, the whole of the child's back takes the strain of the impact, not just the neck. In Sweden, where the recommendation is for children to sit rear facing until age four, research shows that this reduces serious injuries by 92 per cent, while forward-facing seats do so by only 60 per cent. Swedish car seats allow children up to 25kg (55lbs) to sit rear facing, which is the highest rear-facing limit in the world. Such seats can be bought online. At present in the UK, it is only possible to buy rear-facing car seats with an upper weight limit of 30–35lbs (about 2–2½ years), so until the regulation changes, you may have to settle for a rear-facing seat with the highest weight limit available.

In-car entertainment

Make long car journeys as enjoyable as possible:
- play CDs of stories and songs
- join in singing songs and reciting rhymes
- point out people, animals, houses, and lorries
- take toys such as finger puppets or an activity centre
- take snacks and drinks
- stop frequently.

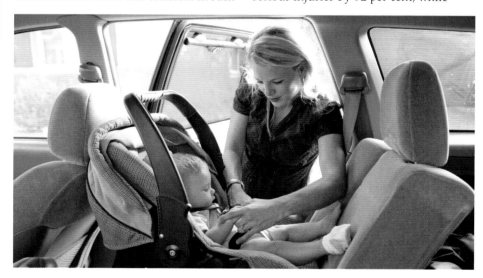

ISOFIX

As car designs vary so much, it is virtually impossible to make a child car seat that can be fitted correctly into all cars. ISOFIX stands for "International Standards Organisation FIX". It is a standard for child-seat installation, intended to make fitting quick and easy. Because ISOFIX creates a rigid link between the child seat and the car, it makes it extra secure. New cars and child seats have ISOFIX points built into them to enable the seat to be simply plugged into the ISOFIX point in the car. The ultimate aim is that any ISOFIX car seat you buy will plug into the ISOFIX point of any car. However, at present you still need to check that the ISOFIX seat you choose is approved for your particular vehicle. Many manufacturers have a fitting list on their website that tells you which cars their seats will fit in, and your car dealer may also be able to advise you on the makes of seats, which fit the ISOFIX points in their vehicles. Ideally, when you are buying a child car seat, ask to try it out in your car before you buy it.

Birth to 12 months (up to 9kg/20lbs)

Safest: A rear-facing infant seat on the back seat, held in place as the manufacturer recommends with the adult seat belt, or on the front seat, provided your car has no air bags (see also page 236). Strap your baby in with the harness. The car seat must conform to European standard number ECE R44-03.

Remember that weight is more important than age or height in determining the suitability of a car seat. It is best to buy from a reputable supplier, who can advise you on which seat is most appropriate for your child.

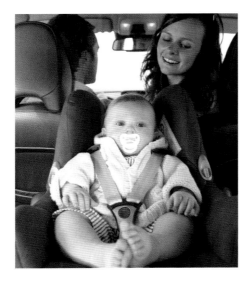

One to four years

Safest: A larger rear-facing seat that allows your child to sit facing rearwards until the age of four years. The seat has improved side impact protection for your child and a head support pad, which increases the length of the backrest, and as such increases the usable height for the child in the seat. The seat is fitted with a sturdier belt system that reduces the impact on the child if a collision should occur. Look for a seat with a recline feature so that it can be used from birth onwards. This will mean that you only make one purchase until your child is old enough for a forward-facing seat.

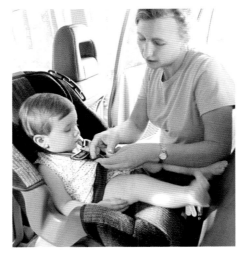

Four to 11 years

Safest: Forward-facing child car seat fitted in the back seat with a purpose-designed anchorage kit. Strap your child in with the harness. Some seats can be held in place with the rear seat belt. For older and larger children (generally aged six years and over, or 22–36kg/48–79lbs), a booster seat or cushion may be appropriate, since an adult seat belt will not fit correctly otherwise. Children of any age are always safer travelling in the back seat than in the front. You can ask your child to decorate his seat with stickers so that he is encouraged to use his own "unique" seat.

Safety in the car

- Make sure the car seat installation conforms to ISOFIX (see facing page)
- Never let any child travel unrestrained. **Always** strap your child into her seat with the safety harness.
- Never travel with your baby in your lap or your arms.
- If your car has air bags, do not put the baby seat in the front passenger seat. Children are always safer in the back seat.
- If you have an accident, replace your seat belts, your child's car seat, and the seat's anchorage kit: they may have been damaged.
- Never buy second-hand car seats, harnesses, or anchorage kits for the same reason.
- Install a mirror on your windscreen so that you can see your child without turning round.
- Put a "BABY ON BOARD" sign on your back window.
- Use a sun-blind when necessary.
- Use booster seats in the back seats for older children.

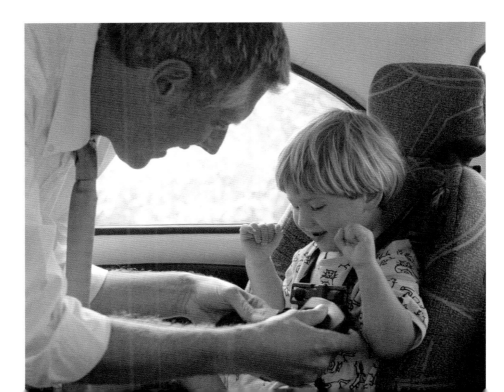

When you have to leave your child

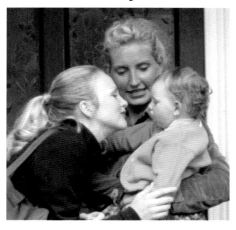

The first time that you leave your baby is a real milestone for you, even if it is just for an hour or two of shopping, a trip to the gym, or a visit to the cinema. Leaving your precious new baby in the care of even the most trusted friend, grandparent, or babysitter can be a real wrench. You may feel a bit guilty because it suddenly seems such a relief to be free, albeit briefly, from the feeling of total responsibility that you have for your tiny infant.

Getting your child used to other people

Babysitters

Nothing is more important during your baby's early months than your ever-loving presence, but eventually he has to learn to lead a separate existence. His eventual transition to school will be easier and his confidence will grow if he has opportunities to explore the world outside his immediate family, and learns to be independent of you, and to make close relationships with other people – grandparents, babysitters, and friends.

It isn't frivolous or selfish to get your baby used to a regular babysitter when he is young. And if you plan to go back to work within a year or so, then it is essential that he gets used to the idea that someone else can be relied on to love and care for him. There are several things you can do to make babysitting easier both for the sitter and your baby.

● Tell your baby what's going to happen, even if he is too young to understand. He will sense your reassurance.

● If you go out in the evening, make sure he knows the babysitter, so that if he wakes he won't be terrified at seeing a stranger.

● Don't introduce any new babysitting arrangement when your baby is tired, hungry, or sick. Pick a time of the day when you think he'll be at his most alert and happiest.

● If you have a new babysitter, don't rush to go out even if you are in a hurry. Spend some time holding him and letting him size up this new person. Let your baby see that you like the babysitter.

● Show the babysitter which toys are his favourites and how to play the games he likes best.

● If the babysitter has to put your child to bed, make sure she knows every detail of his bedtime routine, so that your child will go to bed happily.

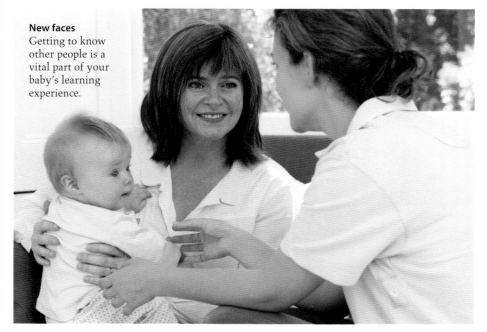

New faces
Getting to know other people is a vital part of your baby's learning experience.

Separation anxiety

At some time, usually between seven months and a year, your baby may start to seem reluctant even to let you out of his sight for a second. He'll cling when you try to put him down, or cry if he is left with anyone else. Don't worry about such behaviour. This "separation anxiety" is normal and means that he recognizes you as separate from him, and realizes how essential you are to him. Even the most clingy baby will eventually become independent. But, meanwhile, patiently accept his dependence on you. If you have to go out, always tell him. Say goodbye confidently, even if you're feeling nervous – your child is sensitive to your emotions and if he senses your anxiety, he may be even more upset. Tell him where you are going, and reassure him that you will be coming back.

Cuddlies and security blankets

By eight or nine months, most children form a strong attachment to a favourite soft toy, blanket, or a special object. This powerful need for something cuddly grows even stronger after the first birthday. The child may carry it around continually during the day, take it to bed at night, cuddling or sucking it for comfort. Eventually, it becomes a kind of talisman, something the child turns to for comfort whenever he is frustrated, frightened, or sad. Your child's cuddly will become grubby, shabby, and eventually probably unsanitary, because your child will be reluctant to let you wash it, as its familiar smell is part of its comforting charm. Don't try to persuade him to give it up. It fulfils a real need. Keep it handy, make sure babysitters know about it, and try to forestall the disaster of losing it by keeping a duplicate somewhere safe.

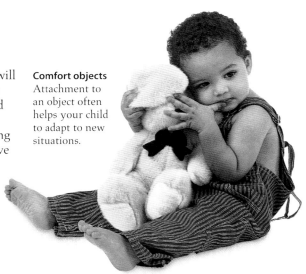

Comfort objects
Attachment to an object often helps your child to adapt to new situations.

Childcare options

Going back to work

Whether you are going back to work because you love your job or whether it is a matter of financial necessity, it is bound to be stressful at first. How smoothly it goes depends almost entirely on the childcare arrangements you make. It will take a little while for everything to settle down, so don't worry too much if the first few days are difficult. Children are pretty adaptable, and most settle down quickly under a new routine. But keep a careful eye on your child during the first few weeks you are back at work. If his behaviour deteriorates or if he seems generally unhappy, you may need to re-think your childcare plans.

Grandparent care

This may be an ideal arrangement provided that the grandparent is willing. It is important that they know and respect your views on childcare – and vice-versa. Problems may arise if you feel that the grandparents are "taking over".

Shared care with a friend or relative

If you intend to work part-time and have a good friend or close relative who also has small children, this may provide a workable solution. It's important to formalize the arrangement and stick to it, so that neither party feels they are being taken advantage of.

Childminder

This is one of the least expensive childcare options. Use a childminder registered with your local authority. A registered childminder may look after three children under five years, and another three under eight years (including her own), in her own home.

A childminder's home is checked by the local authority for suitability and police checks are carried out on members over 16 in their household. But you also need to talk to the minder yourself, to make sure that she is the kind of person you want to care for your child. It may be difficult to find a place for a very young baby.

Nursery care

Private nurseries offer full day care, usually from around 7am to 6pm, and usually stay open during holiday periods. Nursery care is expensive, but there is a fairly high ratio of staff to children and a stimulating environment. Most have a separate baby area for children under the age of two.

Nanny care

This is the most expensive option, but you may be able to split the cost by sharing with another family. Having a nanny means your child has one-to-one care in his or her own home. A qualified nanny will have a childcare qualification such as an NNEB diploma. Always see her registration documents and childcare qualification certificates, and never forget to check references before offering a job.

N.B. An au pair is a mother-helper, not a mother-substitute. Au pairs are untrained and will have little or no childcare experience. He or she is not a suitable person to take sole charge of a baby or young child. Should an au pair who is unfamiliar with the country take care of your child, make sure she knows the emergency numbers.

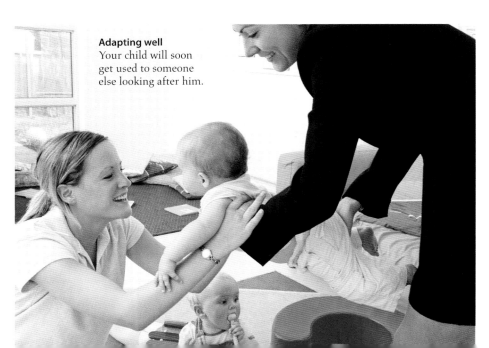

Adapting well
Your child will soon get used to someone else looking after him.

Growing and learning

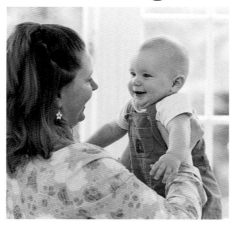

Watching your child grow and learn is a rewarding experience. Every stage brings something new: at first it's rolling over, sitting, crawling, walking. Once he's mastered those, he will learn to talk, and will refine his co-ordination and dexterity. Although there's nothing so thrilling as watching him take his first steps, the next year will bring some subtler achievements that will fill you with pride. Throughout these pre-school years, your child needs your attention and stimulation.

The first six months

During these months you will see your baby develop a real personality, and he will reward you with plenty of enchanting smiles and gurgles. Although there are a lot of toys aimed at this age group, he needs – and loves – your company most of all. When he's wakeful, talk and smile with him. Plenty of stimulation in the form of things to look at, sounds to hear, and textures to explore is vital, too. You don't need expensive toys: old photographs, rattles, and non-glass mirrors will all do just as well.

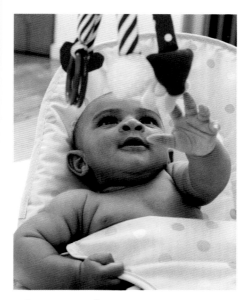

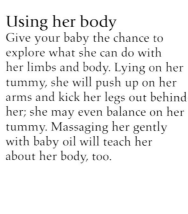

Using her body
Give your baby the chance to explore what she can do with her limbs and body. Lying on her tummy, she will push up on her arms and kick her legs out behind her; she may even balance on her tummy. Massaging her gently with baby oil will teach her about her body, too.

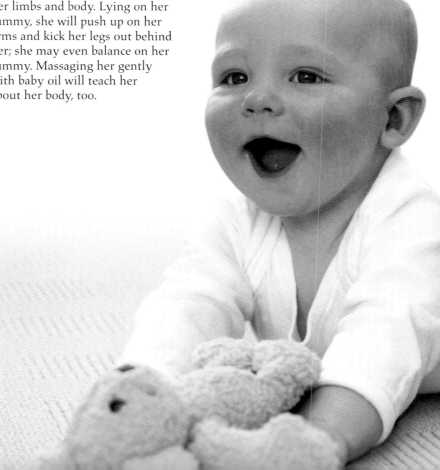

Objects and noises
At around six weeks, let your baby spend some of his wakeful times in a bouncing chair on the floor. (Before this, he will enjoy lying on the floor on a blanket.) If you show him something colourful that makes a noise, he'll show his interest by wriggling around. He may be able to hold something light if you put it in his hand, and soon he'll reach out clumsily to grab things.

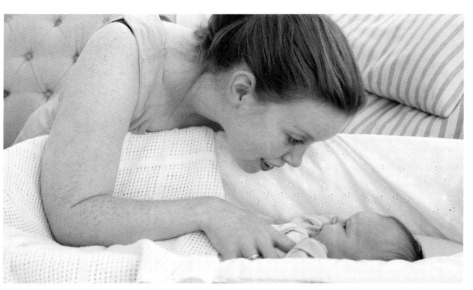

Learning about each other

During the first couple of months of life your baby can't focus beyond about 25cm (10in), so bring your face close when you talk to her, and exaggerate your expressions and smiles. It's this eye contact that helps your baby become a person, and shows her what building a loving relationship is all about.

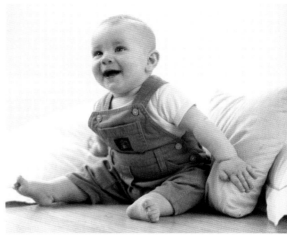

Rolling

Some time during these six months, your baby will learn to roll over, from front to back first, then from back to front. It will give him a great sense of achievement: he's beginning to make his body move for him. Remember that even before he's learnt to roll he can fall off things, so never leave him unattended on a high surface, not even the bed.

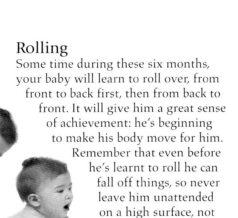

Learning to sit

As your baby gets more control over his body, help him learn to sit by surrounding him with cushions. They will help him balance, and protect him if he topples over.

Premature babies

Your premature baby will probably reach all his developmental milestones later than other babies. Remember that in reality he has two "birthdays": one is the day he was born, but the more important one for the first few months is the date on which he was expected to be born. If you take those missing weeks in the womb into account, you will almost certainly find that his progress is not slow at all. Take him to the clinic for regular monitoring; he should have caught up with other children born at the same time by the age of two.

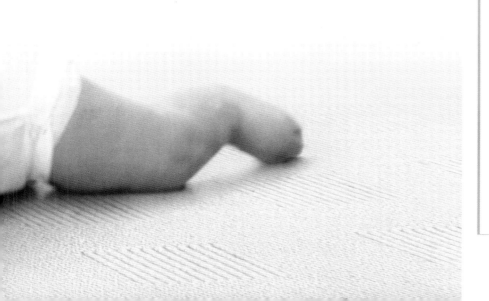

Stepping stones chart

Babies don't all develop at the same rate, or learn a particular skill at a particular time. But because everything they learn acts as a "stepping stone" to the next stage of development, they do acquire skills in the same order. The chart below shows the "stepping stones" in various areas of your child's development – physical skills, manual dexterity, sight, hearing and speech, and social behaviour and play. Your child may learn to do something either earlier or later than the average age given in the chart.

Stepping stones in child development

Age	Physical movements	Manual dexterity	Hearing, vision, and speech	Social behaviour and play
One month	Lies on back with head to one side. When held sitting his head falls forwards with back curved. Held standing on hard surface presses down feet, straightens body, and makes reflex "stepping" movements.	Hands normally closed, but if open will grasp a finger if it touches his palm.	Startled by loud noises. Turns head and eyes towards light. Eyes will follow a dangling toy held 15–20cm (6–8in) away and moved slowly from side to side.	Stops crying when picked up and spoken to. Looks at mother's face intently when she feeds or talks to him.
Three months	Lies on back with head in mid-line. Kicks vigorously. Held sitting can hold head erect and steady. Placed face down lifts head and upper chest well up. Held standing with feet on hard surface sags at knees.	Watches movements of own hands, and begins to clasp and unclasp hands. Holds rattle placed in his hand for a few moments, but can't look at it at the same time.	Alert, and interested in people's faces. Moves head to look around. Eyes converge as a toy held above his face is moved nearer. Smiles at mother's voice. Vocalizes when spoken to. Turns head and eyes towards a sound.	Smiles at 5–6 weeks. Recognizes and begins to react to preparations for bath, feeds, etc. by smiles, coos, and excited movements. Responds with obvious pleasure to friendly handling, tickling, being talked or sung to.
Six months	Raises head when lying on back. Sits with support. When hands are grasped can pull himself up. Rolls over, front to back. Placed face down lifts head and chest up. Held standing takes his weight and bounces.	Stretches out both hands to grasp interesting objects. Usually uses both hands to scoop up an object, sometimes uses just one hand. Shakes rattle, and looks at it at the same time. Takes everything to mouth.	"Sings" and chats to himself using single and double syllables, such as ka, muh. Turns to mother's voice at once. Screams if annoyed. Recognizes and responds to various emotional tones of mother's voice.	Laughs, chuckles, and squeals aloud in play. Still friendly with strangers, but sometimes shows some anxiety, especially if mother is out of sight. When he drops a toy, he forgets about it.
Nine months	Sits alone for 10–15 minutes on floor. Progresses on floor by rolling or squirming. Tries to crawl on all fours. Pulls self to standing with support, but can't lower himself. Held standing steps purposefully on alternate feet.	Examines objects by passing them from one hand to the other. Stretches out one hand to grasp small objects. Will hold out toy to adult, but can't yet let go unless pressing against hard surface. Grasps spoon while being fed.	Shouts to attract attention, listens, and shouts again. Babbles tunefully, using long strings of syllables, e.g. dad-dad. Understands "no" and "bye-bye". Imitates adult noises, like cough, brrr, etc. Watches people and activities with interest.	Looks after toys falling over edge of pram or table. Can find partially hidden toy. Plays "peek-a-boo". May be wary of strangers, clinging to known adult and hiding face.

Age	Physical movements	Manual dexterity	Hearing, vision, and speech	Social behaviour and play
12 months	Sits well. Crawls rapidly. Pulls self to standing. Walks round furniture. Walks with one or both hands held. Stands or walks alone for some time.	Picks up small objects with thumb and index finger. Points at things he wants. Holds spoon but cannot use it alone. Drinks from cup with little assistance.	Responds to own name. Babbles loudly. Shows that he understands familiar words and commands associated with gestures, "clap hands" etc.	Shows affection to familiar people. Tries to help with dressing. Throws toys, watches them fall. Waves and claps hands. Puts cubes in and out of box.
15 months	Walks with feet apart. Goes from standing to sitting by collapsing backwards, or falling forwards on hands. Crawls upstairs. Bends over to pick up toys.	Builds tower of two cubes after being shown. Grasps crayon and imitates scribble. Brings spoon to mouth to lick. Holds cup when given, and gives it back.	Speaks 2–6 familiar words, and understands more. Obeys simple commands, e.g. "shut the door". Looks with interest at pictures in a book, and pats pages.	Helps more constructively with dressing. Easily upset. Depends on mother's reassuring presence. Can push big-wheeled toy on level ground.
18 months	Walks well. Runs stiffly, can't run round obstacles. Carries toys. Walks upstairs with helping hand. Creeps backwards downstairs. Sits on stairs, bumps down a few steps.	Picks up tiny objects with pincer grasp. Preference for one hand obvious. Scribbles with crayon with preferred hand. Builds tower of three cubes after being shown.	Jabbers, uses 6–20 words, and understands more. Sings and tries to join in rhymes. Enjoys picture books, points at and recognizes coloured items. Turns two pages at a time.	Takes off shoes, socks, and hat. Does not take toys to mouth. Plays contentedly alone, but likes to be near adult. Emotionally depends on familiar adults, especially mother.
Two years	Runs safely. Walks backwards. Pulls wheeled toy. Climbs on and off furniture. Goes up and down stairs holding rail, two feet to a step. Sits on wheeled toy and moves forward with feet.	Builds tower of four or five cubes. Draws circles and dots. Can imitate vertical line. Identifies familiar adults in a photograph after being shown once.	Turns pages one by one. Uses 50 plus words. Puts two or more words together to make sentences. Refers to himself by name. Asks names of objects. Joins in rhymes and songs.	Follows mother around, and copies what she does. Plays simple make-believe games. Plays near other children, but not with them. Has tantrums when frustrated, but easily distracted.
Two and a half years	Walks upstairs alone, and downstairs holding rail, two feet to a step. Climbs easy climbing frame. Jumps with two feet together. Kicks a large ball. Sits on tricycle and steers, but can't yet pedal.	Can build tower of seven or more cubes, and line up blocks to form a "train". Can draw a horizontal line and circle when shown how. Eats skilfully with spoon, and may use a fork.	Uses 200 plus words. Knows full name. Uses "I", "me", and "you." Always asks questions beginning "what?" and "how?"Can say a few nursery rhymes. Recognizes self in a photo, once shown.	Rebellious and throws tantrums if frustrated. Less easily distracted. Enjoys make-believe play. Likes to watch other children play, and may join in for a few minutes. Has little idea of sharing toys.
Three years	Walks alone upstairs with alternating feet, downstairs with two feet to a step. Climbs with agility. Rides tricycle. May walk on tiptoes. Sits with feet crossed at ankle.	Eats well with fork and spoon. Washes hands. Pulls pants up. Builds tower of nine cubes or more. Draws man with head and some features. Paints with large brush. Uses scissors.	Can give full name, sex, and often age. Holds simple conversations and speaks of past experiences. Listens to stories, and demands favourites. Can match 2–3 primary colours.	Less prone to tantrums. Helps adults in activities. Enjoys floor play with bricks etc. Plays with other children. Understands taking turns. Friendly with younger siblings.

The second six months

Your baby will cram a great deal into these months. He will sit up unsupported, he may crawl, and even stand or walk by his first birthday. It won't be steady progress, and not every child goes through each stage. This is the age when he learns to explore every new thing by putting it in his mouth. From now until around three years old, make sure your child never gets hold of any small, dangerous objects.

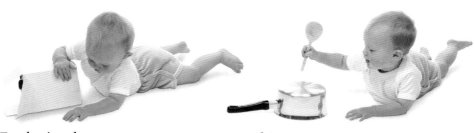

Exploring boxes
Don't be surprised if your baby finds the boxes his toys arrive in just as fascinating as the toys. Check for and remove any staples, and make sure there aren't any sharp edges.

Making noises
A wooden spoon and a saucepan make a perfect drum – your baby will love banging away and listening to the loud noise he creates.

Sitting up
Your baby will lean forwards and splay her legs out wide and straight, when she first learns to balance sitting up. (Put a cushion behind her until she's steady.) Now she has both hands free to explore.

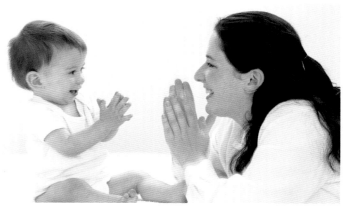

"Pat-a-cake"
Give your baby a small cube in each hand, and clap your hands together as he claps his. He will enjoy this little play.

Crawling
Getting about on all fours is a great achievement. He may not use each leg in the same way: a lop-sided shuffle with one knee and the other foot is quite normal.

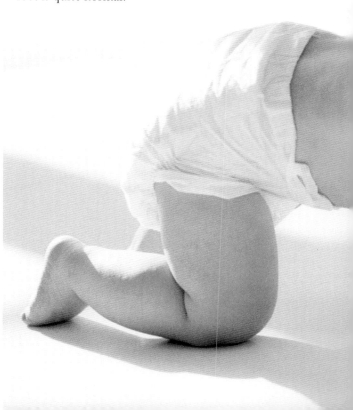

Water play
Show your baby how water feels on his hands. Sieves and plastic jugs make good substitutes for toy buckets.

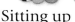

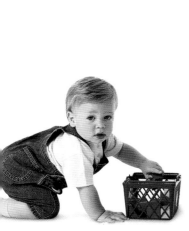

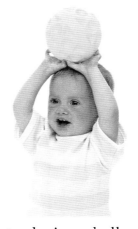

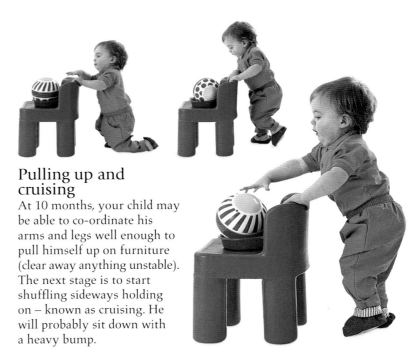

Boxes and objects

Give your older baby a box and some empty cotton reels or brightly coloured blocks, and he will happily take them out one by one, then put them back in again.

Introducing a ball

At seven months, your baby may be fascinated to see a ball rolling around but surprised when he accidentally makes it move. By a year, he may be able to pick it up and throw it.

Pulling up and cruising

At 10 months, your child may be able to co-ordinate his arms and legs well enough to pull himself up on furniture (clear away anything unstable). The next stage is to start shuffling sideways holding on – known as cruising. He will probably sit down with a heavy bump.

Playpens and babywalkers

A **playpen** can be a useful safe place if you have to leave your mobile child alone for a few moments – to answer the door, for example. Never leave him in it for more than a few minutes as he will get bored and frustrated. A **babywalker** is a chair on wheels that your baby can propel around using his feet. It may delay learning to walk by weakening his incentive to get around himself. **Never** leave your baby alone in a walker. It can tip easily, particularly on shallow steps down between rooms.

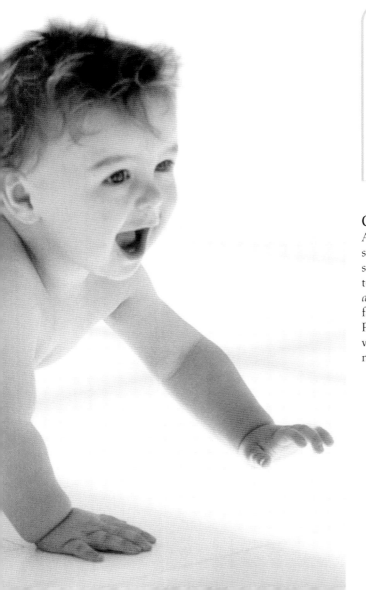

Climbing stairs

As soon as your child shows interest in the stairs, for his own safety teach him how to go up *and* down on all fours, facing into the stairs. Fit a stair gate for when you're not watching.

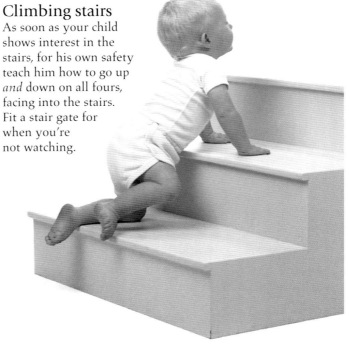

The second year

First steps and first words will probably be your child's most exciting and significant achievements during his second year. Handedness becomes apparent around the middle of this year: he will show a preference for one hand, and once he starts to draw and paint, this will become more marked. Although he'll amuse himself for short periods, you're still his essential and most valued playmate, and his most effective teacher, too.

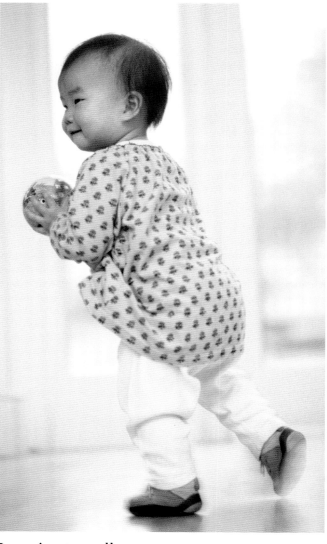

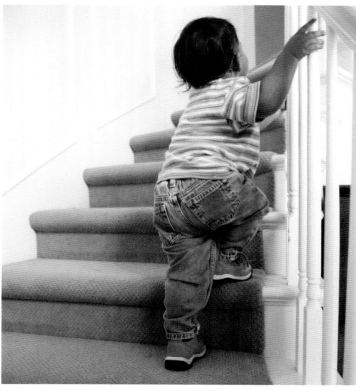

Using stairs

Towards the end of this year, your child may grow confident and skilful enough to go up and down the stairs upright and facing forwards.

Learning to walk

Once your child has taken her first hesitant steps unsupported, it will only be a few days before she's waddling about enthusiastically, though unsteadily. She'll keep her feet wide apart, and her arms out for balance. Let her go barefoot as often as possible: she only needs shoes for walking about outdoors.

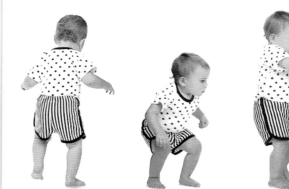

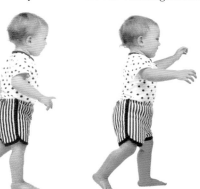

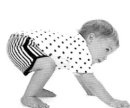

First steps will be unsteady

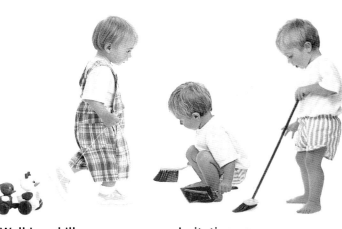

Building a tower
From about two years, your child will be able to build a tower of four or even five blocks.

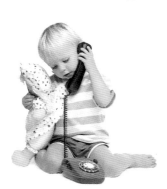

Walking skills
A pull-along toy improves his sense of balance.

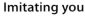

Imitating you
Copying you is how your child learns – and "helping" is always a favourite game. Toy tools make it easy for him to join in.

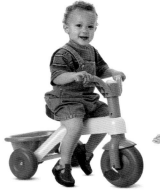

Greater mobility
At around two years, a stable ride-on toy will improve his co-ordination and confidence, and provide a new challenge.

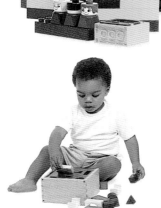

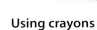

Using crayons
Introduce non-toxic crayons from about two years. He'll scribble now; soon he'll make up and down strokes.

Learning shapes
Sorting shapes into their correct holes is a challenging lesson. Give plenty of praise, when he gets it right.

Practising speech
A telephone and doll are two invaluable toys for practising the art of communication by copying what you do.

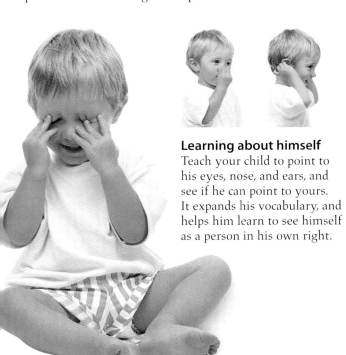

Learning about himself
Teach your child to point to his eyes, nose, and ears, and see if he can point to yours. It expands his vocabulary, and helps him learn to see himself as a person in his own right.

Learning to talk
Your child will say his first word – probably "dada" or "mama" – some time around his first birthday, and from then on he may learn roughly two or three new words a month. By the age of two, he may be able to string two words together – "me go", for example – and will have about 200 words in all. You can help him to improve his vocabulary by:
● talking to him
● continuing to include picture books and rhymes in your playtimes
● listening to him, being interested in what he's saying, and trying to understand
● not interrupting him to make him repeat things "properly" – he won't get the pronunciation right at first
● using adult language when you talk back to him, so he can hear the words spoken correctly
● being clear and direct: "Put the brick on the top" is less muddling than "Let's see if we can get this nice red brick on top of the other".

The third year

During this year, your child may surprise you with his burgeoning imagination that can make an absorbing game out of anything. Don't waste money on expensive kits and toys that can only stifle his creativity. A big cardboard box makes a house, a car, a boat, a spaceship – then when it gets tatty, you can throw it away and get another one (remove any staples). A sheet draped over two chairs is a haven, a tent, a house – anything he can think of. Towards the end of this year, your child might join a playgroup, and start to play with other children in a constructive way. You'll notice that he's becoming open to suggestion and reason when you want him to do things.

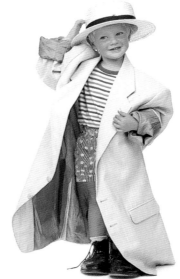

Dressing up
The "let's pretend" game is fun at any age. Your old clothes, shoes, handbags, and hats are all ideal items for a dressing-up box, and much more fun to play with than the special child-size outfits available in the toyshops.

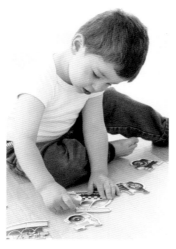

Irregular shapes
Jigsaws demand concentration, dexterity, and visual understanding. If he gives up quickly, try giving him a simpler one.

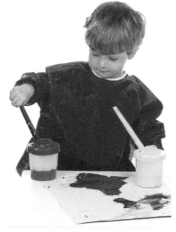

Colour and paint
Painting is a good way to learn about colour and texture. Give him thick brushes and non-spill pots, and protect his clothes.

Imaginary friends
Dolls and teddies will become friends to your girl or boy, and she will want to control their lives in the way you control hers.

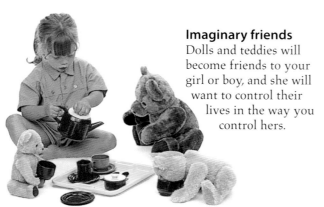

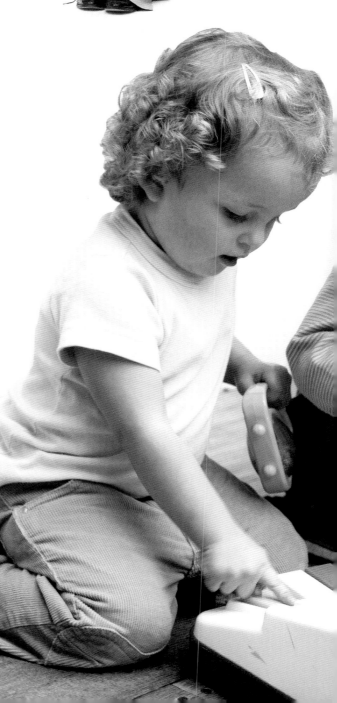

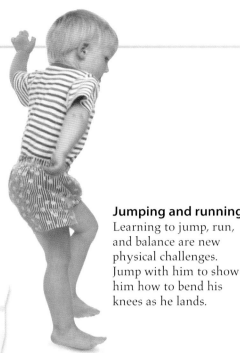

Jumping and running
Learning to jump, run, and balance are new physical challenges. Jump with him to show him how to bend his knees as he lands.

Using her hands
Help your child refine her hand movements. She can screw and unscrew small objects now, and will enjoy using pastry cutters to make shapes out of play dough or your pastry.

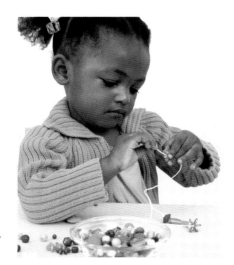

Playing together
A sandpit is always fun. Show your child how to use buckets and shovels, and teach her not to throw sand. She will soon find her own level of creativity. Cover the pit when not in use to stop dogs and cats fouling it.

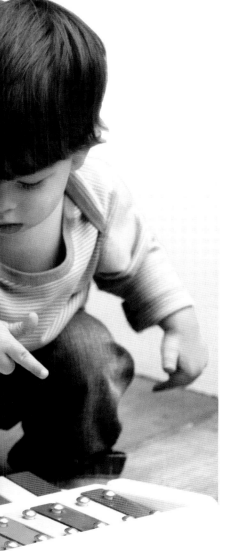

Sharing and playing
It takes time for children to learn to take turns and share toys. Set your child a good example – it's easiest if he learns to share with you first. Some time around the age of two and a half to three, your child will start to play *with* other children for the first time, sharing his toys amicably and joining in a common project. This is the ideal age to introduce him to a playgroup: the more your child is with others of his own age, the more quickly and easily he will learn to join in – and to fit in.

You can provide plenty of good play opportunities yourself: a sandpit, a paddling pool, interlocking plastic bricks, dressing up, making Christmas decorations – all these are great ways for children to learn to play together constructively. Your supervision is vital throughout the pre-school years, to keep a check on safety or to step in if tempers start to fray.

Games to play with your baby

Most parents realize how important it is to talk to their baby, but not everyone finds it easy to do this without feeling embarrassed or self-conscious. That's one reason why the games that parents traditionally play with their babies are so important. They provide a natural way for you to interact with your baby. Many of them involve simple repetitive rhymes and songs that even a baby quickly learns to recognize and that will help to stimulate his own language development. Here are some favourite games to play with your young child.

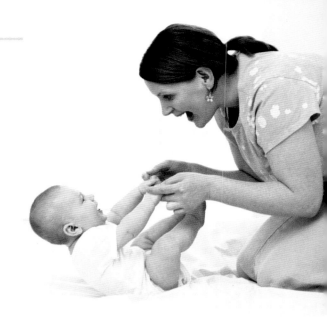

Tickling and touching games

Games that involve you lovingly handling his body are fun for your baby, and you will be surprised at how soon he will learn to understand and respond when you start to play one of them. When you sing "The wheels on the bus", you can involve his whole body, his legs becoming the wheels, his arms the opening and closing doors, and the wipers. He will enjoy having his toes wiggled in "This little piggy", and having you lightly run your fingers from his toes to his head for "All the way home". In games such as "Round and round the garden", and "There was a little mouse that lived just there", he will be overcome with excitement at anticipation of the tickly ending.

Hiding and finding games

Search-and-find games such as the "Hunt the thimble" type games primary school children play can be fascinating right from babyhood. A baby's first "treasure hunt" is to see you hide one of his toys under a blanket or towel right in front of him, and then, when you say "Where did the toy go?" make the discovery that the hidden toy is actually still there, under the blanket. You can step up the excitement by using three towels – which one is the toy under? To find it, your baby has to follow rudimentary rules – the toy is under a towel, not somewhere else quite different – and to remember under which towel his toy has gone.

"Peek-a-boo" is an immensely popular variation on this. The surprise of seeing your face dip out of sight and then come back into view can send your little one squealing with pleasure. You can try playing it with your baby in a "bouncer": as he twirls around you'll disappear, then he'll shout delightedly as he bounces around to face you again. And even if your baby loved it when he was only six months old, he will still enjoy variations on this search-and-find game later on. As he grows older, he'll imitate you and may "hide" from you behind his hands or under a towel. He'll pass through a stage where he thinks you can't see him simply because he can't see you. This is normal and can be fun when you turn it into a game.

Activity games

Games that involve bouncing on a parent's knee, such as "Ride a cock horse", "This is the way the ladies ride", and "Ride a horse to Boston", can be as boisterous or as gentle as the baby's age and temperament dictate. Your baby will very quickly learn to indicate when she wants to do it again – and when she has had enough. Remember to give her some time to relax after a boisterous game by cuddling her quietly.

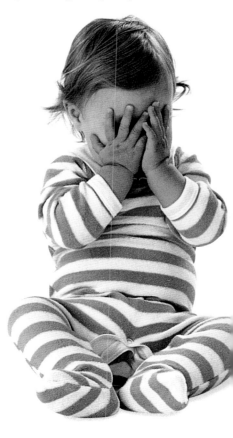

Singing and language games

Nursery rhymes and songs are part of your child's heritage. A few of the many excellent CDs of music and songs for small children are invaluable on car journeys. Best of all though is to sing to your baby yourself. All babies seem to love being sung to. Singing lullabies to your baby, such as "Twinkle, twinkle little star", and "Rock-a-bye baby", can help soothe her. She will enjoy the rhythm and rhymes of these and other lullabies. In finger play songs, such as "Incy Wincy Spider", the action of your hands can reinforce the meaning of the songs and help your baby to remember them.

Songs are one of the best ways to encourage your baby's language development and help her to understand and identify the world around her. "This little piggy" for example, explores the concepts of going and coming, and opposites ("went to market", "stayed at home", "had roast beef", "had none"). "Old McDonald had a farm" will teach her about animals and animal noises.

In her third and fourth years, your child will start to appreciate rhyming and nonsense rhymes. You can reduce her to helpless laughter with your own nonsense variation on a song she knows well ("Hickory dickory dee, The mouse ran up the tree...") and you will find she will very soon start imitating you and making up her own versions.

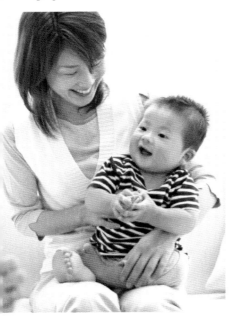

Playing catch

All children seem to love a game of simple catch. Sit down on the floor, with your baby directly opposite to you, and gently roll a soft ball or wheeled toy towards him. He may pick the toy up and want to return it to you. Alternatively, he may simply want to hold the toy and examine, or even chew it. He may puzzle you by holding out the toy for you to take and then pull it back again. This is quite common – although he's learned to grasp something, he may not yet have learnt to let it go. Don't try to pull the toy away from him. Just tell him what a nice toy it is, and keep on chatting to him.

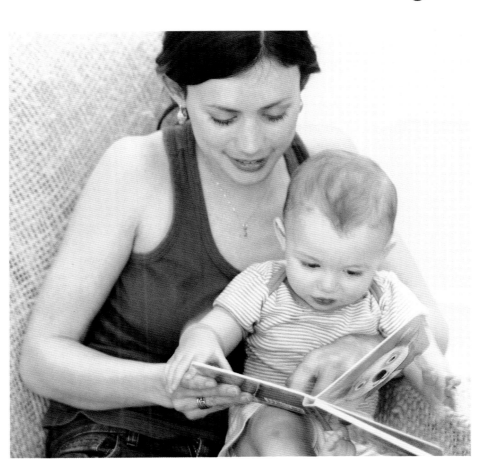

Reading

Your baby will like to have you read to him long before he has any idea of what reading is all about. He will enjoy the physical closeness as he sits on your knee, and is cuddled. Your baby will like the sound of your voice as you talk to him about the pictures in the book. He will like the bright colours of the pictures themselves. To begin with, reading is just another opportunity for you to spend time with your baby and talk to him. But eventually, he will understand what it is you are talking about.

Becoming a person

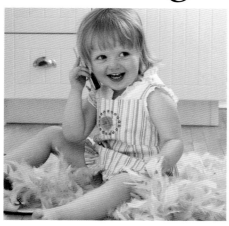

Your baby soon shows her own particular temperament, but her personality is also shaped by your responsiveness. Showing her how special she is to you, and treating her as an individual with her own wishes will help her become confident. Toddlers are easily frustrated, and at times you will need all your tact to help her without making her feel that you're taking over. Watching as she explores and discovers the world around her should make these pre-school years enormously rewarding for you.

Getting along together

Learning to get along well together in pre-school years is a process of adjustment for both of you. Your child has to learn the boundaries of acceptable behaviour, while you may have to adapt your own natural style as a parent, which may not always make you tolerant, consistent, and fair. Your child needs you to show her, not just tell her, how to behave well. Thoughtfulness, politeness, and kindness – all this she will only learn by copying you, when you show the same behaviour to her.

How to handle your child

Your child will respond best to you and do as you say more willingly if you can be both affectionate and firm. It isn't easy to get the balance right.

● Be consistent in what you say and do. If your child is smacked when she is naughty, she will hit other children when she is cross with them.
● "Dos" work better than "Don'ts". "Hang your coat up so no one will tread on it", elicits a more positive response than "Don't drop your coat on the floor".
● Say please and thank you, when you ask her to do something.
● Agree with your partner about what you will allow, and back each other up.
● Try to persuade rather than coerce. If she's in the middle of some absorbing activity, try telling her "Let's finish this, and then it'll be time to go to bed", rather than "Clear away those toys, now it's bedtime".
● Don't be too restrictive. Try listening to the way you talk to your child. Do you find you're nearly always issuing orders: "Stop that", "Do as you're told", "Don't touch"?
● If you were unreasonable over something, say so, and apologize.

● Don't assert your authority unnecessarily – avoid a clash of wills.
● Always explain *why* she mustn't do something as well as *what* she mustn't do, even if she's too young to understand.

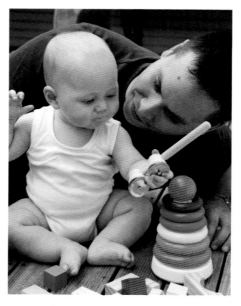

Learning for herself
Give your child help when she needs it, but don't take over – it's her toy, and she needs to feel she can succeed.

Rules to keep your child safe

Until your child has reached at least two and a half, you can't expect her to understand reasons for not doing things, nor to remember what she mustn't do. It's your responsibility to make sure her curiosity can't lead her into much danger, and that the important rules are enforced.

For example, "You must never go out of the garden on your own" is an abstract rule that your toddler cannot comprehend, much less remember when she's busy playing or absorbed in her toys. You can only keep an eye on her, and make sure that she doesn't stray out by putting a secure catch on the garden gate.

According to research, fire, falls, poisoning, and strangulation pose the biggest risk to children. Childproof your home to minimize any dangers. Make sure smoke detectors, which also detect carbon monoxide, are installed and regularly tested. Remove toys from the stairway, fix a stair gate and a handrail by the stairs. Never hang toys on your baby's pram or cot where she can reach them, don't let flexes trail, and put socket covers over electrical sockets. A stair gate across the kitchen door may be the best way to keep her safe when you're cooking.

Loving and spoiling

You may worry that the normal affection you give your child will spoil him. It won't. He needs your love, combined with plenty of attention. But you can spoil him by being over-lenient when he misbehaves. Letting him get his own way through tears and tantrums will not help him in his relations with friends and adults.

If you go out to work, you may find yourself "making up" to your child for not being there by lavishing toys on him. Toys can't take your place, and you may be giving him unrealistic expectations of what you can afford. Instead, when you can be around, give him your time, your love, and plenty of attention.

Showing your love
Your child will prefer your love and attention to any toys. Don't worry about spoiling him with love, you can't.

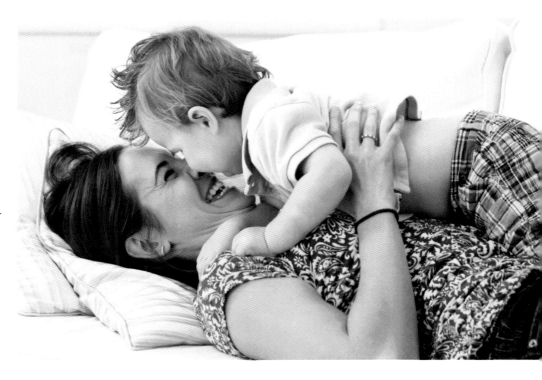

Developing a sense of identity

At around the age of 18 months or so, your child begins to realize that he is a separate person. He will start to refer to himself by name, and he will enjoy looking at photos of himself, too. From now on, he will want to take charge of his life more and more, and assert his own wishes and personality. You can help him foster this determination to do things for himself and nurture his burgeoning sense of identity.

Encouraging independence

● Make things easy. From age two onwards, organize his possessions, so that he can do as much as possible for himself. Buy clothes that are easy to manage, so he can dress and undress himself as much as possible; put a step by the washbasin so he can wash his hands without your help; and fix a low peg so he can hang up his own coat.
● Encourage him to help you. "Helping" is a game at the moment, not a chore. Simple jobs, like unpacking the shopping or laying the table, make your child feel he's achieved something, and show him that helping is part of family life.
● Let him make his own decisions. The opportunity to make simple decisions gives your child the feeling that he has some control over his own life. So let him choose which T-shirt he wants to wear, or how his room is arranged, or where he'd like to go for a walk.

Helping your child to feel special

Your child, just like every child, needs to feel that he's special – that you love him and that he is worth loving. It's this message that helps to make him emotionally strong and able to cope away from the security of home. There are plenty of little ways you can show how special he is to you:
● Don't forget to say you love him, or be too busy to give a hug or a cuddle when he wants one.
● Respect his feelings and respond to his needs. When he's miserable, he needs to cry and be comforted. Saying "Don't be a crybaby" is denying him the right to feel sad.
● Praise him and be enthusiastic about each fresh achievement.
● Listen and show interest when he talks to you.

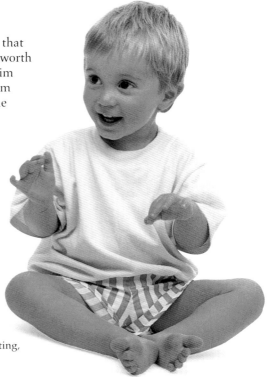

Becoming a person
Try to appreciate your toddler for the lively, fascinating, and independent individual he is fast becoming.

Good and bad behaviour

When they are well and happy, children usually behave acceptably. But every child has off-days, and every child wants to test her limits – and yours – by seeing how far she can go. Bad behaviour is often an effective way of gaining your attention, too. The time of greatest conflict will probably come at some stage during her third year: tears and tantrums often go hand in hand with being two years old.

Dealing with bad behaviour

Act quickly, pick your child up and remove her from the source of the trouble with a firm "NO". At the same time, distract her attention with some other activity or toy.

Most types of bad behaviour, tantrums, whingeing, and whining for example, are simply best ignored. If your child never manages to elicit a response from you, and is never allowed to win any arguments by such behaviour, she will soon stop. Just be calm, and carry on as normal. If necessary, put her outside the room until she calms down.

Rewards for good behaviour

It's very easy to give your child more attention when she behaves badly, and less when she behaves well and you feel you can relax. But rewarding your child with praise, affection, or a story on your lap when she behaves well is much more effective. You will encourage the behaviour you want, and teach her a very useful lesson in life – that being nice to people works much better than being nasty.

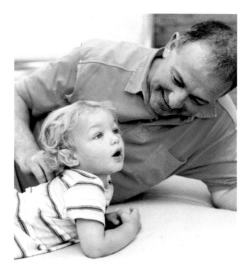

Appreciate good behaviour
Make sure you recognize and praise your child's good behaviour.

Punishments

Until she is about two years old, the question of "punishing" your child should not even arise. Very young children cannot make the connection between what they do and how you react. So punishment is unfair, and it won't work – when she repeats the "bad" behaviour, she won't remember that she was punished for it last time. When your child is above two years of age, she will begin to understand the difference between right and wrong, and also that actions have consequences. Often just looking or sounding cross will be enough of a punishment. But always make sure that your child knows that while you don't like what they are doing, you still love them just as much.

Should I smack my child?

Smacking is often a sign that you have reached the end of your tether. It's not a good way to deal with bad behaviour, and it doesn't deter your child from doing the same thing again. What is more, you are teaching her that physical force is an acceptable way to make people do what you want.

How to avoid getting to the end of your tether

However clever you become at managing your child, there will always be days when her behaviour seems completely unbearable, and you know you are close to losing control.

The solution is simple: take your child out. Whatever the weather, a trip to the park, the shops, or a friend's house will distract both of you from your respective moods, and help you recover your sanity and sense of humour.

Being firm

You needn't be angry or upset when you discipline your child, just consistent, so your child gets the clear message that she's never allowed to behave in that way.

Dealing with aggressive children

All small children fight occasionally, especially when they are bored or tired, and boys are often more aggressive than girls. When the fights get out of hand, step in quickly:
- separate the fighting children
- distract them by introducing some other game or a change of scene
- don't take sides – it's nearly always impossible to work out the rights and wrongs of any situation.

If your child bites another child:
- give all your attention and concern to the bitten child
- remove the biter straightaway, and put her somewhere else, safe but alone, for a few minutes.

Your child is bound to snatch and grab when she first starts to play with other children, but with help from you she will soon learn to share. It helps to get your child used to being with other children from an early age, so ask your health visitor about local toddler groups, where your child can meet other children of her age. A few children will continue to be very rough and aggressive, and their behaviour will eventually make them unpopular. For your child's sake, help her to be gentle with others:
- give her a good model to follow by always trying to be gentle, patient, and loving towards her
- make it clear through the way you act that it's your child's behaviour you dislike, not her
- always step in and stop your child immediately if she starts to hit another child; be firm, but don't shout or be aggressive yourself
- never let her get her own way by behaving aggressively or unpleasantly.

If your child's behaviour continues to worry you, and you can't seem to find a way to deal with it, seek advice from your doctor or health visitor.

Childhood habits

Many small children develop habits such as thumb-sucking, head-banging, breath-holding, hair-twirling and pulling, nose-picking, and nail-biting, which they resort to usually when they are angry, frustrated, bored, or simply in need of comfort. These habits are common and harmless, but they often worry parents. Although children usually grow out of them by the time they are four, sometimes they can be hard to break.

Thumb-sucking and dummies

About half of three year olds suck their thumbs, and a few still do so when they are six or seven. Persistent thumb-suckers may gradually push their front teeth forwards. Continually sucking a cuddly or blanket may have the same effect. However, unless the habit continues after the age of six, when the second set of teeth come in, the distortion won't be permanent. Sucking a dummy is less likely to distort the teeth, so if your baby shows signs of being a habitual thumb-sucker, it might be worth offering her a dummy. You may be able to encourage a persistent thumb- or dummy-sucker to give up the habit by offering a small reward.

Head-banging, rolling, and rocking

Some time in their first year, many children develop a habit of rocking rhythmically on all fours in their cot, rolling their heads from side to side, or banging their heads on the head-board.

Usually they'll do this as they are going off to sleep or as they wake up, and often the rocking is violent enough to move the cot across the floor. Although this is alarming to watch, and to listen to, you really do not need to worry about it. Infants and young toddlers who do this seldom hurt themselves, although they may damage the furniture. These rhythmic behaviours nearly always disappear by the time the child is three or four.

Some toddlers develop an equally worrying habit of banging their head on a hard surface during the day, usually to express frustration or boredom. Again, the child won't hurt herself, apart from the odd bruise. It's usually best to take no notice, although you may want to offer the child a pillow to soften the impact. If you ignore the habit, it will eventually disappear.

Head-banging or rocking that starts in older children, or persists after the age of four, needs to be taken more seriously. Discuss with your doctor; it may mean that your child has some emotional problem.

Breath-holding attacks

A few young children deal with pain or frustration by holding their breath. They may do this for up to half a minute, and sometimes they will even pass out. Immediately when this happens, the child automatically starts to breathe again, and no harm is done; but the child quickly discovers this is

a splendid way to gain attention. Ignore the attacks as much as possible, and they will probably have stopped by the time your child is four.

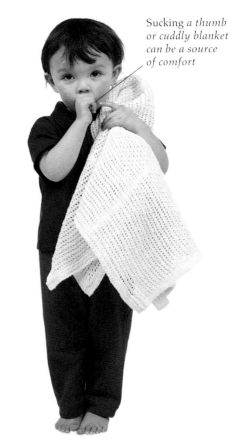

Sucking a thumb or cuddly blanket can be a source of comfort

Thumb-sucking
Many toddlers suck their thumbs. Try to discourage the habit once the second set of teeth have come through.

"Bad dreams" and night terrors

Even a child as young as one year old may have nightmares about something that has frightened her during the day, even though she doesn't yet understand what a dream is, and certainly couldn't tell you about it. If a very young child wakes from a nightmare, simply cuddle and comfort her until she calms down.

By the time she is two years old she may try to tell you about it, and you can reassure her that it was "only a dream", although she won't yet really understand this concept. By three or four, she will have a much better idea of what is "real" and "not real". But she will still need you to soothe her fears and make it clear that you won't let anything bad happen to her. It may reassure her to have a night-light in her room, and for the door to be left ajar.

A few children, however, have night terrors, which are quite different from nightmares. Nightmares usually occur in the second half of the night when the child is sleeping lightly, and dreams are at their most plentiful. A night terror will start much earlier, usually between one and four hours after the child has gone to sleep, when she is sleeping very deeply. You will hear your child screaming or moaning as if in terror, but when you rush in to her, she won't seem to recognize you, may push you away, and scream even more if you try to hold her. This is because she is not properly awake, and if left alone will quite quickly go back to sleep. So don't try to wake her or even hold her. Simply wait beside her so that you're there if she does wake. In the morning, she will have no memory of what happened, and be none the worse for it.

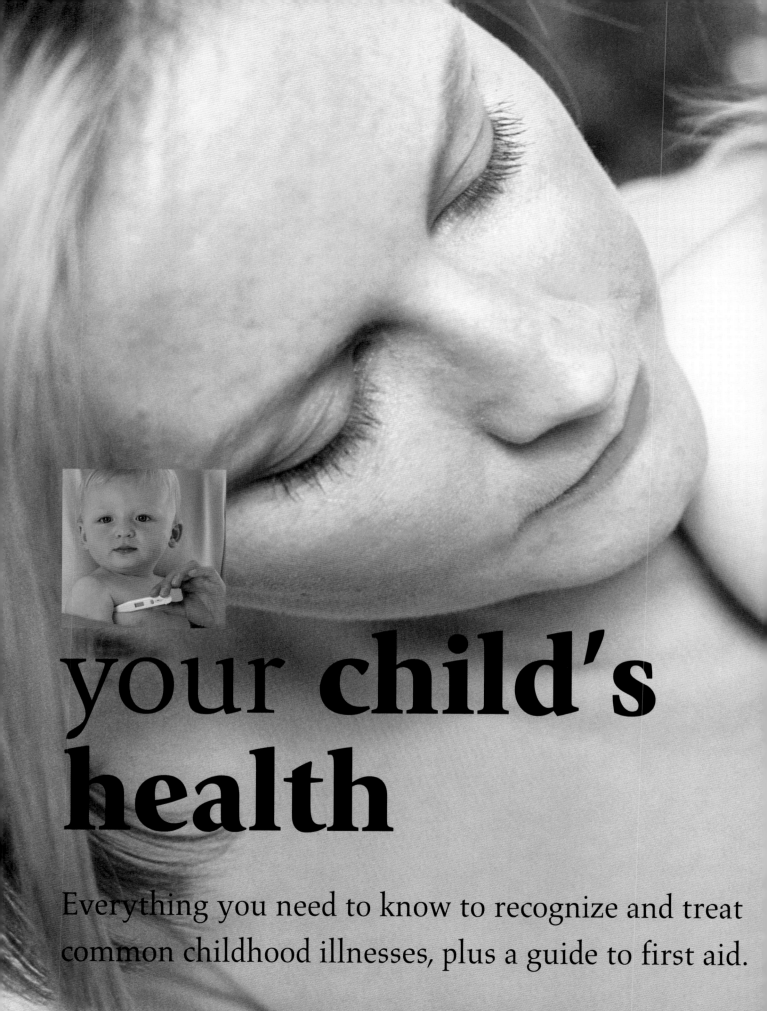

your child's health

Everything you need to know to recognize and treat
common childhood illnesses, plus a guide to first aid.

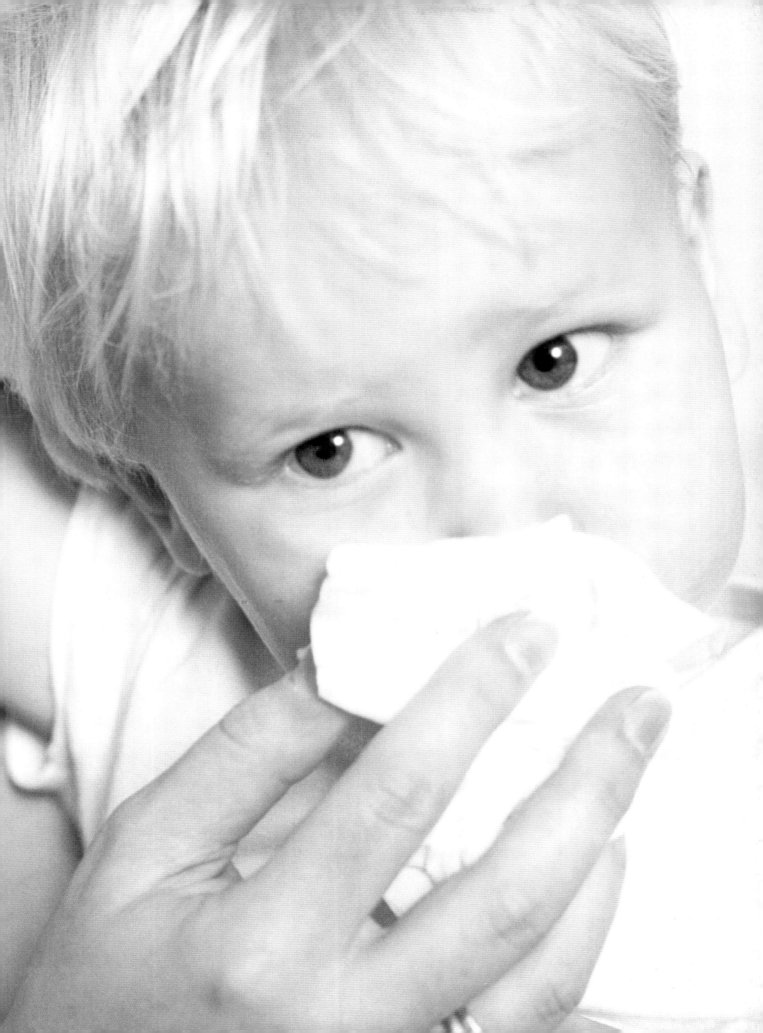

The first three months

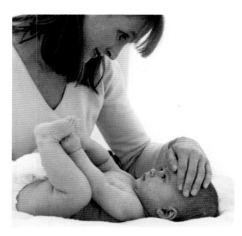

Babies are born with natural immunity which protects them against many infections for about six months. But for the first three months, it's best to seek medical help straightaway if you think your baby is ill. The symptoms listed here relate to the most common health problems that affect babies under three months, and will guide you to the relevant section (see pages 182–5). Pages 186–7 cover illnesses for children of all ages. Remember, however, that only a doctor can give you a definite diagnosis.

Emergency

Call for an ambulance or go to the nearest accident and emergency department if your baby:
- brings up green vomit
- has a body temperature higher than 39°C (102.2°F) for more than half an hour
- vomits AND cries uncontrollably as if in great pain
- is breathing very noisily or rapidly
- has a taut, bulging fontanelle when he isn't crying

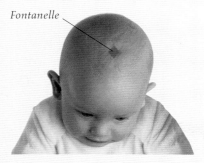

Fontanelle

- has purple spots on his skin that don't fade if glass is pressed against it
- passes stools containing blood and mucus, which resemble redcurrant jelly.

Loss of appetite

If your baby does not want to feed, but seems generally contented and well, there is no need to worry. If he refuses two feeds in succession, or does not demand a feed for six hours, **call your doctor now.**

☎ Seek medical help

Call your doctor now if your baby seems unwell or shows one of these symptoms:
- cries more than usual, or his crying sounds different from usual over a period of about an hour
- seems abnormally listless, quiet, or drowsy
- refuses two successive feeds, or does not demand a feed for more than six hours
- seems particularly irritable or restless.

Crying

If you fail to calm your baby after an hour or so, or if his crying sounds unusual, **call your doctor.** If your baby cries inconsolably for two or three hours at about the same time each day, but shows no other signs of illness, he might have colic (see page 118). This may continue for several weeks, but will resolve itself without any treatment.

Slow weight gain

If your baby does not seem to be gaining weight at the normal rate (see charts on pages 254–7), consult your doctor or health visitor. Occasionally an underlying illness can make a baby grow more slowly than normal.

Premature babies

Babies who were very small at birth, or who were born a month or more before their due date, are more vulnerable to infections during their first weeks. Until your baby is older and has put on weight, try to keep him away from anyone who has a cough or cold, and, if possible, don't take him into public places for the first two or three months.

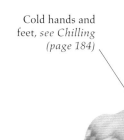

Cold hands and feet, *see Chilling (page 184)*

Areas of dry, flaking skin *mean that your baby's skin needs moisturizing, so avoid soap and rub unperfumed aqueous cream into the dry areas*

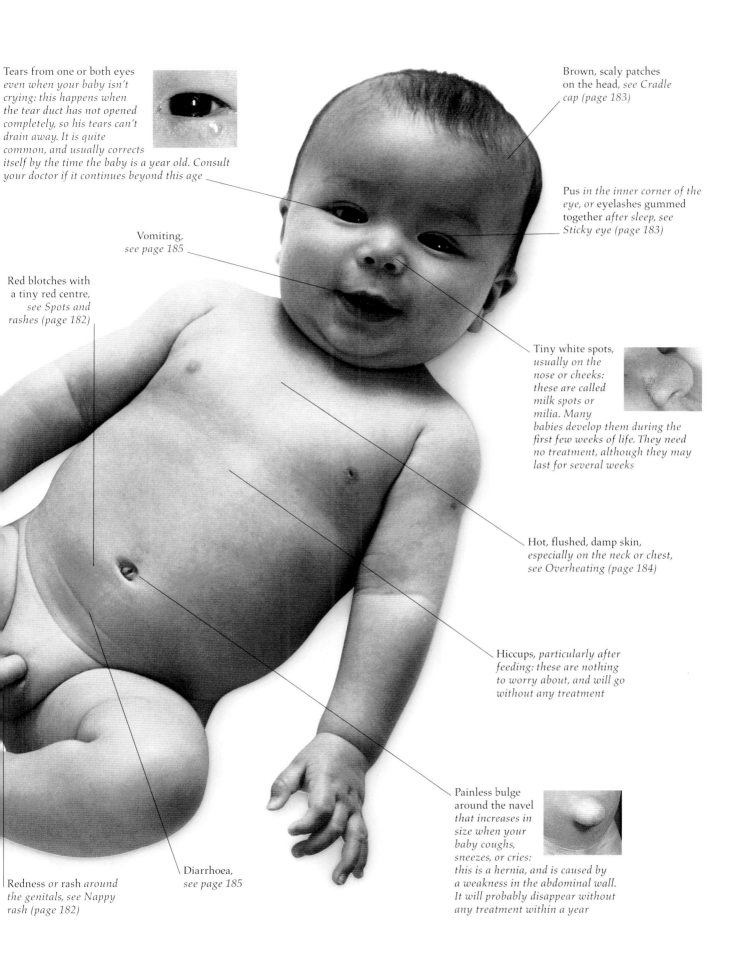

Tears from one or both eyes *even when your baby isn't crying: this happens when the tear duct has not opened completely, so his tears can't drain away. It is quite common, and usually corrects itself by the time the baby is a year old. Consult your doctor if it continues beyond this age*

Vomiting, *see page 185*

Red blotches with a tiny red centre, *see Spots and rashes (page 182)*

Brown, scaly patches on the head, *see Cradle cap (page 183)*

Pus *in the inner corner of the eye, or eyelashes gummed together after sleep, see Sticky eye (page 183)*

Tiny white spots, *usually on the nose or cheeks: these are called milk spots or milia. Many babies develop them during the first few weeks of life. They need no treatment, although they may last for several weeks*

Hot, flushed, damp skin, *especially on the neck or chest, see Overheating (page 184)*

Hiccups, *particularly after feeding: these are nothing to worry about, and will go without any treatment*

Painless bulge around the navel *that increases in size when your baby coughs, sneezes, or cries: this is a hernia, and is caused by a weakness in the abdominal wall. It will probably disappear without any treatment within a year*

Redness or rash *around the genitals, see Nappy rash (page 182)*

Diarrhoea, *see page 185*

Spots and rashes

What are they?

Many newborn babies go through a spotty stage in the first few weeks, so don't worry unnecessarily if your baby develops a few spots – they don't usually mean that she is ill in any way. One of the most common rashes in young babies is called newborn urticaria (erythema toxicum). Newborn urticaria usually appears during the first week of your baby's life, and will generally disappear without any treatment.

What can I do?

If your baby has newborn urticaria (see symptoms box), simply ignore the spots. Unlike urticaria in older children, which may require treatment, newborn urticaria will disappear on its own within about two or three days, so it is not necessary to put any lotions or creams on the spots. Don't be tempted to alter your baby's feeds in any way – the spots are not due to milk disagreeing with her.

Symptoms

- Red blotches with a tiny red centre, which come and go on different parts of the baby's body, and last only a few hours.

☎ Seek medical help

Call your doctor now if the spots are flat, pink, dark red, or purplish (a petechial rash). Consult your doctor as soon as possible if:
- a spot has developed a pus-filled centre
- you think a spot has become infected.

Nappy rash

What is it?

Nappy rash is an inflammation of the skin on a baby's bottom. It may occur if your baby has been left in a dirty nappy for too long, because as urine and faeces are broken down ammonia is released, which burns and irritates her skin. It can also be due to an allergy to soap powder used when washing fabric nappies. A similar-looking rash may be caused by thrush, which can affect the mouth (see page 213), as well as the nappy area. Thrush usually starts in the creases at the top of the legs.

Symptoms

- Red, spotty, sore-looking skin in the nappy area
- smell of ammonia.

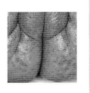

What can I do?

1 Change your baby's nappy frequently, and clean and dry her bottom thoroughly at each change (see pages 150–1). Inside fabric nappies, use an extra-absorbent type of liner.

2 Whenever possible, let your baby lie on a nappy with her bottom exposed to the air. Don't use plastic pants or wraps over fabric nappies until the rash subsides, because these prevent air circulating to her bottom.

3 Look for white patches inside your baby's mouth. If you see any, she may have thrush (see page 213).

4 Don't use biological powder or fabric conditioner to wash her nappies, as they can trigger an allergy. Rinse her nappies thoroughly.

5 Use a nappy rash cream (available at most chemists), and apply it when you change your baby's nappy, to soothe and heal the skin.

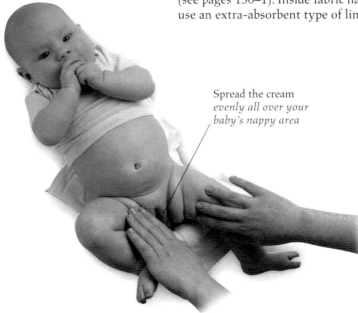

Spread the cream evenly all over your baby's nappy area

☎ Seek medical help

Consult your doctor or health visitor as soon as possible if:
- the rash lasts longer than two days
- you think your baby has thrush.

What might the doctor do?

The doctor may prescribe an antibiotic cream if the rash is infected, or an anti-fungal cream if your baby has thrush.

Cradle cap

What is it?
Thick, brownish, crusty patches on a baby's scalp are known as cradle cap. Sometimes it may spread to the baby's face, body, or nappy area, producing a red scaly rash. Although it looks unsightly, cradle cap is harmless and doesn't seem to distress the baby. It generally clears up by the age of about two years.

Symptoms
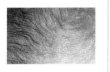
- Brownish, scaly patches on the scalp.

☎ Seek medical help
Consult your doctor as soon as possible if the rash spreads and:
- seems to irritate your baby
- looks infected or begins to ooze
- does not clear up after five days.

What can I do?
1 Rub the cradle cap scales on your baby's head with baby or olive oil to soften them. Leave the oil on for 12 to 24 hours, then brush your baby's hair gently to loosen the scales. Finally, wash her hair – most of the scales should simply wash away.

2 If the rash spreads, keep the affected areas clean and dry. Don't use soap, baby lotion, or baby bath liquid – ask your chemist for an emulsifying ointment instead.

What might the doctor do?
If the condition persists, or if the rash looks infected or starts to ooze, your doctor may prescribe an ointment to be rubbed gently on the area.

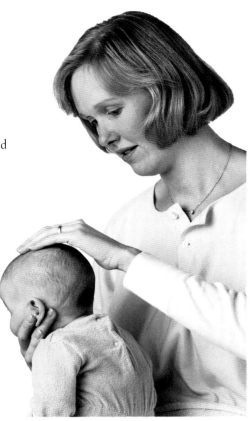

Sticky eye

What is it?
This is a very common mild eye infection caused by blood or fluid getting into your baby's eye during birth. If your baby develops any of these symptoms after she is two days old, she may have conjunctivitis (see page 209).

Symptoms
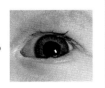
- Eyelashes gummed after sleep
- pus in the corner of the eye.

☎ Seek medical help
Call your doctor now if your baby has a bad discharge of yellow pus. **Consult your doctor as soon as possible** if:
- your baby develops symptoms of sticky eye after first two days of life
- It does not clear up after three days.

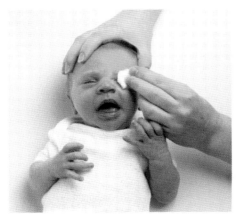

What can I do?
Clean your baby's eyes twice a day with cotton wool dipped in warm boiled water. Wipe outwards from the inner corner of her eye, and use a fresh piece of cotton wool for each eye.

What might the doctor do?
If the doctor thinks your baby has conjunctivitis, he may, in some cases, prescribe antibiotic eye drops.

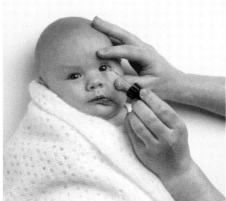

To administer eye drops
Swaddle your baby in a blanket with her arms inside and hold her on your lap in the crook of your arm, or ask someone to hold her for you. Apply the drops to the inner corner of her eye.

Chilling

Why are babies at risk?
For the first few weeks of his life, your baby will be unable to regulate his body temperature very efficiently. If he becomes too cold, his body temperature will drop and he may become dangerously chilled quite quickly. Babies who were born prematurely are particularly vulnerable to serious chilling.

Symptoms
First signs
- Crying and restless behaviour
- cold hands and feet.

Signs of serious chilling
- Quiet and listless behaviour as the baby gets colder
- cool skin on chest and stomach
- pink and flushed face, hands, and feet.

☎ Seek medical help
Call your doctor now if your baby:
- shows signs of serious chilling
- has a body temperature below 35°C (95°F).

What can I do?

1 Warm your baby up by taking him into a heated room and feeding him. Once he has become chilled, it doesn't help just to pile on extra clothes or blankets.

2 Take your baby's temperature (see page 193). If it is below 35°C (95°F), he is dangerously chilled, so **call for an ambulance immediately**.

How can I prevent chilling?
Keep the room your baby sleeps in at about 16–20°C (65–68°F). When you undress and bathe him, the room should be warmer still. Be sensible about taking your child out in cold weather – wrap him up well, and don't stay out for too long. Make sure his head, hands, and feet are well covered; particularly his head, as a lot of body heat is lost through the head. Never leave him to sleep outside in his pram on a cold day. Dress your baby according to the temperature of the environment, and adjust his clothes as the temperature changes.

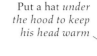

Put a hat *under the hood to keep his head warm*

In cold weather
Dress your baby in an all-in-one outdoor suit, or wrap a shawl over his other clothes, and use mittens and booties. Keep an eye on him to make sure he's not getting too hot.

Overheating

Why are babies at risk?
Overheating is as dangerous for young babies as chilling, especially if they are feverish or unwell. Overwrapping of babies at night is thought to be one of the factors that contributes to cot death (see page 123).

What can I do?

1 Take your baby to a cooler place and remove a layer of clothing.

2 Take your baby's temperature (see page 193) and, if it is raised, offer him plenty of fluids to prevent dehydration.

Symptoms
- Restless behaviour
- hot, sweaty skin
- raised temperature.

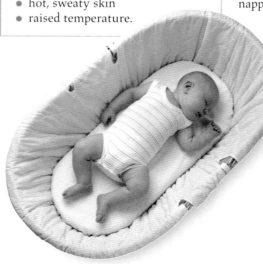

How can I prevent overheating?
Dress your baby according to the weather. On very hot days, he can sleep in just a nappy and a vest, but always remember the danger of chilling (see above). Never leave him to sleep in the sun, his skin will burn easily. Provide shade of some sort, and check him frequently as the sun moves round.

☎ Seek medical help
Call your doctor if your baby's temperature does not return to normal within one hour.

Vomiting

Why do babies vomit?

All babies regurgitate a small amount of milk during or just after a feed, usually due to wind. This "possetting" is perfectly normal, and does not mean that your baby is ill, but until you are used to it, you may think that he is vomiting. If your baby vomits, he will bring up most of his feed. This is less likely to happen in a breastfed baby.

Frequent vomiting, especially if your baby also has diarrhoea, may be caused by gastroenteritis (see page 222). This is extremely serious in a young baby because the loss of fluids can make him dehydrated very quickly.

Forceful vomiting

Sometimes a baby vomits with great force, so that the vomit shoots across the room. If your baby does this at two successive feeds, **consult your doctor as soon as possible.** The most likely reason is that he has brought back part of his feed with a large burp of wind. However, if it happens after every feed, especially if he is hungry all the time, he may have a condition called pyloric stenosis, in which the outlet from the stomach becomes blocked – if your baby has this, he will need a minor surgery to treat the problem.

What can I do?

Continue to feed your baby as usual, but to replace fluids lost through vomiting give your baby small, frequent drinks of cooled, boiled water. You may find that he does not want to take the water at first, if he is used to the taste of breast milk or formula, but be persistent. You can also ask your chemist for an oral rehydration powder that is suitable for babies. It must be mixed according to the manufacturer's instructions. Don't make it up any stronger or weaker. Don't attempt to make your own rehydration solution from salt and sugar at home.

If your baby is vomiting, and is not keeping fluids down, see your doctor urgently. Although vomiting and diarrhoea are not often dangerous in adults and older children, they can cause a young baby to become dehydrated very quickly and so require prompt attention. Don't give your baby any anti-nausea medications, or change your baby's formula unless your doctor has advised it. Breastfed babies should continue to be breastfed.

☎ Seek medical help

Call your doctor now if:
- your baby vomits and shows any other signs of illness
- your baby vomits the whole of two successive feedings.

Emergency

Call for emergency help immediately if your baby:
- vomits all his feeds in an eight-hour period
- has a dry mouth and lips
- has a dry nappy for more than six hours
- brings up green vomit
- has sunken eyes or a sunken fontanelle
- is abnormally drowsy.

What might the doctor do?

The doctor may prescribe a powder to be mixed with water for your baby to drink. If your baby has lost a lot of body fluid, the doctor might send him to hospital, where he may be given liquid through a drip.

How can I prevent an upset stomach?

If you are bottle-feeding your baby, sterilize all the feeding equipment, and throw away any unfinished feeds. When making up feeds, cool them quickly under cold running water and store in the fridge. Never keep a feed warm for a long period.

Diarrhoea

What is it?

Until babies start eating solid food, they will usually pass fairly runny stools a few times a day. If your baby passes watery, and possibly greenish, stools frequently, he has diarrhoea. This is a serious condition in a young baby, since there is an increased danger that he may become dehydrated quite quickly.

What can I do?

It is important to prevent your baby from becoming dehydrated, so make sure that he has plenty to drink. Offer your baby cooled, boiled water between his normal feeds.

If you are concerned that your baby is becoming dehydrated despite your efforts to get him to drink, contact your doctor straightaway.

☎ Seek medical help

Call your doctor now if your baby has fever or is passing blood in the stool, or has had diarrhoea for six hours **and** other symptoms, or if diarrhoea lasts more than 24 hours, or if he may be dehydrated (see emergency box, above).

Diagnosis guide

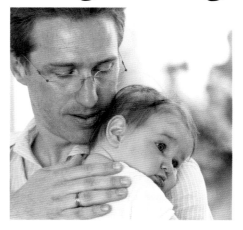

If your child is unwell, try to identify her symptoms by referring to the guide below. If she has more than one symptom, look up the most severe one. This gives you a possible diagnosis and refers you to a section covering the complaint, which contain a brief explanation of the nature of the illness, with information about how you can help your child, and advice on whether you need to call a doctor. Bear in mind that only a doctor can give an accurate diagnosis.

General symptoms of illnesses

All children suffer from minor illnesses at some stage. The following are the most common symptoms babies and young children develop when they are ill.

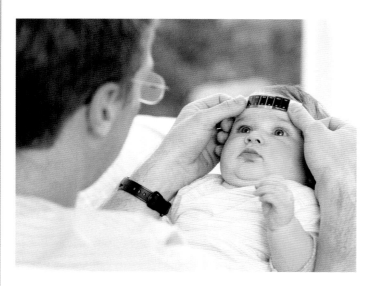

Fever
A raised temperature (fever) may mean that your child has an infection, so you should check for other signs of illness. However, healthy children may get a slight fever during energetic play or in very hot weather, so check your child's temperature again after she has rested for about half an hour. If it is still over 38°C (100.4°F), she may have an infection.

Changed behaviour
If your child is less lively than usual, more irritable, whiney, or simply unhappy, she may be ill.

Unusual paleness
If your child looks much paler than usual, she may be ill.

Hot, flushed face
This may be a sign of a fever.

Loss of appetite
Although a child's appetite varies from meal to meal, a sudden loss of appetite may be a sign of illness. If your baby is under six months old and has refused two successive feeds, **call your doctor now.** If your child goes off her food for more than 24 hours, look for other signs of illness (see chart).

Part of body	Symptoms	Page reference
Eyes and ears	• Eyes looking in different directions	See "Squint" p.210
	• Red, sore, or sticky eyes or eyelids	See "Eye problems" pp.209–10
	• Itchy eyes, especially if accompanied by runny nose or sneezing	See "Colds and flu" pp.200–1
	• Aversion to bright light, especially if accompanied by fever, headache, and stiff neck	See "Meningitis" p.208
	• Earache, partial deafness, discharge from ears, itchy ears	See "Ear problems" pp.211–12

Part of body	Symptoms	Page reference
Skin, hair, and teeth	• Sore mouth • Itchy head or tiny white grains in the hair • Red lump, perhaps with pus-filled centre • Red raw skin • Spots or rash • Spots or rash accompanied by sore throat or fever • White or brown lump on sole of foot/dry, painless lump anywhere on the body • Red, tender skin • Areas of very itchy, dry, red, scaly skin • Sore around the mouth	See "Thrush" p.213 See "Lice and nits" p.232 See "Spots and boils" p.226 See "Chapped skin" p.229 See "Skin problems" pp.226–32 or "Insect stings" p.252 See "Infectious illnesses" pp.203–8 See "Warts and verrucas" p.230 See "Sunburn" p.229 or "Burns and scalds" p.245 See "Eczema" p.228 See "Cold sores" p.230 or "Impetigo" p.231
Brain and nerves	• Momentary lapses of attention • Loss of consciousness, combined with stiffness and twitching movements	See "Epilepsy" p.233 See "Epilepsy" p.233
Bones, muscles, and joints	• Puffy face, swollen glands at the angle of the jaw-bone and on the side of the neck • Stiff neck accompanied by fever and headache	See "Mumps" p.206 See "Meningitis" p.208
Lungs and airways	• Runny or blocked nose, sneezing • Swollen glands accompanied by sore throat • Sore throat • Sore throat accompanied by fever and general illness • Sore throat accompanied by a rash • Sore throat accompanied by puffy face • Breathing difficulty, wheezing, rapid breathing • Whooping cough	See "Colds and flu" pp.200–1 See "Tonsillitis" p.214 or "German measles" p.203 See "Throat infections" p.214 See "Colds and flu" pp.200–1 See "German measles" p.203 See "Mumps" p.206 See "Coughs and chest infections" pp.215–9 See "Whooping cough" p.207
Digestive organs	• Stomach pain • Stomach pain accompanied by nausea, vomiting, or diarrhoea • Abnormal-looking faeces • Diarrhoea • Constipation • Intense itching around the anus • Vomiting or nausea • Vomiting with great force	See "Dealing with a tummy ache" p.220 See "Gastroenteritis" p.222 See "Diarrhoea" p.223 See "Diarrhoea" p.223 See "Constipation" p.221 See "Threadworms" p.232 See "Vomiting" p.222 See "Forceful vomiting" p.185
Urinary organs	• Pain when urinating, odd-coloured urine, frequent urination • Sore tip of penis/painless bulge in the groin or scrotum • Intense itching around the vagina • Soreness, itching, or redness around the vagina, vaginal discharge	See "Urinary system infections" p.224 See "Genital problems in boys" p.225 See "Threadworms" p.232 See "Genital problems in girls" p.225

First signs of illness

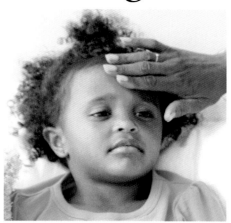

Even if your child has no definite symptoms, you will probably know when he is not feeling at his best. He may look pale, be more clingy than usual, cry or whine, or seem very irritable. He may be off his food. When your baby is teething, don't assume that the symptoms are due to this. All symptoms should be taken seriously in a baby under a year old – babies can become ill very quickly. If your child is over a year old, keep a check on how his symptoms progress over the next few hours.

Calling the doctor

If you think you know what is wrong with your child, read the relevant section among complaints covered on pages 200–33. This advises you whether you need to call the doctor. As a general rule, the younger the child, the more quickly he should be seen by a doctor. If you are unsure what to do, phone your doctor and describe your child's symptoms to him, and tell him his age. The doctor will tell you what to do, and will know whether your child needs medical attention.

Alternatively, you can call NHS Direct, which is a health advice service run by nurses, who are available 24 hours a day to provide help and information.

Degree of urgency

Whenever you are instructed to call the doctor, you will be told how quickly your child needs medical help.
- **Call for emergency help immediately:** this is a life-threatening emergency. So call for an ambulance, or go to the nearest hospital emergency department.
- **Call your doctor now:** your child needs medical help now, so contact your doctor straightaway, even if it is the middle of the night. If he can't come immediately, call for emergency help.
- **Consult your doctor as soon as possible:** your child needs to be seen by a doctor within the next 24 hours.
- **Consult your doctor:** your child should be seen by a doctor within the next few days.

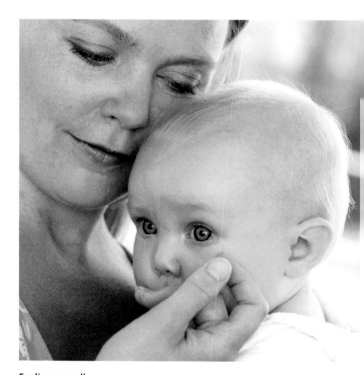

Feeling unwell
Your child may become more clingy, and demand extra attention when he is ill.

Symptoms

The most common early symptoms of illness in children are:
- raised temperature – 38°C (100.4°F) or more
- crying and irritability
- vomiting or diarrhoea
- refusal to eat or drink
- sore or red throat
- rash
- swollen glands in the neck or behind the jaw.

Emergency

Call for emergency help immediately if your child:
- is breathing very noisily, rapidly, or with difficulty
- has a convulsion
- loses consciousness after a fall
- is in severe, persistent pain
- has a fever and is unusually irritable or drowsy
- has a rash of flat, dark red or purplish blood-spots (petechial rash)
- screams with pain and turns pale when he screams.

Checking for symptoms
What can I do?

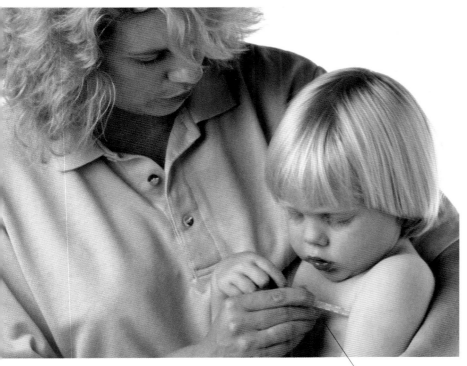

1 If you think your child is feeling unwell, or if he looks as though he has a fever, take his temperature with an aural, digital, or strip thermometer (see page 193). A temperature of 38°C (100.4°F) or above can be a symptom of illness.

Tuck the end *of the digital thermometer into your child's armpit*

Q&A

"Is my child in pain?"

If your baby is in pain, his crying may sound quite different from normal. When a baby or a small child cries or complains of pain, it can be difficult to discover where the pain is, and even more difficult to ascertain how bad it might be.

Serious pain will affect your child's behaviour, so watch him to find out how severe his pain is. Does it make him cry or stop him sleeping, eating, or playing? Does his face look drawn or his colour changed? Would you know that he had a pain even if he didn't tell you? If not, his pain probably isn't too severe.

If your child is in pain, give him the recommended dose of paracetamol syrup or ibuprofen suspension (not aspirin). Consult your doctor if the pain continues.

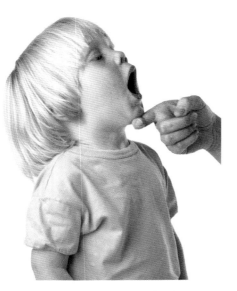

2 Check whether your child's throat is inflamed or infected, but don't try to examine the throat of a baby under a year old. Ask your child to face a strong light and open his mouth. If his throat looks red or has creamy spots, he has a sore throat (see Throat infections, page 214).

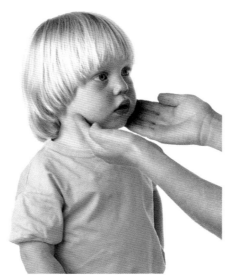

3 Feel gently along your child's jaw-bone and down either side of the back of his neck. If you can feel tiny lumps under the skin, or if any of these areas seem swollen or tender, your child has swollen glands, which is a common sign of illness.

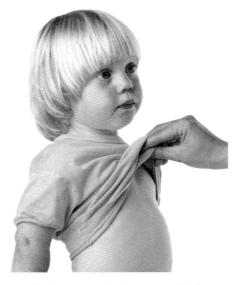

4 Check to see whether your child has a rash, particularly on his chest and behind his ears – the most common areas for a rash to start. If he has a rash and a fever, he may have one of the common childhood infectious illnesses (see pages 203–8).

The doctor's examination

The doctor will ask you about any symptoms you have noticed in your child and how long he has had them, and will then examine your child. If your child is old enough to understand, explain what will happen when he visits the doctor. If the doctor suspects any particular illness, he may do other investigations as well as, or instead of, those shown below.

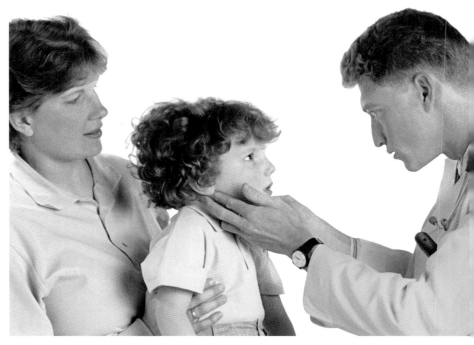

1 The doctor will feel the glands that lie along your child's jaw-bone, down the back of his neck, and in his armpits and groin. These may become swollen during an infectious illness.

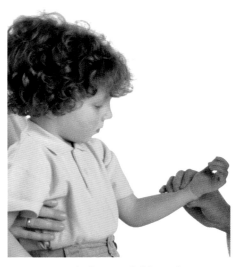

2 He may feel your child's pulse to check if his heart is beating faster than usual. This is often a sign of a raised temperature. The doctor may also take your child's temperature.

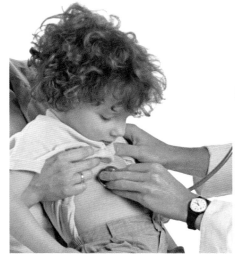

3 By listening to your child's chest and back through a stethoscope, and asking your child to breathe deeply, the doctor will check the health of his heart and lungs.

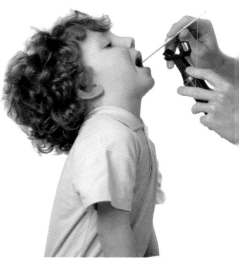

4 If your child has a sore or inflamed throat, the doctor will examine his throat using a small torch, pressing his tongue down with a spatula.

5 The doctor may ask your child to lie on the examining couch so that he can gently feel his abdomen. He will check for swelling or tenderness in any of the internal organs.

Questions to ask the doctor
Don't hesitate to ask the doctor about anything that is worrying you. In particular, find out:
• how long your child may be ill, and what symptoms to expect
• whether he is infectious, and whether you should isolate him, particularly from small babies and pregnant women
• how you can make your child more comfortable while he is ill.

Going to hospital

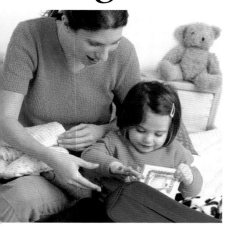

It can be terrifying for a child to go to hospital, especially if she is separated from her parents. If your child is under two, all she really needs at this age is your presence. If your child is over two, playing with a favourite toy may help: explain that teddy goes to the hospital to be made better by helpful people and soon teddy comes home again. Keep your explanations simple but truthful; your child will feel let down and mistrustful if you promise something won't hurt, and then it does.

Visiting your child

Hospital staff know how important it is for a parent to be with a child to comfort and reassure her, and should make it easy for you to visit her at any time. Many provide accommodation so that you can stay with your child – find out about this before her admission. She won't find the hospital so frightening if you continue to care for her as you would at home, so ask the nurses whether you can still bathe and feed her.

If you can't stay in hospital with your child, visit her as often as you can, and bring brothers and sisters to see her. Even if she cries when you leave, don't feel that she might settle better without your visits. It would only make her feel even more anxious, unhappy, and abandoned. Make a special effort to be with her for the first day or two, and when she has any unpleasant procedures such as injections, or is having stitches removed.

What to pack

Your child will need the items pictured here while she is in the hospital. Pack nappy changing equipment as well, if necessary. Label everything, particularly her toys, so that they don't get misplaced. Pack soap, a face flannel, a sponge, her toothbrush and toothpaste, her brush, comb, and a towel. Pack your own bag if you are staying overnight in the hospital with your child.

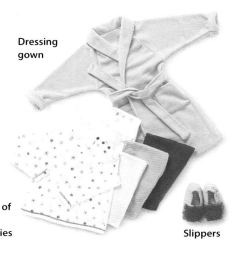

Dressing gown

Slippers

Three pairs of pyjamas or three nighties

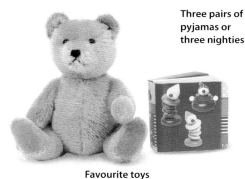

Favourite toys

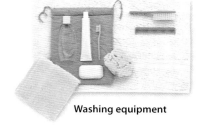

Washing equipment

Having an operation

If your child is old enough to understand, it will help to explain what will happen on the day of her operation. Ask the doctor how the anaesthetic will be given (it may be injected or inhaled through a mask). If inhaled through a mask, you will be allowed to stay with your child while she is given the anaesthetic, and also be allowed in the recovery room after she wakes up. Try to be with her after the operation since she may be frightened.

1 Warn your child that she will not be allowed to eat or drink anything on the day of her operation.

2 Tell your child that she will be dressed up for the operation in a hospital gown, and will wear a bracelet with her name on it.

3 While she is still in the ward, your child may be given a "pre-medication" (pre-med) to make her sleepy.

4 Tell your child that she will walk or be wheeled in her bed to the anaesthetic room, where she will be given an anaesthetic. She will fall asleep.

5 Warn your child that she may vomit when she wakes up.

6 If your child has stitches, discourage her from scratching them. It will hurt only momentarily when they are removed.

The child with a temperature

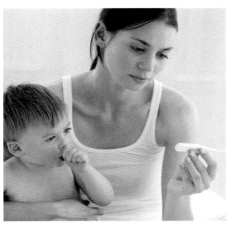

In children, body temperature above 37.5°C (99.5°F) may be a sign of illness. However, a slightly raised temperature is not a reliable guide to her health. Fluctuations in temperature are common and not a cause for concern, but if your child's high temperature persists she may be ill, so check for other signs of illness. Babies and children can be ill with a normal or below normal temperature between 36°C (96.8°F) and 37°C (98.6°F), and some children can have a slight fever without being ill.

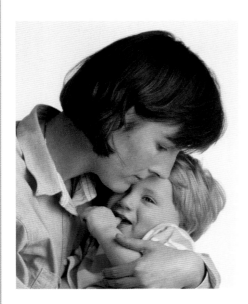

Signs of fever
Your child may have a fever if she:
- complains of feeling unwell
- looks pale, and feels cold and shivery
- looks flushed and her forehead feels hot.

Feel your child's forehead with your cheek if you think he has a fever – don't use your hand because, if it is cold, your child's skin will feel warm by comparison. If his forehead feels hot, take his temperature.

☎ Seek medical help
Call the doctor now if your child:
- has a raised temperature, as well as other signs of illness
- is under three months old, and has a temperature of 38°C (100.4°F)
- is between three and six months old, and has a temperature of 39°C (102°F)
- has a temperature of over 39.4°C (103°F), or over 39°C (102°F) if she is under a year old, and you can't bring it down
- has a fever for 24 hours.

Choosing a thermometer

The best thermometers for babies and young children are the digital thermometer, the ear thermometer, and the temperature indicator strip.

Safe and easy to use, the digital and ear thermometers give an accurate reading. Although they are more expensive than other thermometers, they are ideal for young children as they read the temperature quickly. Always keep spare batteries.

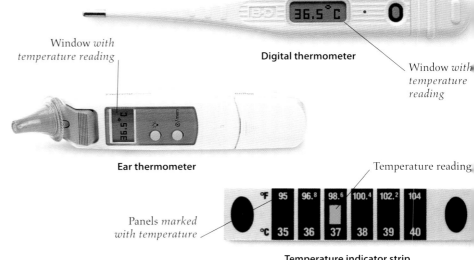

Window *with temperature reading*

Digital thermometer

Window *with temperature reading*

Ear thermometer

Temperature reading

Panels *marked with temperature*

Temperature indicator strip

Taking your child's temperature

When your child is unwell, take her temperature reading every two to three hours. Never use the old-style mercury thermometers, especially in a child's mouth, since they can break easily. These are no longer available to buy. A digital thermometer is safe to put into a young child's mouth, but if she can't hold it correctly under her tongue, place it in her armpit. Placed under her arm, the thermometer gives a reading 0.6°C (1°F) lower than her true temperature. The ear thermometer is also suitable for young children as long as they are able to sit still. The temperature indicator strip is the easiest way of taking a young child's temperature, but the reading is less accurate than that of a digital thermometer. A reading of over 37.5°C (99.5°F) is considered as a high temperature.

Using a digital thermometer

Underarm

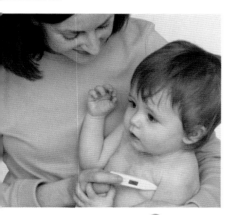

1 Sit your child on your knee and lift her arm. Switch the thermometer on and tuck the end of it into her armpit.

2 Bring your child's arm down, and fold it over her chest. Hold the thermometer firmly in place for the recommended time – usually between 10 seconds and two minutes. Then remove the thermometer from under your child's arm.

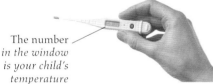

The number *in the window is your child's temperature*

3 Read your child's temperature in the window of the thermometer. Switch the thermometer off, then wash it in cool water and dry it.

By mouth

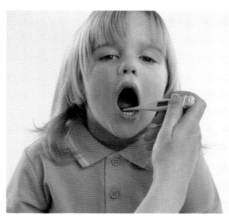

Switch the thermometer on, and ask your child to open her mouth. Place the thermometer under her tongue, and ask her to close her mouth. Wait for about three minutes.

Using an indicator strip

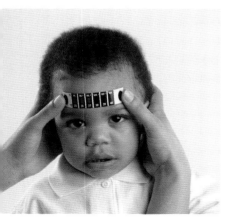

Hold the indicator strip on your child's forehead for about 15 seconds. The highest panel that glows indicates your child's temperature.

Using an ear thermometer

Make sure a clean lens filter is in place. Pull the ear back gently, and insert the thermometer until the ear canal is sealed off. Press the button on top of the thermometer for one second, then remove the thermometer and read your child's temperature.

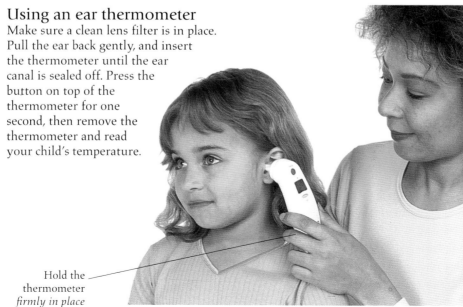

Hold the thermometer *firmly in place*

Bringing down a fever

Keeping him comfortable

If your child has a fever, make sure that he has plenty of fluids but don't cold sponge him – this won't help reduce his fever.

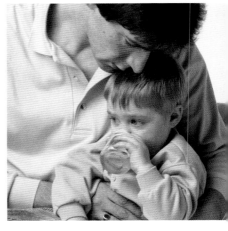

1 If your child's temperature rises to 38°C (100.4°F) or above, give him the recommended dose of paracetamol or ibuprofen suspension. Check his nappy – if it remains dry for longer than usual, it may be a sign of dehydration. Don't give paracetamol or ibuprofen suspension to a baby under three months old, unless your doctor advises it.

2 Your child may sweat profusely as his temperature falls, so give him plenty to drink to replace the lost fluid. If your child has a low-grade fever that isn't affecting his behaviour, don't give him any medication to lower his fever.

Keeping her cool

Do not overdress your child. In fact, if your child has a fever try to keep her cool, but not so much that she shivers. Never try to "sweat" the fever out of her. When body temperature is rising, it's imperative to use light bedclothes and keep her in light clothing, so as not to increase the fever.

1 Keep your child cool by removing her top layer of clothing.

2 Change her bedding and pyjamas when her temperature is normal again, to make her comfortable.

3 Monitor your child's temperature at regular intervals. If it continues to rise and gets above 39.4°C (103°F), **call your doctor now.**

Monitor your child
Stay close to your child and make sure that she doesn't get too cold.

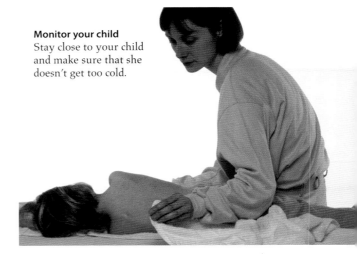

Febrile convulsions

A rapid rise in temperature can cause a convulsion in children, in which they lose consciousness and go rigid for a few seconds, then twitch uncontrollably.

What can I do?

Place your child carefully on the floor with her hand in line with her body or slightly lower (the recovery position, see page 241) and stay with her, but do not try to restrain her in any way. Call your doctor.

How can I prevent febrile convulsions?

If a tendency to have febrile convulsions runs in your family, keep your child's temperature as low as you can when she is ill. Follow the cooling methods shown above, and try not to let her temperature rise above 39°C (102.2°F). Your doctor may instruct you to give her a dose of paracetamol or ibuprofen suspension when she shows the first signs of illness, to stop her getting a fever.

Delirious children

Some children become delirious when they have a high fever. If your child is delirious, she will be very agitated, and may even hallucinate and seem extremely frightened. This delirious state is alarming, but it isn't dangerous for your child. Stay with her to comfort her. When her body temperature drops, she will probably fall asleep, and will be back to normal when she wakes up.

All about medicines ✳ 195

All about medicines

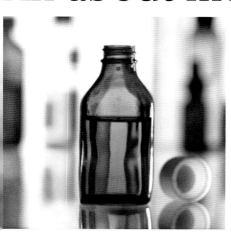

Most minor illnesses get better on their own, with or without treatment. However, if a medicine is necessary your doctor will tell you how often your child should take it, and for how long. Follow the directions carefully. Never mix a medicine into your baby's feed or your child's drink, since he may not finish it. If the doctor prescribes a course of antibiotics, your child must take the full course. If it is later diagnosed as a viral illness, the doctor will suggest stopping the antibiotics mid-course.

Giving medicine to babies

Always shake the bottle before pouring out the medicine and measure the dose exactly. If your baby cannot yet sit up, hold him as if you were going to feed him. If he can sit up, sit him on your lap, and tuck one of his arms behind your back. Put your hand firmly on his other arm to prevent him from struggling. If this doesn't work, ask another adult to hold him still while you give him medicine. You can prevent a baby from wriggling by swaddling him firmly. Keep some tissues handy.

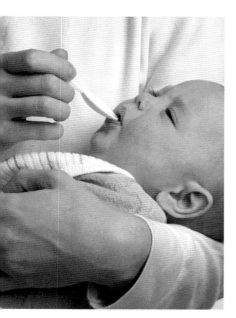

Medicine spoon
Measure your baby's dose, and pour half into another spoon. Keep both spoons nearby, then pick up your baby. Hold him so that he can't wriggle, then pick up one spoon, and rest it on his lower lip. Let him suck the medicine off, then repeat with the rest of the dose.

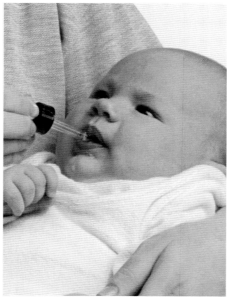

Medicine dropper
Measure the dose in a measuring spoon, then suck some of it into a plastic dropper. Put the dropper into your baby's mouth, and squeeze the medicine in. Give the rest of the dose. Don't use a dropper for a baby under four months old – he could choke. Don't use a glass dropper as it could break.

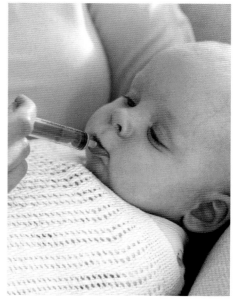

Syringe
Draw up the correct dose into the syringe, then pick up your baby, and rest the mouthpiece of the syringe on his lower lip. Tilt it slightly so that the medicine runs into your baby's cheek when you gently depress the end of the syringe (easiest method for babies).

Giving medicines to children

Most medicines for children are made to taste fairly pleasant, but if your child dislikes the taste, the following tips may help.

● Have your child's favourite drink ready to take away the taste of the medicine, and try bribery – a small treat or reward may help.

● Tell your child to hold her nose so that she can't taste the medicine, but never do this forcibly for her.

● If your child is old enough to understand, explain why she has to take the medicine – if she knows that it will make her feel better, she may be more inclined to take it.

● If you find it impossible to get medicine into your child, ask the doctor if he can prescribe it with a different flavour or in a different form.

Medicine and safety

Make sure that your child can't help herself to any medicines in your home.

● Keep all kinds of medications out of her reach, preferably in a locked cabinet.

● Always make sure that the medicines you buy have child-proof lids or packaging.

● Don't pretend to your child that her medicine is a soft drink.

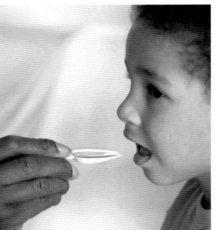

Medicine and tooth decay

Try to clean your child's teeth after giving her medicine. This is because many medicines for children contain sugar, and may cause tooth decay. If your child has to take medicine over a long period, ask your doctor or pharmacist whether a sugar-free alternative is available.

A taste tip
If your child does not like the taste of the medicine, pour it onto the back of her tongue – it won't taste so strong, because her taste buds are at the front.

Warning

Never give aspirin to your child unless advised to do so by your doctor; give her paracetamol syrup instead. A few children who have been given aspirin have developed a serious illness called Reye's syndrome. Give the correct dose, and buy the right strength and product for her age and weight. Don't give paracetamol for more than 48 hours, unless your doctor has advised this. If your child vomits and develops a high fever while she is recovering, **call for emergency help immediately.**

Giving nose drops

Children

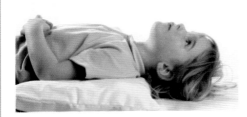

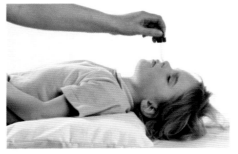

Babies

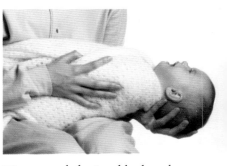

1 Place a small pillow or cushion on a bed, and help your child to lie on his back with the pillow beneath his shoulders and his head dropped back. If your child is likely to wriggle as you give him drops, ask an adult to help you by holding his head.

2 Put the tip of the dropper just above your child's nostril, and squeeze out the prescribed number of drops. Don't let the dropper touch his nose – if it does, wash it before using it again. Keep your child lying down for about a minute.

Wrap your baby in a blanket, then lay her on her back across your knee, so that her upper back is supported. Keep your left hand beneath her head to support it, then give the drops as instructed for a child.

Giving ear drops

Children

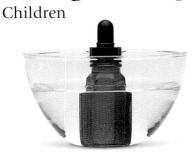

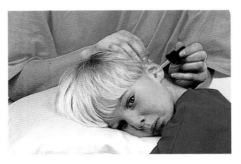

Babies

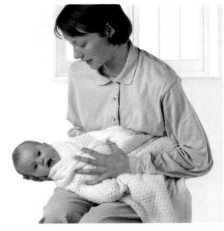

1 Most children find ear drops too cold as they are squeezed into their ears, so ask your doctor whether you can warm them up (some medicines deteriorate if they are warmed). To warm the drops, place the bottle in a bowl of warm, **not hot,** water for a few minutes. Before giving to your child, check the temperature on the inside of your wrist.

2 Ask your child to lie on his side with the affected ear uppermost. Then place the dropper close to his ear, and gently squeeze the prescribed number of drops into the ear canal. Keep your child lying down for about a minute, and place a piece of cotton wool very lightly in his ear to prevent excess liquid running out down his neck.

Wrap your baby and lay her on her side across your lap. Support her head with one hand, then give the ear drops as instructed for a child.

Giving eye drops

Children

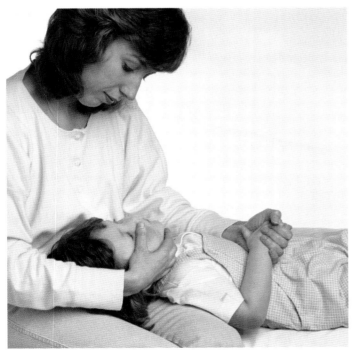

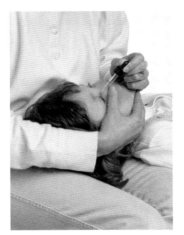

Babies

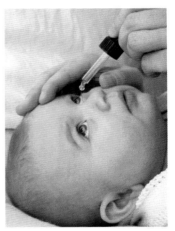

1 Bathe your child's affected eye with cotton wool dipped in warm, boiled water, then ask your child to lie on her back across your knee, or with her head in your lap. Put one arm around your child's head with your palm against her cheek, then tilt her head so that the affected eye is slightly lower than the other. Draw her lower eyelid gently down with your thumb.

2 Hold the dropper carefully over the gap between the lower lid and the eye, angling it so that it is out of your child's sight. If necessary, ask someone to hold her head steady. Gently squeeze out the prescribed number of drops, being careful not to touch the eye or the lid. Even if she cries, enough of the medicine is likely to stay in her eye.

Always choose a time when your baby is relaxed, then swaddle her, and lay her on a firm surface or across your knee. Give the drops as prescribed for a child.

Eye ointment

If your child is prescribed an eye ointment, gently squeeze out a small amount into the outer corner of her eye.

Caring for a sick child

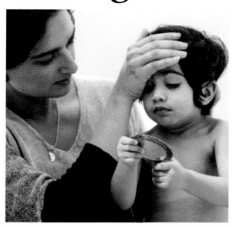

While your child is feeling ill, she may demand a great deal of attention, and may be irritable and easily bored. When ill most children need a lot of extra cuddling and reassurance. Keep your baby with you during the day, so that you can check on her frequently. Let your child lie down in the sitting room, so that she is near you. At night, sleep in the same room as her if she is very unwell, so that you are nearby if she needs you. Many children vomit when they are ill, so keep a small bowl nearby.

Eating and drinking

Your child will probably have a smaller appetite than usual while she is ill. Don't worry if she doesn't want to eat much for a few days – it won't do her any harm. Allow her to choose her favourite food, and offer small helpings. Let her eat as much or as little as she wants: when she is feeling better, her appetite will return. Babies may demand feeds more frequently than usual, but take very little milk each time. Be patient if your baby behaves like this – she needs the comfort of feeling close to you as she suckles. Drink is much more important than food while your child is ill. Make sure that she has plenty to drink – about 1½ litres (3 pints) a day, especially if she has a raised temperature, or has been vomiting or has diarrhoea – to make sure that she doesn't get dehydrated.

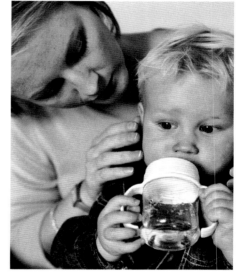

Giving your child a drink
Let your child choose her favourite drink – it doesn't matter whether it is a fizzy drink, fruit juice, milk, or water.

Encouraging your child to drink
If it is difficult to persuade your child to drink enough, make her drinks seem more appetizing by trying some of the ideas suggested below.

An unusually shaped straw *will appeal to her*

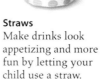

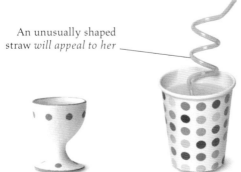

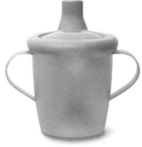

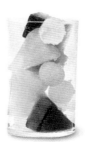

Small container
Offer frequent small drinks from a doll's cup or an egg cup, rather than giving large amounts.

Straws
Make drinks look appetizing and more fun by letting your child use a straw.

Teacher beaker
Offer drinks in a teacher beaker, which will help avoid spills while she is in bed.

Ice cubes
For a child over a year old, freeze diluted fruit juice into cubes, then let her suck the cubes.

Ice lolly
Your child may prefer an ice lolly – the "drink on a stick". Try to avoid ones with artificial colouring.

Sickness and vomiting

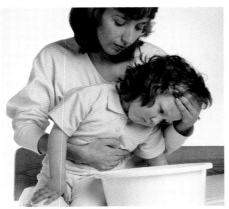

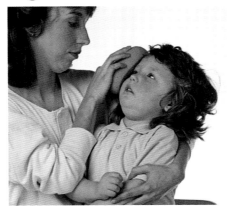

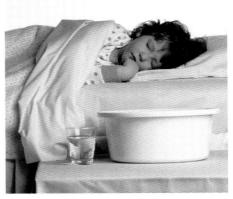

1 Hold your child while she is vomiting to comfort her. Sit her on your lap leaning over a bowl. When she begins to retch, support her head with one hand on her forehead, and put your other hand over her stomach, just below her rib cage.

2 After she has finished vomiting, do your best to reassure your child. Then sponge her face and wipe around her mouth. Give her a few sips of water, let her rinse her mouth out, or help her to clean her teeth, to take away any unpleasant taste that she may have.

3 Let your child rest after vomiting; she may want to lie down for a while. Wash out the container and put it within easy reach, in case she vomits again. If your child vomits frequently, she may have gastroenteritis (see page 222). Wash hands to prevent the spread of infection.

Comfort and entertainment

Staying in bed

There is no need to insist that your sick child stays in bed, although if she is feeling very ill she will probably prefer to stay there. If she wants to get up, make sure that she is dressed in cool, loose clothes, and that the room she is playing in is well ventilated, but not draughty. However, your child may want to lie down and go to sleep during the day, even if it isn't her usual naptime. If she doesn't want to be left alone, let her snuggle up with a pillow, a duvet, and her favourite cuddly toy on the sofa in the sitting room, or make up a bed for her wherever you are (a folding guestbed is ideal). In this way, your child still feels like she is a part of the family, and does not get too bored or lonely.

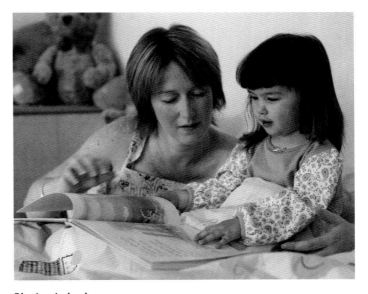

Playing in bed
If your child feels like staying in bed, but wants to sit, prop her up on her bed. Give her a picture book and read to her.

Entertaining your child

Try to keep your child occupied so that she doesn't get too bored, but remember that she will probably act younger than her age while she is feeling unwell. She won't be able to concentrate for very long, and she won't want to do anything too demanding. Bring out an old favourite toy that she hasn't played with for a while. If you give her small presents to keep her entertained and cheer her up don't be tempted to buy toys that are advanced for her age. Babies will enjoy a new mobile or a rattle that makes a new sound. Quiet activities such as interlocking building bricks, felt pictures, simple jigsaws, crayons or felt tip pens, a kaleidoscope, or Plasticine are ideal for sick toddlers and children. Protect the bedding with a towel if your child wants to play with something messy while she is in bed. She might enjoy a CD player with her favourite songs or music, too. Remember that she will probably want more of your company than usual, so be prepared to spend some more time with her, looking at her books, and drawing pictures for her to colour in. She will be happier if you are within her sight, even if not actively playing with her.

Colds and flu

All children get colds and the flu. As soon as your child comes into contact with other children, she may get one cold after another – some children under six may have up to seven a year. As she grows older, your child develops resistance to many of these viruses.

Emergency

Call for emergency help immediately if your child develops a rash of dark, purplish-red spots (see page 208). Doctors refer to this as a petechial rash.

☎ Seek medical help

If your child has been feeling absolutely miserable, and especially if she is not yet one year old, **consult your doctor as soon as possible** if she has:

- a temperature over 39°C (102.2°F)
- wheezy, fast, or laboured breathing
- earache
- a throat so sore that swallowing is painful
- a severe cough
- not improved after three days.

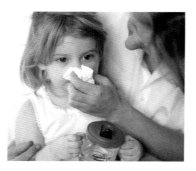

Wiping your child's nose
If your child has a runny nose, dab it gently with a tissue to prevent it becoming sore from frequent wiping. Remember to throw the tissue away immediately, to avoid spreading infection.

Colds

What are they?

Perhaps the most common of all illnesses, a cold is a viral infection that irritates the nose and throat, so children don't catch a cold simply by being cold, by going out without wearing a coat, or by getting their feet wet. While it is not a severe illness, a cold should be taken more seriously in babies and children than in adults, because of the risk of a chest or ear infection developing. If your child develops a rash in addition to the symptoms of a normal cold, contact your doctor to determine what the rash could be.

Symptoms

- Runny or blocked nose and sneezing
- slightly raised temperature
- sore throat
- cough.

What might the doctor do?

If your baby has trouble sucking because her nose is blocked, your doctor may prescribe nose drops to be given just before a feed.

Nose drops

Use these only if your doctor has prescribed them, and never use them for more than three days. When overused, they can increase mucus production, which will make your child's nose even more blocked.

What can I do?

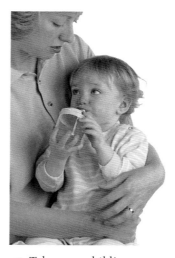

1 Take your child's body temperature (see page 193), and give her a children's syrup containing paracetamol to bring it down if necessary. Make sure she has plenty to drink, but don't force her to eat if she's not hungry. A drink before bedtime may help to keep her nose clear at night.

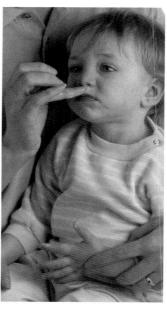

2 Spread a barrier cream, such as petroleum jelly, under your child's nose and around her nostrils if the area has become red and sore from a constantly runny nose or frequent wiping.

Flu

What is it?

Flu (also known as influenza) is a very infectious illness caused by hundreds of different viruses. It tends to occur in epidemics every two or three years, when a new strain of the virus appears to which people have not yet developed immunity. The flu season begins every year in late autumn and early winter. The peak season for flu in the northern hemisphere is from November through March. If your child has caught flu she will develop symptoms a day or two later, and will probably be sick for about three or four days. She may be sick enough to want to stay in bed, and could remain weak for several days after her temperature has gone down. A few children develop a chest infection, such as bronchitis or pneumonia (see pages 218–9), after having flu.

Symptoms

- Raised temperature
- headache
- ache all over the body
- feeling shivery
- runny nose
- cough
- sore throat.

What can I do?

Take your child's temperature (see page 193), and if necessary, give her paracetamol or ibuprofen suspension to reduce fever (see page 196). Offer her plenty of cooled water – it's important that she has plenty to drink. See your doctor if the paracetamol fails to bring her temperature down. You may want to use a humidifier in your child's room to make the air easier for her to breathe.

"Should I have my child vaccinated against flu?"

A vaccination may be a good idea, even for healthy children, so discuss it with your doctor. It will protect your child from the illness for about a year. The flu vaccine is especially important for children with ongoing health problems, such as heart, kidney, or lung disease. Because new strains of the virus develop every two or three years, the vaccine (which can only be made from the existing forms of the virus) does not give lifelong protection from the illness.

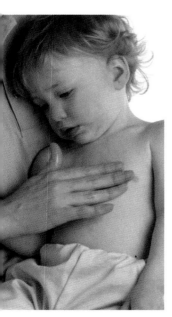

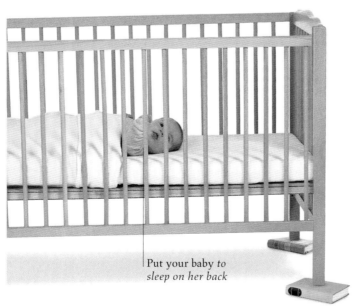

Put your baby to sleep on her back

3 If your child has a cold, sit her on your lap and use menthol inhalation or a menthol rub. This will ease her cough and help her to settle before bed.

4 She will be able to breathe more easily if you raise the head of the cot slightly. Place a book under the legs of the cot so that your baby's head and chest are slightly raised. Never prop up the mattress as this is considered unsafe practice.

5 Make sure that the air in your child's room isn't too dry, since breathing very dry air can be uncomfortable. Use a humidifier if you have one, to add moisture to the air.

Sinusitis

The sinuses are air-filled cavities in the bones of the face. The lining of the nose extends into them, so they can easily become infected after a cold. This infection, sinusitis, often seems like a cold that won't go away, with nasal congestion, cough, and bad breath. These sinuses don't develop until age three or four, so for younger children, sinusitis isn't a problem. Sinusitis is, however, often misdiagnosed in children. At the first sign of nasal congestion or runny nose many parents (and doctors) think that the child is suffering from a sinus infection. Instead, these children often just have a common cold, and do not require treatment.

Having your child immunized

You should start the immunization programme at birth and continue throughout childhood. The vaccines she will be given contain harmless versions of the germs that cause the most severe infectious diseases. These make the body produce special proteins (antibodies) that will protect your child from that disease in the future.

Why should my baby be immunized?
Some parents decide against immunization because they are worried about possible risks, or because they think that it is unnecessary. However, if fewer immunizations are given, these potentially serious diseases will affect an increasing number of children.

What are the risks?
Immunizations may make your child mildly unwell for a short time, but more serious side effects are extremely rare. Nearly all children are able to be immunized – the few reasons for not vaccinating a child include a severe reaction to a previous dose. Do not take her to be immunized if she has a feverish illness. However, there is no need to postpone immunization if she has some minor infection, such as a cold, or is simply off-colour.

What are the after-effects?
Within 12–24 hours of immunization, your baby may have a slight fever and possibly some sickness or diarrhoea, and may feel miserable for up to 48 hours. If her temperature rises, give the recommended dose of paracetamol syrup.

She may develop a small, hard lump at the injection site. This will go in a few weeks, and is nothing to worry about. If she develops any other symptoms, becomes "floppy" and less responsive than usual, her crying sounds unusual, her temperature rises above 38°C (100.4°F), or she has a febrile convulsion (fit), **call your doctor.**

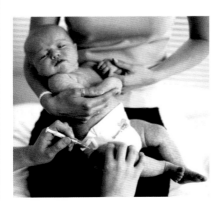

Having an injection
Hold your baby firmly on your lap while she has the injection, to comfort her and keep her as still as possible. The practice nurse usually gives the injection into the top of the baby's thigh.

Immunization programme

Age	Vaccine	How given
at birth	Tuberculosis (BCG) **(given to babies especially likely to come in contact with TB)**	1 injection
2 months	Diphtheria Tetanus Whooping cough (pertussis) Polio Hib*	1 injection
	Pneumococcal infection (PCV)	1 injection
3 months	Diphtheria Tetanus Whooping cough (pertussis) Polio Hib*	1 injection
	Meningitis C	1 injection
4 months	Diphtheria Tetanus Whooping cough (pertussis) Polio Hib* Meningitis C	1 injection
	Pneumococcal infection (PCV)	1 injection
12 months	Hib* Meningitis C	1 injection
13 months	Measles Mumps Rubella	1 injection (MMR)
	Pneumococcal infection (PCV)	1 injection
3½–5 years, Pre-school booster	Diphtheria Tetanus Whooping cough (pertussis) Polio	1 injection
	MMR	1 injection
Girls aged 12–13 years	Cervical cancer caused by human papillomavirus types 16 and 18 (HPV)	1 injection
School leavers	Diphtheria Tetanus Polio	1 injection

*Hib: *Haemophilis influenzae* type b, a bacterium that can cause one type of meningitis and other serious childhood diseases.

Infectious illnesses

Now that most children are immunized, many of these diseases have become much less common. If your child catches one of them, she will probably be immune for the rest of her life. Since most of these infectious diseases are caused by viruses, there are no medicines to cure them, but most children recover quickly and uneventfully. There is little point in trying to isolate your child when she has an infectious illness, unless she has rubella (see below), but it is a good idea to inform the parents of any children she has recently been in contact with.

Warning

If your child has a raised temperature while she is ill with one of these diseases, **do not** give her aspirin to bring the fever down, unless advised by the doctor, since it can cause a very serious disease called Reye's syndrome (see page 196). You can give your child paracetamol or ibuprofen suspension instead.

Emergency

Call for emergency help immediately if your child has an infectious disease and develops any of these signs:
- unusual and increasing drowsiness
- headache or stiff neck
- convulsions
- rash of flat, dark red or purplish blood-spots.

Rubella (German measles)

What is it?

Rubella was once common, but has become rare because of routine immunization (see opposite). It is a mild illness, so your child may feel perfectly well, and may not stay in bed. She will develop symptoms two to three weeks after she has been infected. Keep her away from others for a few days after the rash appears.

What can I do?

1 Take your child's temperature (see page 193) and, if necessary, give her paracetamol syrup to reduce her fever.

2 Make sure that your child has plenty to drink, especially if she has a raised temperature.

Symptoms

Days 1 and 2
- Symptoms of a mild cold
- slightly sore throat
- swollen glands behind the ears, on the sides of the neck, and on the nape of the neck.

Day 2 or 3
- Blotchy rash of flat, pink spots appearing first on the face, then spreading down the body
- slightly raised temperature.

Day 4 or 5
- Fading rash, and general improvement.

Day 6
- Your child is back to normal.

Day 9 or 10
- Your child is no longer infectious.

☎ Seek medical help

Call for emergency help immediately if your child develops any of the emergency signs above. **Consult your doctor as soon as possible** if you think your child has rubella, but do not take her to the doctor's surgery in case she comes into contact with a pregnant woman who is not immune.

What might the doctor do?

Your doctor will confirm that your child has rubella, but there is no treatment for it.

Rubella and pregnancy

While your child is infectious, keep her away from any women who might be pregnant. Although rubella is a mild illness, it can cause defects in a developing baby if a pregnant woman catches it.

Measles

What is it?
Measles is a very infectious illness that causes a rash, fever, and a cough, and sometimes more serious complications, such as pneumonia and inflammation of the brain. It will become a rare disease if widespread immunization is achieved.

What can I do?

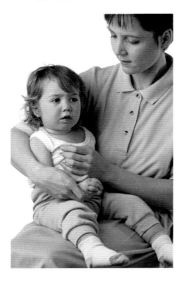

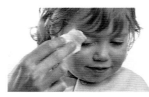

1 Try to bring down her temperature (see page 194) and give plenty of fluids. She may feel very miserable and want to stay in bed.

2 If her eyes are sore, bathe them using a cotton wool dipped in cool water. Keep her room dark if this makes her more comfortable.

What might the doctor do?
Your doctor will confirm the diagnosis and keep a check on your child. He will treat any complications if they develop.

Symptoms
Symptoms develop 10–14 days after infection.

Days 1 and 2
- Runny nose, dry cough, and red watering eyes
- steadily rising temperature.

Day 3
- Tiny white spots, like grains of salt, in the mouth.

Days 4 and 5
- Dull red rash of slightly raised spots appears, first on forehead and behind the ears, gradually spreading to rest of the face and trunk. After two or three days, the rash fades and other symptoms disappear.

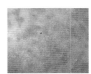

☎ Seek medical help
Call for emergency help immediately if your child develops any of the signs on page 203. **Consult the doctor as soon as possible** if you think your child has measles. Call him again if:
- your child is no better three days after the rash develops
- your child's temperature rises suddenly
- her condition worsens after she seemed to be improving
- she has earache or her breathing is noisy and difficult.

Roseola infantum

What is it?
Roseola is a mild illness that is very common in early childhood. It is characterized by a high fever that lasts for about three days, followed by a rash of pink spots. Most children will have had it by the time they are two.

What can I do?

1 Call your doctor if your child's temperature is 39°C (102.2°F) or above. In some cases, febrile fits may follow the high temperature. Follow the protocols given on page 194.

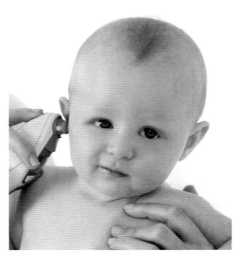

2 Try to bring down the fever to make your child more comfortable (see page 194). Paracetamol may bring his temperature down briefly.

3 Make sure your child has plenty to drink so that he is always adequately hydrated.

Symptoms
Symptoms appear 5–15 days after the incubation period.

Days 1 to 4
- High temperature
- sometimes a mild cold or cough.

Days 4 to 8
- Temperature returns to normal
- rash of pink, slightly raised spots appears over head and trunk
- rash fades, and the child is back to normal.

☎ Seek medical help
Call for emergency help immediately if your child develops any of the emergency signs listed on page 203.

Chickenpox

What is it?

Chickenpox is a very infectious illness, characterized by a rash of itchy spots that turn into fluid-filled blisters. It is usually accompanied by a slight fever. Your child may not feel very ill, but if he has a lot of spots he may itch all over. Symptoms appear two to three weeks after your child has been infected. It is a very common childhood illness. In later life, the chickenpox virus may be reactivated and cause shingles, so a child may catch chickenpox after contact with an adult who has shingles. Rarely, chickenpox can cause complications for a pregnant woman or her unborn baby.

Symptoms

Days 1 to 4
- Groups of small, red, very itchy spots with fluid-filled centres, appearing in batches first on the child's chest, abdomen, and back, later elsewhere on the body
- fluid within the spots becomes white and cloudy
- slight temperature.

Days 5 to 9
- The spots burst, leaving small craters
- scabs form over the spots and drop off after a few days.

Day 10
- Your child is back to normal.

Day 11 or 12
- Your child is no longer infectious and is safe to come into contact with other children and adults, although he still remains a high risk to pregnant women.

☎ Seek medical help

Call for emergency help immediately if your child develops any of the signs listed on page 203. Consult your doctor as soon as possible if you think your child has chickenpox, and call him again if he has any of the symptoms listed below:
- very severe itching
- redness or swelling around any spots, or pus oozing from the spots – this means they have become infected
- temperature of 39°C (102.2°F) or more
- rashes affecting area around the eyes
- infection persisting beyond nine days.

What can I do?

1 Take your child's temperature (see page 193), and give him the recommended dose of paracetamol syrup to bring it down if it is raised. Give him plenty of fluids to drink if he has a fever. Although your child may not feel very ill, try to make sure that he has plenty of rest as this will aid his recovery.

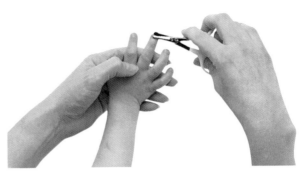

2 Try to discourage your child from scratching the spots, since it can infect them, and also cause scarring when they heal. Cut your child's fingernails short and keep them clean, so that the spots are less likely to become infected if he does scratch them. Put scratch mitts on him.

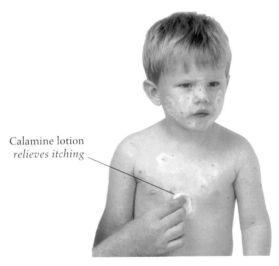

Calamine lotion *relieves itching*

3 Try to relieve your child's itchiness. Dab the spots gently with cotton wool dipped in calamine lotion.

4 Give your child lukewarm baths with a handful of bicarbonate of soda dissolved in the water to help reduce itching.

5 If your child is very itchy, he will probably find loose cotton clothes the most comfortable.

What might the doctor do?

Your doctor will confirm the diagnosis, and may prescribe an antihistamine cream or medicine to relieve your child's itching if it is very severe. If any of the spots have become infected, he may prescribe an antibiotic cream.

Mumps

What is it?

Mumps is an infection that was quite common among children until routine immunization was introduced. It causes swollen glands, particularly the glands just in front of and below the ears. Occasionally, mumps also causes inflammation of the testicles, but this is rare in a boy before puberty.

What can I do?

1 Give paracetamol syrup to bring his temperature down, and hold a cold compress to his swollen glands.

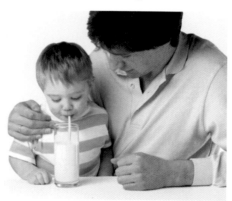

2 Give plenty of cold drinks, but avoid acidic drinks, such as fruit juice. Let your child drink through a straw, if it hurts him to open his mouth.

Symptoms

Symptoms appear 14–24 days after the infection.
● Raised temperature
● one or two days later, the child develops painful swelling on one or both sides of the face. This lasts for four to eight days.

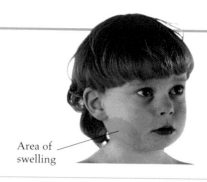

Area of swelling

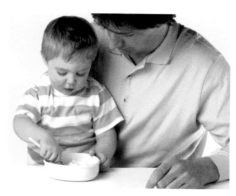

3 If it hurts your child to swallow, give him liquid or semi-liquid foods, such as ice cream and soup.

4 Keep him away from unimmunized teenagers and young adults, and from women in the first 16 weeks of pregnancy when mumps carries a slightly increased risk of miscarriage.

☎ Seek medical help

Call for emergency help immediately if your child develops any of the signs listed on page 203. **Consult your doctor as soon as possible** if you think your child has mumps, and call him again if he develops bad stomach pain or a red testicle.

What might the doctor do?

Your doctor will confirm that your child has mumps, and treat any complications if they develop.

Erythema infectiosum (Slapped cheek disease)

What is it?

Erythema infectiosum is a mild, and mildly infectious, illness that usually occurs in small outbreaks in the spring, and mostly affects children over the age of two years. It is also sometimes called "fifth disease". The disease is characterized by a bright red rash that suddenly appears on both cheeks, hence its other name of "slapped cheek disease".

What can I do?

Give your child paracetamol syrup to reduce the fever. Make sure he drinks plenty of fluids, and apply a cold compress on the site. If your child has a blood disorder (for example, sickle-cell anaemia or thalassaemia), consult your doctor. Erythema infectiosum can sometimes cause severe illnesses in such children. If your child has Erythema infectiosum, keep him away from any women who might be pregnant. Although once the rash appears he is unlikely to be infectious, the disease can, in rare circumstances, lead to miscarriage, if contracted during pregnancy.

Symptoms

Symptoms appear 4–14 days after the infection.

Day 1
● Bright red cheeks, with a contrasting pale area around the mouth
● mild fever
● joint pain.

Days 2 to 5
● Blotchy, lace-like rash spreading over trunk and limbs.

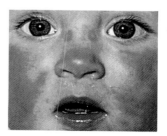

Days 7 to 10
● Rash fades. Your child is no longer infectious. The rash may recur over the next few weeks or months, particularly if your child is exposed to sunlight.

Whooping cough

What is it?

One of the most serious childhood diseases, whooping cough (also known as pertussis), is characterized by a severe and persistent cough. It is caused by a bacterial infection. It is highly infectious, so keep your child away from babies and children who have not been immunized. Immunized children can get a mild form of the illness. A few children with whooping cough develop a secondary infection, such as bronchitis or pneumonia (see pages 218–9).

What can I do?

1 Stay with your child during any coughing fits, because he may become very distressed. Sit him on your lap, and support him gently as he leans slightly forwards. Keep a small bowl nearby so that he can spit out any phlegm that he coughs up, and in case he should vomit. Clean the bowl thoroughly with boiling water afterwards, to make sure that the infection doesn't spread to the rest of the family.

2 If your child often coughs and vomits after meals, offer him small meals at frequent intervals, just after a coughing fit if possible.

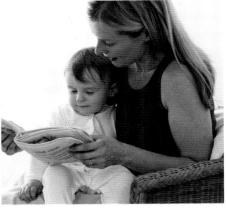

3 Keep your child entertained – he will have fewer coughing fits if his attention is distracted, but don't let him get too excited or over-tired, as this may bring on a coughing fit.

4 Sleep in the same room as your child, so that you can be with him if he has a coughing fit at night.

5 Don't let anyone smoke near your child, and don't give him any cough medicines.

Symptoms

Week 1
- Symptoms of a normal cough and cold
- slight temperature.

Week 2
- Worsening cough, with frequent coughing fits lasting up to a minute, after which your child has to fight for breath
- if your child is over 18 months, he may learn to force breath in with a "whooping" sound
- vomiting after a coughing fit.

Weeks 3 to 10
- Cough improves, but may worsen if your child gets a cold
- your child is unlikely to be infectious after the third week.

Emergency

Call for emergency help immediately if your child turns blue during a coughing fit.

☎ Seek medical help

Consult your doctor as soon as possible if you suspect that your child has whooping cough.

What might the doctor do?

The doctor may prescribe an antibiotic. Although it won't cure your child's cough, it may reduce its severity, and make your child less infectious. This is particularly important if you have a baby who is at risk of catching whooping cough from an older brother or sister who already has the disease. However, the antibiotic is only really effective if it is given right at the beginning of the infection.

Nursing a baby

Whooping cough is dangerous in babies, because they may not be able to draw breath properly after coughing. Your baby will need careful nursing, and may be admitted to the hospital. Your child may receive intravenous antibiotics to treat infection or reduce lung inflammation. Sedatives may be prescribed to allow your child to rest while his breathing is carefully monitored. He may find feeding difficult if he vomits frequently, so abandon your regular feeding schedule and offer a feed as soon as he has calmed down after coughing or vomiting.

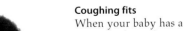

Coughing fits
When your baby has a coughing fit, sit him on your lap, and keep rubbing his back. Stay with him until he has stopped coughing and is breathing normally again. Then cuddle to comfort him, and put him down to sleep on his back as usual.

Rub his back *when he has a coughing fit*

Meningitis

What is it?

Meningitis is an inflammation of the tissues covering the brain. It can be caused by an infection with bacteria or viruses. Viral meningitis is more common than bacterial meningitis, and is also less serious. It can be caused by several different viruses, and tends to occur in winter epidemics. Viral meningitis is more likely to affect children over five years old. Bacterial meningitis is quite rare, but it can be life-threatening. In Britain, the Hib vaccination has wiped out one type of bacterial meningitis. Unfortunately there are others, of which the most common is called Group B meningococcal bacteria. Two other strains of these bacteria, Group A and Group C, also cause the disease, but are rarer. There is now a vaccination for meningitis C (see page 202). Although bacterial meningitis can occur at any age, it is most common in children under the age of five.

The early symptoms of bacterial and viral meningitis are very similar, too, and can easily be mistaken for those of flu. However, the symptoms of bacterial meningitis are usually more severe. It can develop very rapidly, so that the child may become seriously ill within a few hours, with increasing drowsiness and sometimes loss of consciousness or convulsions.

Meningitis rash

Some children with meningitis develop a characteristic rash of tiny blood-spots under the skin, which can appear anywhere on the body. The spots are flat, pink, dark red, or purple. They look like pinpricks at first, but if untreated, grow bigger until they look like fresh bruises.

What can I do?

Call your doctor now, or take your child to the nearest accident and emergency department if she seems abnormally drowsy or has any two of the symptoms listed in the emergency box below.

What might the doctor do?

The doctor may send your child to hospital for a lumbar puncture test to confirm the diagnosis.

If viral meningitis is diagnosed no treatment is necessary except painkillers, and your child will recover completely within a week or two.

Bacterial meningitis will be treated with antibiotics and, if convulsions occur, with anticonvulsant drugs. If the disease is picked up early and treated promptly, most children recover completely. Rarely, the disease may be fatal, and in a few children it may cause some brain damage, especially if treatment is delayed.

The meninges

Three protective layers, known as the meninges, cover the brain and spinal cord. Meningitis occurs when the meninges become infected by viruses or bacteria.

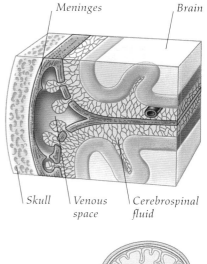

Meninges *Brain*

Skull *Venous space* *Cerebrospinal fluid*

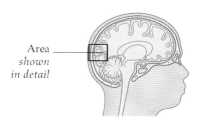

Area shown in detail

Emergency

Call for emergency help immediately if your child has two or more of the following symptoms:
- vomiting and refusing feeds
- stiff neck
- restlessness and irritability, especially when picked up (this can be due to limb or muscle pain)
- tense or bulging fontanelle
- purple-red rash that does not fade when pressed
- fever with cold hands and feet – a temperature of 38°C (100.4°F) or more in babies under three months, and of 39°C (102.2°F) or more in babies between three and six months
- rapid or unusual breathing patterns
- skin that is extremely pale, blotchy, or turning blue
- a high-pitched moaning cry
- shivering
- floppiness and listlessness, or stiffness with jerky movements
- abnormal drowsiness, or your child being less responsive, vacant, or difficult to wake.

Older children may also have:
- severe headache
- dislike of bright light and loud noise.

If your child has a dark, purplish rash, check to see whether it fades when pressed. To do this, press the side of a glass on to the rash. If the rash is still visible through the glass it may be a purpura rash, which requires immediate medical attention. Take your child to the nearest accident and emergency department.

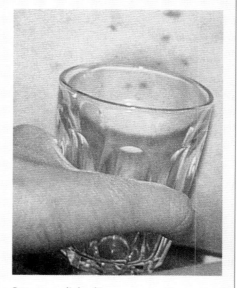

Purpura on light skin

Eye problems

Most eye disorders clear up quickly with treatment, but all problems affecting the eye should be taken seriously. Eye infections spread easily, so give your child her own face flannel and towel. Use a clean tissue to dry each eye. Keep your child's hands clean and try to stop her rubbing her eyes – this helps to prevent the infection from spreading.

3 If your child has dandruff, wash her hair with an anti-dandruff shampoo. Use an anti-cradle cap shampoo for a baby, and wash her scalp gently.

> ☎ **Seek medical help**
> **Consult your doctor as soon as possible** if:
> - your child's eyes are sticky
> - there is no improvement after about a week of home treatment.

> **Emergency**
> **Call for emergency help immediately** if your child has any injury that has damaged her eye, or if she cannot see clearly after an injury.

What might the doctor do?
The doctor may prescribe a cream to soothe your child's eyelids, or an antibiotic ointment.

Blepharitis

What is it?
Blepharitis is an inflammation of the edges of the eyelids, which usually affects both eyes. Many children with dandruff get blepharitis.

> **Symptoms**
>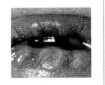
> - Red and scaly eyelids
> - irritation in the eyes.

What can I do?

1 Use warm, boiled water to wash your child's eyelids, using fresh cotton wool for each eye. Hold the warm pad over the closed eyelid for about 5–10 minutes, then rub it gently over the closed eyelid to help loosen any crusting. Do this twice a day using fresh warm water each time.

2 Gently clean the eyelids with a cotton bud, using warm water mixed with a small amount of baby shampoo, or with a teaspoonful of sodium bicarbonate dissolved in a cup of water.

Conjunctivitis

What is it?
Also known as "pink eye" because the white of the eye turns pink, conjunctivitis is an inflammation of the lining of the eye and eyelids. It can be caused by a virus or by bacteria, although it is milder when caused by a virus. If your child's eyelids are gummed together with pus when she wakes up, she probably has bacterial, rather than viral, conjunctivitis. If your baby develops any of the symptoms in the first day or two of life, see Sticky eye (p.183).

What can I do?

1 Try to find out whether your child's symptoms are caused by something other than conjunctivitis. She might have an allergy such as hay fever, or she may have a speck of dust or an eyelash in her eye. If she has an allergy, her eyes may be itchy and watering, as well as red and sore.

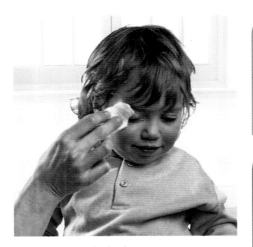

2 If you think she has conjunctivitis, dip a cotton wool ball into some warm, boiled water and bathe both of her eyes, using fresh cotton wool for each one. Start with the infected one, and wipe from the inside corner to the outside. Wash your hands before and afterwards.

> **Symptoms**
>
> - Bloodshot eye
> - gritty, sore eye
> - discharge of pus
> - eyelids gummed together after sleep.

> ☎ **Seek medical help**
> **Consult your doctor as soon as possible** if you think your child has conjunctivitis or if her eyes are bloodshot and sore.

What might the doctor do?
The doctor may prescribe antibiotic drops or ointment for a bacterial infection, which will cure it. Viral conjunctivitis needs no treatment, but may last a few weeks.

Stye

What is it?

A stye is a painful, pus-filled swelling on the upper or lower eyelid. It is caused by an infection, usually bacterial, at the base of an eyelash.

Some styes simply dry up, but most of these come to a head, and then burst within about a week, relieving the pain. Styes are not serious and you can treat them at home. Try to stop your child from touching the stye to prevent the infection from spreading.

Symptoms

● Red, painful swelling on the eyelid
● pus-filled centre appearing in the swelling.

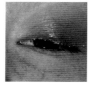

What can I do?

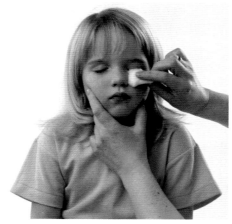

1 Dip some cotton wool in hot, but not boiling, water, squeeze it out, and press it gently onto your child's stye. This will help to bring the stye to a head more quickly, and encourage the release of pus. Repeat this for two or three minutes, three times a day until the stye bursts.

2 When the stye bursts and releases the pus, the pain is relieved. Wash the pus away very gently with cotton wool that has been dipped in warm, boiled water. The swelling will go down very soon.

☎ Seek medical help

Consult your doctor as soon as possible if:
● the stye does not improve after about a week
● your child's whole eyelid is swollen
● the skin all around your child's eye turns red
● your child also has blepharitis (see page 209).

Squint

What is it?

Normally, both eyes look in the same direction at the same time, but in a child with a squint one eye focuses on an object while the other does not follow it properly.

A newborn baby's eyes do not always work together correctly, so intermittent squinting is common. This is nothing to worry about. But if your baby's eyes don't move together by the time he is three months old, talk to your health visitor. He may have a squint.

Squinting may be constant, but in some children, it comes and goes. However, children do not grow out of a squint, so it is essential to have it treated. The younger the child, the more successful the treatment.

Symptoms

● Eyes looking in different directions.

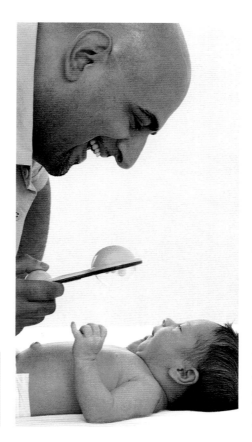

How can I check for a squint?

When your baby is about three months old, hold a toy 20cm (8in) from his face, and move it slowly from side to side. Check that his eyes work together to follow the moving object.

☎ Seek medical help

Consult your doctor if you think your child has a squint.

What might the doctor do?

The doctor will check your child's vision and may give him a patch to wear over his stronger eye for several hours each day, so that he is forced to use his weak or lazy eye. A toddler may need to wear glasses. If your child is under two, this treatment will probably cure his squint within a few months. If your child has a severe squint caused by muscle weakness, he may need to have an operation to correct the defect and straighten his eyes.

Ear problems

Most ear problems in small children arise from an infection of the outer or middle ear. Acute middle ear infections may cause severe pain and pus may build up behind the ear-drum, causing it to burst. (The hole should heal within a few weeks.) Occasionally, the infection may spread into the bone behind the ear.

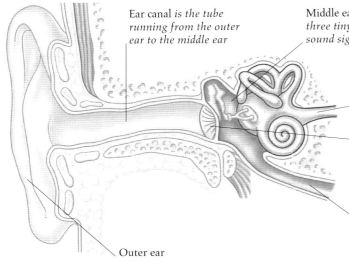

Ear canal *is the tube running from the outer ear to the middle ear*

Middle ear cavity *contains three tiny bones that transmit sound signals to the inner ear*

Auditory nerve *takes sound signals to the brain*

Ear-drum *vibrates in response to sound waves*

Eustachian tube *leads to the back of the throat. It is much shorter in children than in adults, making it prone to blockage*

Outer ear

Anatomy of the ear
Each ear consists of three parts. From the outer ear (the only visible part), a slightly curved canal leads to the ear-drum. Behind this is a cavity, the middle ear, in which lie three small bones, which transmit sound vibrations to the inner ear, the part of the ear that contains the structures concerned with hearing and balance.

Outer ear infection

What is it?
The skin lining the outer ear canal becomes inflamed when your child has an outer ear infection. This may happen if he swims a lot in chlorinated water, or because he has poked or scratched his ear, and it has become infected. Children with eczema are especially prone to such infections if they get water in their ears.

What can I do?

1 Give your child the prescribed dose of paracetamol syrup to relieve the pain.

2 Make sure that water doesn't get into the affected ear at bathtime, and just sponge his hair clean. Don't let your child go swimming until the infection clears up.

☎ **Seek medical help**
Consult your doctor as soon as possible if you think your child has an outer ear infection.

What might the doctor do?
Your doctor will probably prescribe antibiotic ear drops to clear the infection. Ask your child to lie on his side and keep still while you squeeze out drops into the affected ear. Keep him in this position for about a minute afterwards.

Symptoms
- Pain in the ear that is worse when the child touches his ear or lies on it
- redness in the ear canal
- discharge from the ear
- itchiness inside the ear.

Wax in the ear
Wax sometimes accumulates in the ear, giving a feeling of fullness or partial deafness. If your child has a lot of ear wax, very gently wipe away any visible wax with cotton wool, but don't poke anything into the ear. If this doesn't help, consult your doctor.

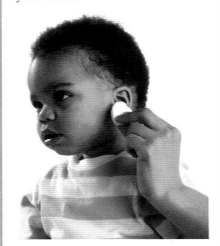

Middle ear infection

What is it?
Earache is commonly caused by an infection of the middle ear. If your child has a middle ear infection, the cavity behind his ear-drum becomes infected or inflamed, usually because an infection has spread from the throat. The tube that runs from the throat to the ear is very short and narrow in a child, and so is obstructed easily. Generally, only one ear is infected.

By the time your child is seven or eight years old, the eustachian tube (see page 211) will have increased in width, making your child much less prone to these infections.

Symptoms
- Very painful ear which may stop your child sleeping
- crying and rubbing or tugging at the ear, if your child can't yet talk well enough to complain of earache
- crying, loss of appetite, and general signs of illness in young babies, especially after a cold
- raised temperature
- partial deafness.

What can I do?

1 To relieve your child's earache, fill a hot water bottle with warm, **not hot,** water, and wrap it in a towel. Then let him rest his ear against it. Don't give a hot water bottle to a baby who is too young to push it away if it is too hot – heat a soft cloth, and hold it against your baby's ear instead.

2 If your child's ear is very painful, and is causing him a lot of discomfort, try giving the recommended dose of paracetamol syrup. This should relieve the pain.

3 If you notice a discharge, don't clear it away or probe his ear – just put a clean handkerchief over his ear. Encourage him to rest his head on the affected side, so that any discharge can drain away.

☎ Seek medical help
Consult your doctor as soon as possible if your child's ear is infected, or has a discharge.

How can I prevent ear infection?
In cold weather, keep your child's ears warm. Use menthol inhalation or a menthol rub whenever he has a cold.

What might the doctor do?
Your doctor will examine your child's ears, and may prescribe an antibiotic. If pus has built up behind the ear-drum, the doctor may prescribe a drug to help it drain away. If this is not effective, your child may need a small surgical procedure.

Glue ear

What is it?
Repeated middle ear infections can lead to glue ear, an accumulation of sticky fluid in the middle ear.

Symptoms
- Partial deafness after repeated middle ear infections.

What can I do?
If you smoke, try to stop. Children of parents who smoke seem to be more prone than others to suffer glue ear.

☎ Seek medical help
Consult your doctor as soon as possible if you think your child has glue ear.

What might the doctor do?
The condition may clear up on its own, so treatment may not be needed. Your doctor may prescribe a decongestant, but a simple operation may be necessary. Under anaesthetic, a hole is made in the ear-drum and a tiny tube (a grommet) is inserted. After several months, it will fall out, the hole will heal, and your child's hearing will be back to normal.

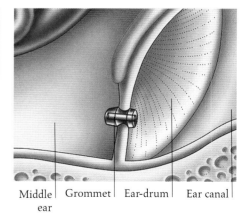

Middle | Grommet | Ear-drum | Ear canal
ear

The grommet is implanted in the ear-drum, to equalize air pressure on either side of it, and to allow the ear to dry out. The grommet is not uncomfortable, and will not affect your child's hearing.

Mouth infections

A baby or child with a mouth infection will have a very sore mouth. Thrush is the most common mouth infection in babies. Children over one are prone to cold sores (see page 230), usually around the lips, but sometimes inside the mouth.

Helping a child with a sore mouth

If your child's mouth is sore, try to make eating and drinking as painless as you can. Allow warm meals to get cool before giving them to your child, since hot food generally hurts more than cold, and offer her plenty of very cold drinks. If she is reluctant to eat or drink, try some of the suggestions given here.

Let your child drink
through a straw or use a teacher beaker, because this may be less painful than drinking from a cup.

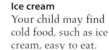

Soup
This is nourishing and easy to eat, and can be served cold. Alternatively, liquidize food, or chop it very small.

Cold drinks
Serve drinks very cold; avoid fruit juice, since it is too acidic.

Ice cream
Your child may find cold food, such as ice cream, easy to eat.

Water

Cheese
Encourage your child to finish meals with cheese and a drink of water to help keep her teeth clean, if she can't brush properly.

Thrush

What is it?

Thrush is an infection caused by a yeast that lives in the mouth and intestines. The yeast is normally kept under control by bacteria, but sometimes it multiplies out of control, producing a sore, irritating rash. It can also cause a rash in the nappy area. Thrush is not a serious infection, and usually clears up with medical treatment.

What can I do?

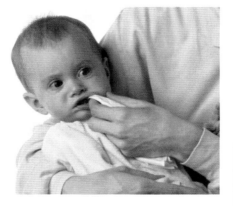

1 Wipe the patches in your child's mouth very gently with a clean handkerchief. If they don't come off easily, she probably has thrush. Don't rub them hard, because if you scrape them off they will leave a sore, bleeding patch underneath.

2 Give your child food that is easy to eat (see above). If you are bottle-feeding, buy a special soft teat and clean it carefully, then sterilize it after each feed.

3 If you are breastfeeding, continue to feed as normal, but take extra care with nipple hygiene. Wash them in water only, not soap, after every feed, and don't wear breast pads. If they are sore or develop white spots, consult your doctor.

☎ Seek medical help
Consult your doctor as soon as possible if you think your baby or child has thrush.

What might the doctor do?

Your doctor may prescribe a medicine to be dropped into your baby's mouth just before a feed, or, for a child over about two, lozenges to suck. If you are breastfeeding, the doctor may prescribe an antifungal cream for your nipples.

Symptoms

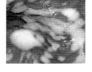

- Creamy yellow, slightly raised patches on the inside of the cheeks, tongue, or the roof of the mouth, which do not come away easily if you try to wipe them off
- reluctance to eat due to a sore mouth
- in babies, a red rash in the nappy area that starts in the creases at the top of the legs.

Throat infections

Sore throats are common in children, and often accompany other illnesses, such as colds or flu. Mild sore throats clear up in a few days, but severe infections, particularly if the tonsils are affected, may give your child a fever, and make swallowing painful.

> ## ☎ Seek medical help
>
> **Consult your doctor as soon as possible** if your child:
> - has such a sore throat that swallowing is painful
> - seems generally unwell and has a fever or rash
> - has infected tonsils
> - has not been immunized against diphtheria.

Sore throat

What is it?
Sore throat is an infection that makes the throat area sore and red. It may be part of a cold or flu (see pages 200–1), or one of the first signs of German measles or mumps (see pages 203 and 206). Children are prone to earache when they have a throat infection (see pages 211–2).

> ## Symptoms
> - Reluctance to eat as it hurts to swallow
> - red, raw-looking throat
> - earache (see page 211–2)
> - slightly raised temperature
> - swollen glands.

What can I do?

1 Ask your child to face a strong light and open his mouth. Examine the back of his throat (see page 189). If it is sore, it will look red and raw, and you may see creamy spots.

2 Gently feel down each side of his neck and just below the angle of his jaw-bone, to check whether his glands are swollen (see page 189).

3 Give your child plenty of cold drinks, and liquidize food if swallowing hurts him. He may find cold food, such as ice cream, less painful to eat than warm food.

4 Take your child's temperature (see page 193), and if necessary give him the recommended dose of paracetemol to bring his fever down.

What might the doctor do?
Most mild sore throats need no treatment, but it is advisable to get medical advice and diagnosis early, especially if the child has a fever or is generally unwell. If the doctor suspects that the infection is caused by bacteria he may prescribe an antibiotic.

Tonsillitis

What is it?
Tonsillitis is inflammation of tonsils, causing a sore throat and other symptoms. The tonsils are glands at the back of the throat, one on either side, which trap infection, and stop it from spreading.

> ## Symptoms
> - Very sore throat
> - red and enlarged tonsils, possibly covered with creamy spots
> - temperature over 38°C (100.4°F)
> - swollen glands on the neck.

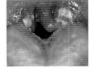

What can I do?

1 Examine your child's tonsils and feel his glands (see page 189). If infected, his tonsils will be large and red, and may have creamy spots.

2 Take his temperature (see page 193). Give him paracetamol or ibuprofen suspension to bring it down, if necessary.

3 Encourage your child to have plenty to drink, especially if he has a fever.

What might the doctor do?
Your doctor will examine your child's throat, and take a throat swab. He may prescribe an antibiotic to clear infection.
    If your child frequently has severe tonsillitis, your doctor may recommend having his tonsils removed. However, this operation is done after a child is four

Coughs and chest infections

Most coughs in small children are a symptom of a cold or flu (see pages 200–1), which produces a dry, tickly cough. If your child finds breathing difficult and coughs up phlegm, he may have a chest infection (see pages 216–9). However, slightly wheezy breathing is normal for a child with a cold, because his airways are narrow and become narrower if they are swollen. A cough may be an early sign of measles (see page 204), and a severe, persistent cough might be whooping cough (see page 207).

Emergency
Call for emergency help immediately if your child:
● has a bluish tinge round his face, mouth, and tongue
● is breathing very rapidly
● is breathing so noisily that it can be heard across the room
● seems to be fighting for breath
● is abnormally drowsy
● is unable to speak or make sounds as usual.

Frequent chest infections
Babies under a year old and children with a long-term chest disorder such as asthma (see page 218) are prone to chest infections. If you smoke, your children are much more likely to develop chest infections than are the children of non-smoking parents.

   If your child has frequent chest infections, your doctor may arrange for tests to find the cause.

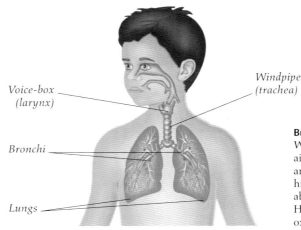

Voice-box (larynx)

Windpipe (trachea)

Bronchi

Lungs

Breathing
When your child breathes in, air is sucked down his windpipe and bronchi (the airways) into his lungs, where oxygen is absorbed into his bloodstream. His blood then carries the oxygen all round his body.

Croup

What is it?
Croup is an inflammation of the voice-box and windpipe, which makes it swell, so that your child finds it difficult to breathe. Attacks of croup tend to occur at night, and usually last about two hours.

Symptoms
● Breathing difficulty
● loud crowing sound as breath is drawn in
● barking cough
● rib recession (sucking in of lower ribs during in-breath).

What can I do?

1 Keep calm, and reassure your child. He is likely to be very frightened, but if he panics, it will be even harder for him to breathe.

2 Create a steamy atmosphere by taking your child into the bathroom and turning on the hot taps. The moist air will soothe his air passages and help him to breathe more easily.

3 Prop your child up on pillows, or hold him on your lap – he will be able to breathe easily in these positions.

☎ Seek medical help
Call your doctor now if your child has difficulty breathing, or if you think he has croup.

4 Make sure he drinks plenty of fluids to prevent dehydration.

5 When the attack has abated, don't allow anyone to smoke near him, and keep a window open to circulate fresh air. Make sure the room doesn't get too cold.

6 Don't give your child any medicine that might make him drowsy.

What might the doctor do?
The doctor will tell you what to do if the croup recurs. If the attack is severe, the doctor might send your child to hospital where he will be carefully monitored and may be given a medicated inhalation.

Cough

What is it?

A cough is a protective reflex action that helps to clear any irritants or blockages from the airways. It can be either a reaction to irritation in the throat or windpipe, or the result of an infection of the respiratory tract. It may also be caused by an obstruction in the airways. A cough will generally disappear of its own accord.

A dry, ticklish cough, without sputum, is rarely serious. It probably means that your child's throat or windpipe is irritated, which may be a by-product of a cold, because mucus dribbles down the throat, and irritates it. Her throat might also be irritated, if she is with adults who smoke. An ear infection can also cause a dry cough. If your child has a moist-sounding cough, and brings up vomit while she coughs, then she probably has a minor respiratory infection. While most coughs like this are not serious, they can be a symptom of bronchiolitis, bronchitis, or pneumonia (see pages 217–9). Coughing only at night could be a sign of asthma (see page 218).

☎ Seek medical help

Consult your doctor as soon as possible if:
- your baby is under six months
- the cough prevents your child from sleeping
- the cough does not improve in three days
- your child has a recurrent cough.

What might the doctor do?

The doctor will examine your child, and listen to her breathing.

If your child has a dry cough, the doctor may prescribe a cough medicine that will help soothe her throat.

If the cough is particularly chesty, the doctor may carry out some diagnostic tests. He may prescribe antibiotics, and perhaps a cough medicine, to make the phlegm easier to cough up.

What can I do?

1 If your child has a sudden attack of coughing, check whether she has inhaled a small object, such as a sweet or a button (see Choking, page 242), but don't put your fingers down her throat to try to hook it out.

2 If your child has a chesty cough, help her to clear the phlegm from her chest when she is coughing. Support her as she leans forwards. Hold a small bowl, and encourage her to spit out any phlegm that she coughs up. However, most young children will swallow their phlegm.

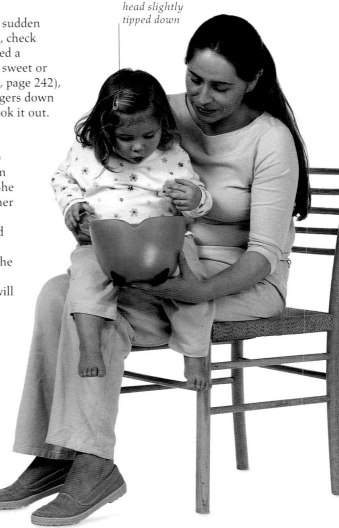

Keep your child's *head slightly tipped down*

3 If your child has a dry cough, a warm drink at bedtime will ease her throat. Ask your chemist for a soothing cough linctus that is suitable for children.

4 Make sure that your child's bedroom is not overheated because this will dry out the air. If the air becomes too dry, it will aggravate her cough.

5 Moisten the air in her bedroom at night by hanging a wet towel near a radiator.

6 Don't allow anyone to smoke around your child.

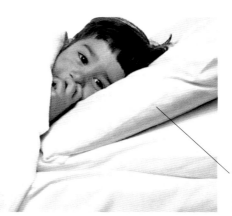

If she is over 18 months *extra pillows will prevent mucus dribbling down her throat at night*

Bronchiolitis

What is it?

Bronchiolitis is a common and usually mild viral illness that causes inflammation of the smallest airways in the lungs, called bronchioles. It occurs in epidemics during the winter. Those most commonly affected are babies under a year old. The risk of a child getting bronchiolitis increases if his parents are smokers, or if he lives in overcrowded accommodation in which viral infections spread more easily.

Your baby may have a runny nose for a day or two, and then suddenly seem much worse, with a fever, dry rasping cough, and rapid or difficult breathing. Mild bronchiolitis usually improves within a week or so.

Symptoms

- Runny nose
- fever
- dry, rasping cough
- rapid or difficult breathing
- wheezing
- feeding difficulties.

What can I do?

1 Give your baby plenty of drinks to make sure that he is getting enough fluids.

2 No drug will alter the course of the illness, but paracetamol suspension especially formulated for babies and children will help bring down his temperature.

3 Increase the humidity in your child's bedroom by hanging a wet towel near a source of heat, such as the radiator. This will help to relieve your child's breathing.

4 Raise the head of your baby's cot or bed slightly by putting a book with a 1.5in (4cm) spine under each leg (see page 201). If your baby is over 18 months, you can give him an extra pillow.

☎ Seek medical help

Consult your doctor as soon as possible if:

- your child is breathing faster than usual, or his breathing is laboured or wheezy
- your child is having difficulty feeding
- your child looks bluish around the lips.

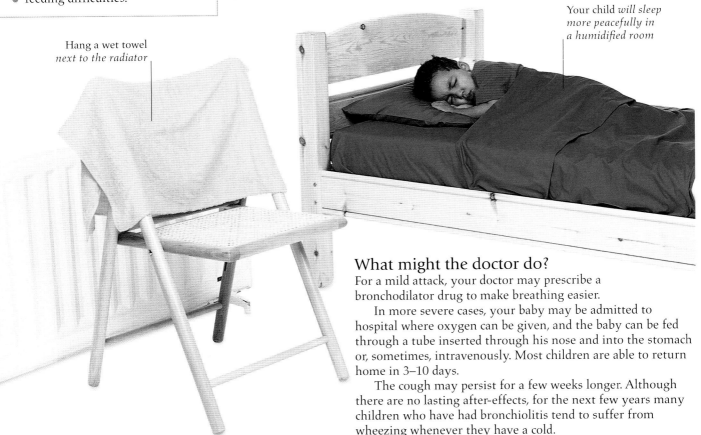

Hang a wet towel *next to the radiator*

Your child *will sleep more peacefully in a humidified room*

What might the doctor do?

For a mild attack, your doctor may prescribe a bronchodilator drug to make breathing easier.

In more severe cases, your baby may be admitted to hospital where oxygen can be given, and the baby can be fed through a tube inserted through his nose and into the stomach or, sometimes, intravenously. Most children are able to return home in 3–10 days.

The cough may persist for a few weeks longer. Although there are no lasting after-effects, for the next few years many children who have had bronchiolitis tend to suffer from wheezing whenever they have a cold.

Bronchitis

What is it?
Bronchitis is an inflammation of the lining of the bronchi (the main air passages leading to the lungs). It usually follows a viral infection, such as a cold, flu, or sore throat, because the infection spreads downwards, but the inflammation may also be caused by a bacterial infection.

Your child probably won't feel particularly ill, but he may have difficulty sleeping if his cough tends to be worse at night.

Symptoms
- Rattly cough
- slight wheeziness
- slight temperature
- runny nose.

What can I do?

1 Help to relieve wheezy breathing, and clear your child's lungs, when he has a coughing fit. Support your child as he leans forwards, and pat his back.

2 Take your child's temperature and, if it is raised, give him paracetamol or ibuprofen suspension. Also give him plenty of water to drink.

3 Raise the head of the baby's cot by placing a book under the legs. When your older child goes to bed, try to prop him up in bed with extra pillows (see page 216).

4 Until your child is feeling better, make sure that he is kept indoors in a warm, though not too hot or stuffy, room.

☎ Seek medical help
Call for emergency help immediately if your child shows any of the emergency signs listed on page 215. **Consult your doctor as soon as possible** if you think your child may have bronchitis, and call him again if he:
- shows no sign of improvement after two days
- coughs up greenish-yellow coloured phlegm.

What might the doctor do?
If your doctor thinks your child has a bacterial infection he might prescribe an antibiotic to eliminate it.

Asthma

What is it?
Asthma is a series of recurrent episodes of narrowing of the tiny airways leading to the lungs, which makes breathing, especially breathing out, difficult. In young children it is usually triggered by colds and viral infections, not by allergies. Mild asthma is common, and children who develop it at a very young age are more likely to grow out of the condition as they grow older.

Symptoms
- Coughing, particularly at night, or after exercise
- slight wheeziness and breathlessness, especially during a cold
- attacks of severe breathlessness, when breathing is shallow and difficult
- feeling of suffocation during an asthma attack
- pale and sweaty skin during an attack
- blue tinge round the lips during a severe attack.

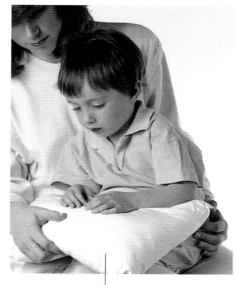

Put a small cushion *on his lap for him to lean on*

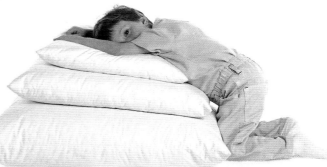

What can I do?

1 Keep calm, and reassure your child. If he has had previous attacks, give him whatever medicine the doctor has prescribed. If this has no effect, **call for emergency help.**

2 Sit your child on your lap, and help him to lean slightly forwards – this makes it easier for him to breathe. Don't hold him tightly – let him settle into the most comfortable position.

3 If your child prefers to sit on his own, give him something to rest his arms on – a table top or pile of pillows, for example – so that he leans forwards.

Pneumonia

What is it?

Pneumonia is an inflammation of the lungs, which causes breathing difficulty. Usually only a portion of the lungs is affected, but in severe cases both lungs may be affected.

In young children, pneumonia is nearly always due to the spread of an upper respiratory tract infection, such as a cold or flu, and is usually caused by a virus, not bacteria.

Occasionally, pneumonia is the result of a tiny amount of food being inhaled into the lungs, causing a small patch of inflammation and infection.

Pneumonia is most common in babies under a year old. Although it is a serious disease, most babies who are otherwise healthy will usually recover completely in about a week, and it will not result in any long-term damage to the lung tissues.

Symptoms

- Deterioration in a sick child
- raised temperature
- dry cough
- rapid breathing
- difficult or noisy breathing.

☎ Seek medical help

Call for emergency help immediately if your child develops any of the emergency signs listed on page 215. **Call your doctor now** if you think your child has pneumonia.

What can I do?

1 Prop your child up with extra pillows in bed, so that he can breathe more easily. For a baby, you might try putting him into a car seat.

2 Take your child's temperature and, if it is raised, try to reduce it by giving him the recommended dose of paracetamol or ibuprofen suspension.

3 Make sure your child has plenty to drink, especially if his temperature is raised. Give your baby cooled, boiled water.

What might the doctor do?

The doctor will advise you how to care for your child, and if the infection is bacterial, he may prescribe an antibiotic. If your child is very ill, he might need to be treated in a hospital.

Emergency

Call for emergency help immediately if your child:
- has a bluish tinge on his tongue or round his lips
- is severely breathless
- does not start to breathe more easily 10 minutes after taking his medicine
- becomes unresponsive.

☎ Seek medical help

Call your doctor now if this is your child's first asthma attack. **Consult your doctor as soon as possible** if you think your child may have asthma.

What might the doctor do?

If your child's asthma is mild, the doctor may recommend a bronchodilator drug that he can inhale whenever he has symptoms. If he has the symptoms daily, a drug to prevent attacks every day may be prescribed.

Preventing asthma attacks

Try to find out what causes your child's asthma attacks by keeping a record of when they occur. Vigorous exercise and over-excitement can bring on an attack. Some other common triggers are shown here.

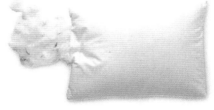

Feather-filled cushions or duvets
Change these for ones with a synthetic filling, and air them regularly.

House dust mites
Reduce house dust by vacuuming and damp sponging, rather than sweeping and dusting. Cover your child's mattress with a plastic sheet. Consider buying special bedding that reduces dust levels.

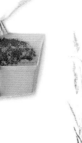

Pollen, especially from grass and trees
Discourage your child from playing in long grass, and keep him inside when the pollen count is high.

Animal fur
If you have a pet, let it stay somewhere else for a while, and note whether your child has fewer attacks.

Cigarette smoke
Don't let people smoke near your child.

Stomach pain

Stomach pain can be a symptom of many disorders, including gastroenteritis and urinary tract infections. It may also be caused by vomiting, and can accompany illnesses, such as tonsillitis and measles.

Your child may complain of a tummy ache if he feels generally unwell, knows he is about to be sick, or if he has a pain elsewhere but can't quite describe its precise location.

Dealing with a tummy ache

What causes stomach pain?
Many children have recurrent bouts of stomach pain when something makes them feel anxious or insecure. Provided that your child's pain is not severe and lasts for only an hour or two, you needn't worry; try to find out what is bothering him, and reassure him.

However, if your child is in severe pain for a few hours you should take it seriously. He might have appendicitis, although this is extremely rare in children under three. Typically, appendicitis pain is felt around the navel for a few hours, then moves to the lower right part of the abdomen.

Waves of severe stomach pain at intervals of about 15–20 minutes in a baby or toddler may mean that his bowel has become blocked.

What can I do?

1 Take your child's temperature. If it is slightly raised, he may have appendicitis, especially if the stomach pain is severe, or seems to be located around his navel. Don't give him a pain killer to ease it, or anything to reduce his temperature.

2 If you think your child may have appendicitis, don't give him anything to eat or drink. Give him some water only if he is thirsty.

3 Comfort your child by giving him cuddles and extra attention.

4 If you don't suspect appendicitis, fill a hot water bottle with warm water and wrap it in a towel. Let your child lie down with this held against his stomach.

☎ **Seek medical help**
Call your doctor now if your child:
● develops any other symptoms
● has stomach pains for longer than three hours.
Consult your doctor if your child has frequent stomach pain.

Wrap the hot water bottle *securely in a towel*

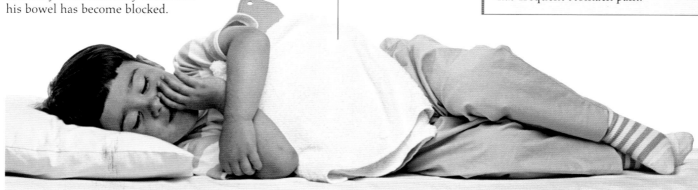

Emergency
Call for emergency help immediately if your baby or child:
● screams with pain at intervals of about 15–20 minutes, and goes pale when he screams
● passes dark red stools that resemble redcurrant jelly
● has severe stomach pain for longer than three hours
● has severe stomach pain combined with a raised body temperature.

What might the doctor do?
The doctor will examine your child to try to find out the cause of his stomach pain. The treatment will depend on his diagnosis, but stomach pain often needs no treatment. If the doctor suspects appendicitis or a blocked bowel, he will arrange for your child to go to hospital for an emergency operation.

Constipation, vomiting, and diarrhoea

A minor change in your child's diet can cause temporary constipation or diarrhoea. Vomiting or diarrhoea may accompany almost any illness, and can also be caused by excitement or anxiety.

Frequent vomiting or severe diarrhoea can quickly make a baby or a young child dehydrated. This is a serious condition and must be treated promptly (see page 222).

Constipation

What is it?
If your child has constipation he passes stools less frequently than usual, and they are harder than normal. Children's bowel habits vary greatly: some children have a bowel movement twice a day, others go only once every two or three days. Whatever your child's regular pattern is, it is quite normal and nothing to worry about unless it suddenly changes.

☎ Seek medical help
Consult your doctor as soon as possible if your child:
- cries or complains of pain when moving his bowels
- has streaks of blood in his stools, or on his nappy or pants
- has constipation for more than three days.

What can I do?

1 Don't worry if your child is temporarily constipated, it won't do him any harm. Don't give him a laxative, because this will upset the normal action of his bowels, and don't add sugar to his bottle.

2 Give your child plenty of fluids to drink, especially if the weather is hot – this will help to soften his stools. Fruit juice will ease his constipation. Don't let your child drink more than 500ml (1 pint) a day.

3 Don't hurry your child when he is sitting on potty, but on the other hand, don't let him remain there for too long.

4 Try to include more fibre in your child's diet (see below). This provides the bulk that facilitates bowel movement.

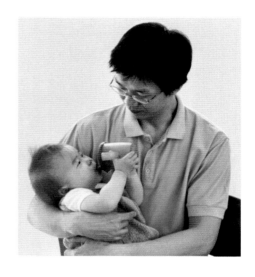

What might the doctor do?
The doctor may prescribe a mild laxative, and give you some advice on your child's diet. If your child has streaks of blood in his stools he could have a small tear in the lining of his anus. This usually heals when the constipation is treated.

Good sources of fibre
Some examples of foods rich in fibre are shown here. Fresh foods are always the best. Wash vegetables and fruit thoroughly, remove pips and strings, and peel for a child under one year old. Purée the food for a baby under eight months (see pages 110–1).

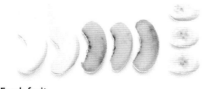

Fresh fruit
Offer your child a variety of fruit, such as slices of peeled pear, peach, and banana.

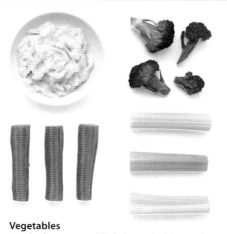

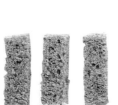

Wholemeal bread

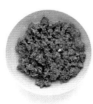

Wholemeal breakfast cereal

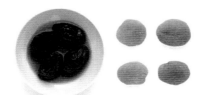

Dried fruit
Prunes and apricots are ideal for young children.

Vegetables
Mashed potato and lightly cooked broccoli are high in fibre. Carrots and celery can be served raw.

Vomiting

What is it?

When your child vomits, she will bring up most of the contents of her stomach. Most cases clear up within 24 hours, but young children and babies can dehydrate rapidly, so make sure your child drinks plenty of fluids.

Babies under about six months old often regurgitate a small amount of their feeds. This is known as "posseting" and is normal – your baby is not vomiting.

Identifying and treating dehydration

Your child may be dehydrated if she shows one or more of the symptoms listed below:
- dry mouth and lips
- dark, concentrated urine
- no urine passed for six hours
- sunken eyes
- sunken fontanelle
- abnormal drowsiness or lethargy.

If your child is dehydrated, or is in danger of becoming so, buy a ready-mixed oral rehydration powder from your chemist. If you are breastfeeding, give rehydration solution before the breastfeed.

What can I do?

1 Hold your child over a bowl and comfort her while she is vomiting (see page 199). Wipe her face afterwards and give her some sips of water.

2 Make sure that your child has plenty to drink – she needs 1–1½ litres (2–3 pints) a day. Make up a rehydration solution from the oral rehydration powder, and offer her a little every hour. If your baby won't take a bottle, try using a teaspoon or a medicine syringe (see page 195).

☎ Seek medical help

Call your doctor now if your child:
- vomits and seems abnormally drowsy
- throws up greenish-yellow vomit
- has vomited repeatedly for more than six hours
- shows any signs of dehydration.

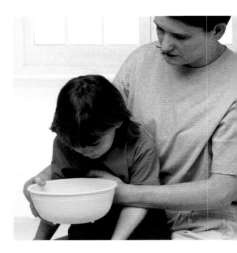

What might the doctor do?

The doctor will examine your child to find out what is making her vomit, and will then treat her according to the diagnosis.

If she shows signs of dehydration, the doctor may recommend persevering with oral rehydration fluids or may arrange for her to be admitted to hospital, where she can be given fluids through a drip.

Gastroenteritis

What is it?

Gastroenteritis is an infection in the stomach and intestines that can be caused by contaminated food. It is serious in babies, because it can dehydrate them very quickly, but it is rare in breastfed babies. A mild attack in a child over two years old is not serious.

Symptoms
- Vomiting and nausea
- diarrhoea
- stomach cramps
- loss of appetite
- raised temperature.

What can I do?

1 Make sure that your child drinks about 1–1½ litres (2–3 pints) a day. Give an oral rehydration solution from your chemist. Oral rehydration is successful in at least 95 per cent of cases.

2 Don't give your child anything to eat until she stops vomiting, then introduce bland foods. Continue your baby's usual milk feeds (see page 185).

3 Take your child's temperature and, if it is raised, give her a dose of paracetamol syrup to reduce it.

4 Let your child wear a nappy again if she has just grown out of them.

5 Make sure that your child washes her hands properly after using her potty and before eating. Wash your own hands after changing her nappy and before preparing food. Sterilize all her feeding equipment.

Note: Breastfed babies should continue to breastfeed.

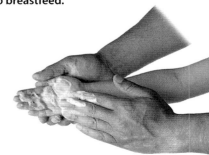

Diarrhoea

What is it?

If your child has diarrhoea, she will pass watery stools more frequently than normal. This may be the result of eating food that is too rich for her or contains more fibre than she is used to. It may also be caused by an infection. Give your child plenty of fluids to prevent dehydration.

☎ Seek medical help

Call your doctor now if your child:
● has had diarrhoea for more than 24 hours
● has blood in her stools
● shows any signs of dehydration (see page 222).

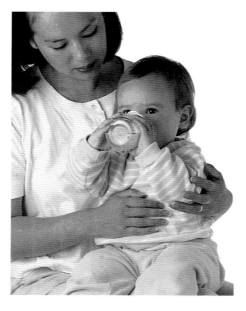

What can I do?

1 Make sure that your child always has plenty of water to drink (see Dehydration, page 222).

2 Put your child in a nappy again if she has just grown out of them. This will prevent any unnecessary soiling.

3 Always pay careful attention to hygiene: wash your hands after changing your baby's nappy and before preparing her food, and make sure that your child washes her hands after using the potty and before eating.

Abnormal-looking faeces

Changes in colour of your child's faeces are probably caused by a change in her diet, so check whether she has eaten anything unusual. Sometimes, though, an underlying illness may account for the different appearance of the faeces.

● **Very pale, bulky faeces** that smell offensive may mean that your child can't digest gluten, a protein found in cereals (coeliac disease). Consult your doctor.
● **Frothy, acid faeces** may indicate that your child can't digest milk properly (lactose intolerance). Consult a doctor.

What might the doctor do?

The doctor will examine your child to find out the cause of her diarrhoea, and will treat her according to the diagnosis. If your child has become dehydrated, the doctor may prescribe oral rehydration fluids to supplement her drinks. If she is very dehydrated, he might arrange for her to be admitted to hospital, where she can be given extra fluids through a drip.

☎ Seek medical help

Call your doctor now if your child:
● is under two and you suspect may have gastroenteritis
● is over two and has had symptoms of gastroenteritis for more than two days.

What might the doctor do?

The doctor will probably treat your child for dehydration and may advise you to give her only liquids for a few days. He may also ask for a sample of your child's faeces.

"What steps can I take to prevent gastroenteritis?"
Sterilize all your baby's feeding equipment for as long as she drinks milk from a bottle (see pages 100–1). Always make a fresh feed for your baby. Never store made-up feeds in the fridge or keep them warm in a vacuum flask, since bacteria thrive in warm conditions.

Be scrupulous about personal hygiene, and pay particular attention to hygiene when preparing food. If you store any cooked food, keep it in the fridge for no longer than two days, and make sure it is piping hot when you reheat it because heat kills the bacteria that could give your child gastroenteritis. Avoid using a microwave, because it tends to heat quite unevenly.

Wash your child's feeding bowls and beakers in very hot water. Dry all the feeding equipment on kitchen paper, not a tea towel.

If you are travelling abroad, ask your doctor or health visitor about any precautions you should take, particularly with regard to water, fruit, and salads. Always take an oral rehydration powder with you – in the event your child is struck down by gastroenteritis, this will help to prevent dehydration.

Q&A

Bladder, kidney, and genital problems

Most urinary system infections are due to bacteria entering the urethra, and spreading up into the bladder. They are quite common in young children, and are usually not serious. Some children are born with minor abnormalities of the urinary system, which make them prone to such infections. Minor infections of the genitals are often part of the nappy rash symptoms (see page 182).

The urinary system
Your child has two kidneys that filter his blood. The clean blood returns to his bloodstream, while the waste product (the urine) drains into his bladder, where it collects until he is ready to urinate.

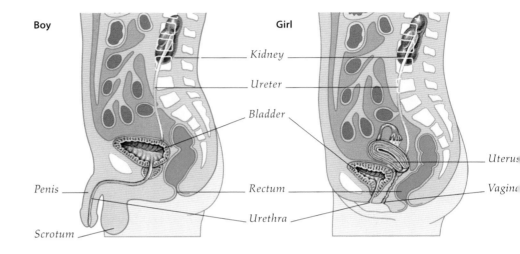

Boy / Girl

Kidney
Ureter
Bladder
Penis
Rectum
Uterus
Urethra
Vagina
Scrotum

Urinary system infections

What are they?
Any part of the urinary system – the kidneys, the bladder, and the connecting tubes – can become infected with bacteria. Infections are more common in girls because the tube from the bladder (the urethra) is shorter than in a boy, and its opening is nearer to the anus, so germs can spread to it more easily.

What can I do?

1 If your child seems unwell, check to see whether her urine looks pink or cloudy. Note whether she is urinating more frequently than usual, and whether it seems to hurt her to pass urine. If your child is still in nappies, you probably won't be able to tell that urination is frequent or painful, but you may notice a change in odour of the urine.

2 Make sure that your child has plenty to drink, to keep her kidneys flushed out.

3 Take your child's temperature and, if it is raised, give her the prescribed dose of paracetamol or ibuprofen suspension to reduce it.

> ☎ **Seek medical help**
> **Consult your doctor as soon as possible** if you think your child has a urinary system infection.

Symptoms
- Urinating more often than usual
- pain when urinating
- pink, red, or cloudy urine
- change in odour of the urine
- raised temperature
- listlessness
- loss of appetite
- abdominal pain.

What might the doctor do?
The doctor will examine your child, and if he suspects an infection will ask you to take a sample of her urine. If your child has an infection, the doctor will prescribe an antibiotic. He may also arrange for special tests or investigations to check her kidneys and urinary tract.

Genital problems in girls

What can go wrong?

A little girl's vagina can become sore due to nappy rash (see page 182), an infection such as thrush (see page 213), or threadworms (see page 232).

If your daughter has a blood-stained or smelly discharge from her vagina, she may have pushed something into it. Newborn girls often produce a white or blood-stained discharge for a few days, and this is nothing to worry about. After this age until just before puberty, a discharge is abnormal, and should be investigated by a doctor.

What can I do?

1 If your daughter's bottom is sore or red, don't use soap when you wash it as this may irritate it even more – just use water, and dry it thoroughly. Always wipe from the front to back, so that germs can't spread forwards from her anus.

2 Allow your child to go without a nappy for as long as possible each day, and don't put plastic pants over her nappies as they prevent air circulating to her bottom.

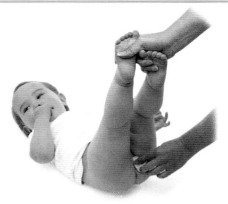

3 If your daughter has a discharge from her vagina, check whether she has pushed something into it. If she has, **consult your doctor as soon as possible.**

Symptoms

- Soreness or itching in or around the vagina
- redness around the vagina
- discharge from the vagina.

> ## ☎ Seek medical help
>
> **Consult your doctor as soon as possible** if your daughter:
> - has a discharge from her vagina
> - still has symptoms after two days of home treatment
> - has pushed something into vagina.

What might the doctor do?

The doctor will examine your daughter, and may take a sample of the discharge. If she has something lodged in her vagina, he will remove it gently. If she has an infection, he may prescribe antibiotics to be taken by mouth, or a cream to be applied to the affected area, depending on the cause of her symptoms.

Genital problems in boys

What can go wrong?

The foreskin, which covers the tip of the penis, can become inflamed or infected (balanitis), often as part of nappy rash (see page 182).

If a swelling develops in your son's groin or scrotum, he may have a hernia (a loop of intestines bulging through a weak area in the wall of the abdomen), which will require medical attention.

What can I do?

Wash and dry his foreskin carefully at each nappy change, and let him go without a nappy for as long as possible each day. Use an enzyme-free washing powder, and rinse nappies and pants well.

How can I prevent inflammation?

Don't try to pull your son's foreskin back – it won't retract until he is at least four. If you try to force it, you may cause his foreskin to inflame.

> ## ☎ Seek medical help
>
> **Consult your doctor as soon as possible** if:
> - your son's foreskin looks red or swollen, or if there is any discharge
> - your son's hernia becomes painful, the bulge grows or changes in any other way
> - you think your son may have a hernia.

Symptoms

Inflamed foreskin
- Red, swollen foreskin
- discharge of pus from the penis.

Hernia
- Soft, painless bulge in the groin or scrotum, which may disappear when your child lies down, and get bigger when he coughs, sneezes, or cries.

Circumcision

This is an operation to remove the foreskin. If you are thinking of having your son circumcised, first discuss it with your doctor. Like any other operation, it carries a small risk, so it is usually done only for religious or medical reasons.

What might the doctor do?

If your son's foreskin is inflamed, the doctor may prescribe an antibiotic cream. If your son has a hernia your doctor will recommend that he has an operation to repair it. If the hernia is painful or tender, the doctor may send him to hospital straightaway for emergency surgery.

Skin problems

Minor skin problems are common in childhood. Most clear up quickly, but some are very contagious, and must be treated promptly. If your child has a rash combined with other signs of illness, she may have an infectious illness (see pages 203–8). For other problems, see below.

Quick diagnosis guide

One or more red spots, or a rash, see Spots and boils, Hives, Heat rash (below and opposite), Insect stings (page 252), or, if dry and scaly, see Eczema (page 228).
Raw, cracked areas, usually on or around the lips, or on the cheeks and hands, see Chapped skin (page 229).
Small blisters or crusty patches on or around the mouth, see Cold sores and Impetigo (pages 230–1).
Hard lump of skin, usually on the hands or feet, see Warts and verrucas (page 230).
Itchy head, see Lice and nits (page 232).
Intense itching around the anus, see Threadworms (page 232).

Dealing with itching

Many skin problems cause itching, and since scratching can make the skin infected, it is important to relieve your child's itchiness.
● Dress her in cotton clothes, since cotton is less irritating to the skin than wool or other fabrics.
● Gently dab the area with cotton wool soaked in calamine lotion, to soothe inflamed or irritated skin.
● Add a handful of bicarbonate of soda in your child's bath.
● Buy cotton scratch mitts for her to wear in bed.

Spots and boils

What are they?

A spot is a small red swelling, usually on the face. A boil is an infection in the skin that causes a large, painful lump, which then festers to produce a head of pus in the middle. Boils are most likely to occur on the face or on pressure points such as the buttocks, but they can appear anywhere on the body.

Don't worry if your child gets occasional spots, but recurrent boils may be a sign of illness.

Symptoms

Spot
● Small, red, painless lump.

Boil
● Painful, red lump that gradually gets larger
● white or yellow centre of pus appearing after a day or two.

☎ Seek medical help

Consult your doctor as soon as possible if:
● your child has a spot that looks inflamed
● your child has a boil in an awkward or painful place
● the centre of pus does not appear three days after the boil first developed
● red streaks spread out from the boil.
● your child gets boils on a frequent basis.

What can I do?

1 If your child gets occasional spots, simply ignore them. They will clear up in a few days without treatment. If she tends to dribble, and the spots appear around her mouth, smear a small amount of barrier cream over the area.

2 If your child has a boil, or a spot that looks inflamed, gently clean it, and the skin around it, with cotton wool and cool boiled water.

3 If it is rubbed by clothing, or is in a painful place such as on the buttocks, cover it with a sterile dry dressing.

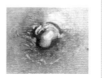

4 The boil will come to a head and burst of its own accord in a few days. Don't squeeze it – this may spread the infection. After it has burst, clean it gently with cotton wool dipped in antiseptic cream, and keep it covered until it has healed.

What might the doctor do?

The doctor may lance the boil and drain away the pus, and might prescribe a cream. If your child has a lot of boils, or if they keep recurring, the doctor may prescribe a course of antibiotics.

Hives

What is it?

Hives (also known as nettle rash or urticaria) is an intensely itchy rash of red patches. The patches usually fade after a few hours, but new ones may appear. A nettle sting is the most common cause, but it can be caused by strong sunshine or by an allergy to certain foods (for example, milk or a citrus fruit) or drugs (for instance, penicillin).

Symptoms

- Itchy rash of raised red patches (weals), sometimes with a pale centre
- welts varying in length from 1mm to 1cm (¹⁄₁₆ to ½in)
- larger weals joining together
- sudden swelling of lips, face, and tongue (Angioedema).

What can I do?

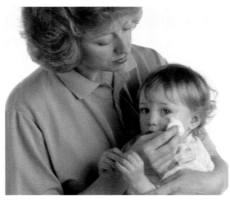

1 Dab your child's rash with cotton wool dipped in calamine lotion. Piriton, an antihistamine available over the counter, will help, although it may make your child drowsy.

2 If the rash is caused by an allergy, try to find out what your child is allergic to, so that it can be avoided in future. Try to remember whether, for example, she has recently eaten a new food.

☎ Seek medical help

Call your doctor now if your child's face, tongue, or throat is swollen. You might use an Epipen, which is an antihistamine already prescribed by your doctor to administer to your child when she has an allergy attack. **Consult your doctor as soon as possible** if:
- the rash does not disappear within four hours
- your child has frequent attacks.

What might the doctor do?

The doctor may prescribe an antihistamine cream or medication. He might also carry out tests to discover the cause of your child's allergy. If your child's face, tongue, or throat is swollen, she might need an injection to reduce the swelling.

Heat rash

What is it?

Heat rash is a faint rash caused by overheating. It is more common in babies than in children, and usually appears on the face or in skin creases, where sweat can gather. It is not a serious disorder, and you can treat it yourself at home.

Symptoms

- Pink rash on the face or in skin creases
- the site may be itchy.

☎ Seek medical help

Consult your doctor as soon as possible if the rash has not faded 12 hours after your child cools down.

What can I do?

1 Take off any heavy bedding and remove a layer of your baby's clothing. Let him sleep dressed in just a vest and nappy.

2 Give him a bath in lukewarm water. Pat his skin dry gently, leaving it slightly damp so that he cools down as his skin dries. When he is dry, dress him in cotton clothing.

3 Take your baby's temperature and, if it is raised, give him the recommended dose of paracetamol or ibuprofen suspension.

How can I prevent heat rash?

Dress your baby in light clothes when the weather is hot, with cotton next to his skin rather than wool or a manmade fibre. Keep him in the shade, or put a sun canopy over him.

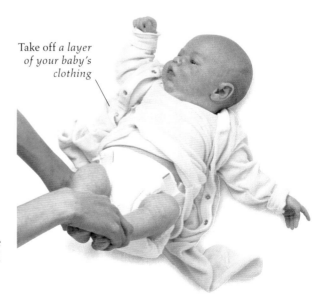

Take off *a layer of your baby's clothing*

What might the doctor do?

The doctor will check that the rash is just a heat rash. If it is, your baby needs no medical treatment. If the rash has another cause, the doctor will treat that.

Atopic eczema

What is it?

Atopic eczema is an allergic condition in which there are areas of inflamed, itchy, red, scaly skin. It most commonly affects the face and skin creases, such as the inside of the elbows and the back of the knees, although it can appear anywhere on the body.

It usually first appears between the ages of three months and two years, then improves as the child grows older. About half of all children with eczema grow out of it by the age of six, and nearly all of them grow out of it by puberty. Your child is more likely to develop eczema if other members of the family suffer from eczema or from any other allergic condition, such as asthma or hayfever.

Symptoms

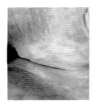

- Itchy, red, scaly, dry patches, usually on the face or in skin creases
- clear fluid oozing from the affected areas.

☎ Seek medical help

Consult your doctor as soon as possible if:
- your child's eczema is very widespread or very itchy
- fluid is weeping from the eczema.

What might the doctor do?

The doctor may prescribe a cream, and if the area is infected, an antibiotic. If your child is allergic to a particular food, your doctor or health visitor can advise you how to give him a balanced diet while avoiding that food.

What can I do?

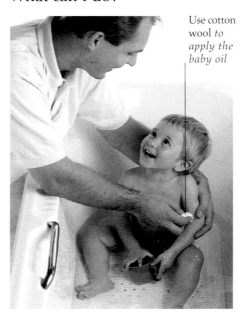

Use cotton wool *to apply the baby oil*

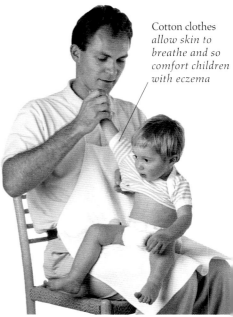

Cotton clothes *allow skin to breathe and so comfort children with eczema*

1 When you give your child a bath, clean the affected areas by wiping them with natural unscented baby oil or aqueous cream, or emulsifying ointment, rather than washing with soap. Rinse well with water.

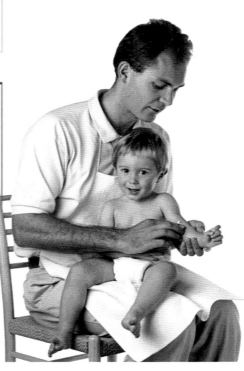

2 After a bath, apply an unscented moisturizing cream to your child's skin, since it may be very dry. Babies' brands are ideal.

3 Dress your child in cotton, rather than wool. In cold weather, put cotton clothing under warmer layers.

4 Try to stop your child scratching the affected areas – put scratch mitts on him at night if this seems to help, and keep his fingernails short.

5 Try to discover the cause of the allergy. Common allergens include foods (especially dairy produce and wheat), animal fur, woollen clothes, and washing powder and fabric conditioner. Anxiety can trigger eczema, so find out if anything is worrying your child.

6 When your child's eczema is bad, keep him away from anyone with chicken pox or a cold sore.

Sunburn

What is it?
Sunburn is sore or reddened skin caused by over-exposure to ultra-violet rays from the sun. The skin becomes hot and tender, and may blister if badly burnt. Babies and young children, especially those with fair hair and blue eyes, are particularly vulnerable to it. Too much exposure to the sun increases the risk of skin cancer in later life.

Symptoms
- Red, sore areas of skin
- blisters appearing on badly affected areas
- flaking or peeling skin a day or two later.

What can I do?

1 Take your child inside or into the shade as soon as his skin begins to look red. Bear in mind that the worst symptoms of sunburn are likely to be delayed for a few hours.

2 Cool any reddened areas of skin with cold water, then apply a soothing after-sun lotion or dab on some calamine lotion.

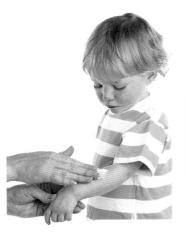

Preventing sunburn
Never leave your baby to sleep in the sun, and try to minimize the amount of time an older child spends playing out in the sun. Make sure that your child wears protective clothing at all times. An old T-shirt can be worn over a bathing suit while swimming. In particular, your child should always wear a hat. Apply Factor 40+ sunscreen **before** your child goes outdoors in the sun, making sure that every part of the body is covered. Re-apply the sunscreen every hour, and always after he has been playing in the water.

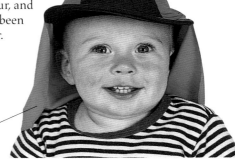

Choose a hat *that protects your child's neck*

☎ Seek medical help
Consult your doctor as soon as possible if:
- your child has a fever and seems unwell
- blisters appear over large area.

What might the doctor do?
The doctor may prescribe a soothing and healing cream.

Chapped skin

What is it?
Chaps are small cracks in the skin that occur when the skin becomes dry after being exposed to cold or hot, dry air. Chapping is not serious, but it can be painful.

What can I do?

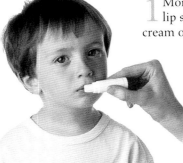

1 Moisturize your child's lips with lip salve, and apply moisturizing cream or Vaseline to his skin.

2 Use baby oil or lotion to wash the area, and keep his hands warm and dry. If your child habitually licks his lips, encourage him to stop as this can cause chapping.

Symptoms
- Tiny cracks in the skin, usually on or around the lips, or on the cheeks or hands
- bleeding if the cracks are deep.

☎ Seek medical help
Consult your doctor as soon as possible if:
- the cracks do not heal after three days
- the cracks become red, sore, or pus-filled.

What might the doctor do?
The doctor might suggest a moisturizer or, if the area is infected, prescribe an antibiotic.

Cold sores

What are they?
Cold sores are small blisters, usually on or around the lips but they sometimes develop inside the mouth or elsewhere on the face. They may be tender and painful.

They are caused by a strain of the herpes simplex virus that, once it has infected a child, lies dormant in the skin and tends to flare up occasionally. So if your child has had a cold sore, he is liable to get others in the future. Strong sunlight or cold winds can trigger a recurrence, and so can a minor illness, such as a cold (which is why they are known as cold sores). Anxiety or emotional stress may also reactivate the virus.

Symptoms
- Raised, red area that tingles or itches, usually around the mouth
- small, painful yellow blisters forming about a day later
- blisters crusting over after a day or two
- fever and general illness during the first attack.

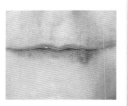

What can I do?

1 At the first sign of a cold sore, hold an ice cube against the affected area for 10 minutes. This may prevent the blister developing.

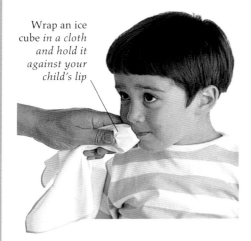

Wrap an ice cube in a cloth and hold it against your child's lip

2 Keep his hands clean, and stop him touching the sore, as he could spread the infection to his eyes.

3 Since cold sores are very contagious, don't let your child kiss other people and, if he tends to put toys into his mouth, don't let him share them with other children until the sore has gone.

4 If your child has ever had a cold sore, protect his lips from strong sunlight with a sunscreen because sunlight can trigger a recurrence.

☎ Seek medical help
Consult your doctor as soon as possible if:
- your child has a cold sore for the first time
- your child's cold sore starts to weep or spread
- your child has a cold sore near his eyes.

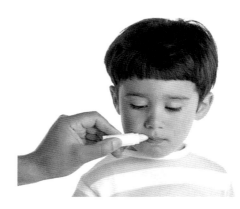

What might the doctor do?
The doctor may prescribe an antiviral cream, which should be applied on the cold sore at the first sign of an attack to make it less severe.

Warts and verrucas

What are they?
A wart is a lump of hard, dry skin; a verruca is a wart on the sole of the foot. They are caused by a virus that invades the skin, and are contagious. Almost all children get occasional warts or verrucas. Warts are not painful, and disappear spontaneously, usually after a few months, so treatment is not necessary. Verrucas tend to be painful because of the pressure put on them whenever the child walks or wears shoes, so they should be treated promptly.

Symptoms
Wart
- Hard lump of dry skin.

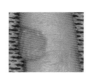

Verruca
- Hard, painful area on the sole of the foot, perhaps with a tiny black centre.

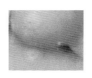

What can I do?

1 If your child has a wart simply ignore it, unless it is on his genitals or by his anus in which case consult your doctor. It will disappear on its own probably after a few months, although some last for a year or more.

Impetigo

What is it?

Impetigo is a bacterial skin infection that may develop when a rash such as eczema or a cold sore becomes infected, although even healthy skin can sometimes become infected with impetigo. It most often affects young children, especially babies.

It usually affects the skin around the mouth and nose, and the nappy area in babies, but it can occur anywhere on the body. Impetigo isn't a serious disorder in children, but in a young baby it can spread over a large area and make him quite ill. It is very contagious, so it is important to have it treated promptly.

Symptoms

- Rash of small, red spots
- blisters forming over the spots
- the spots burst, then form large brownish-yellow scabs
- fever and general illness in a young baby.

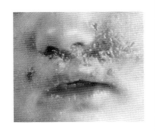

What can I do?

1 Keep your child's flannel and towel separate from those of the rest of the family, and wash them frequently so the infection doesn't spread.

2 Try to keep him from touching the affected area – don't let him suck his thumb or pick his nose, as this could spread the infection.

3 If your doctor has prescribed a cream, remove the crusts each day before applying it by wiping them with damp cotton wool. Don't rub hard, but persevere until the crusts loosen.

4 Pat the area dry with a tissue or paper towel and throw it away immediately, so that the infection can't spread.

5 Keep your child away from other children, especially young babies, until he has had 48 hours of treatment.

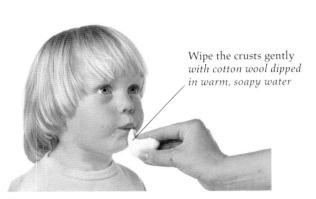

Wipe the crusts gently *with cotton wool dipped in warm, soapy water*

☎ Seek medical help

Call your doctor now if your baby is under three months old and suddenly develops widespread impetigo. **Consult your doctor** if you think your child has impetigo.

What might the doctor do?

The doctor may prescribe a cream and tell you to wipe away the crusts (see left) before applying it. If the infection is widespread, he may prescribe an antibiotic.

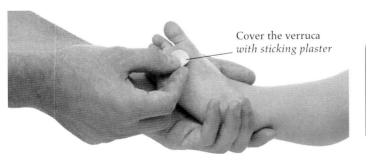

Cover the verruca *with sticking plaster*

2 If your child has a verruca, try an over-the-counter remedy from your chemist. Remove dead skin from the surface of a verruca by rubbing with a pumice stone. Cover a verruca with sticking plaster if your child goes swimming.

☎ Seek medical help

Consult your doctor if:
- your child's warts multiply
- your child has a wart on his genitals or anus
- your child has a verruca.

What might the doctor do?

If home treatment is not successful, your doctor may refer your child to the out-patient's department at hospital, where the wart can be burnt or frozen off under local anaesthetic. Warts sometimes recur even after they have been treated.

Lice and nits

What are they?
Lice are tiny insects that infest the hair, and make the child's head itchy. Their minute white eggs (nits) cling to her hair roots. Lice spread very easily from one head to another, so treat the whole family if your child picks up lice. Tell your friends to check their children's heads, and tell the staff at your child's toddler group or nursery school. Keep her at home until she is free of nits.

Symptoms
● Itchy head
● tiny white grains firmly attached to the hairs near the roots
● red bite marks under the hair.

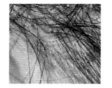

What can I do?

1 Wash the hair in the normal way. Put on plenty of conditioner. This makes the hair slippery and the lice easier to remove.

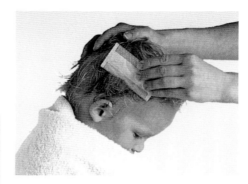

2 Comb the wet hair from the roots, using a special fine-tooth nit comb. Wipe the comb with a tissue between each stroke to remove lice. Repeat this treatment every three or four days for two weeks to eradicate all the lice.

3 Seal your child's hats, brush, and comb in a plastic bag and leave for at least 10 days – the nits will die.

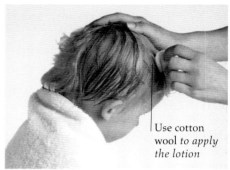

Use cotton wool to apply the lotion

4 As an alternative to wet-combing, ask your health visitor to suggest a lotion that will kill the lice and nits. You can then comb them off. If you use this method, it is important to follow the instructions carefully. You can also use the lotion to clean your child's brush and comb.

Threadworms

What are they?
Threadworms are tiny, white thread-like worms, about 1cm (½in) long, which infect the gut. They can enter the body in contaminated food, and then live in the bowels, coming out at night to lay eggs around the anus, and causing intense itchiness. They are common in children, and are harmless, although the itching may be very uncomfortable. In little girls, the worms may crawl forwards to the vagina. The eggs are easily transferred, so it is sensible to treat the whole family if your child is infected.

Symptoms
● Intense itching around the anus, which is usually worse at night
● intense itching around the vagina
● tiny white worms in the faeces
● worms around the anus.

What can I do?

1 Try to prevent your child scratching, since she might inflame the skin around her anus or vagina.

2 Keep her fingernails short, and discourage nail-biting or thumb-sucking which could re-infect her.

3 Make sure that the whole family washes their hands thoroughly after going to the lavatory and before eating. Use a nail brush to clean the nails properly.

4 If your child no longer wears nappies, make sure she wears close-fitting pants or knickers in bed. Change and wash her pants and nightwear daily, rinse well at a normal 40°C temperature.

5 Give her regular baths or showers, and wash around her anus and vagina first thing every morning to get rid of any eggs laid overnight.

Hygiene measures
The eggs can survive for two weeks outside the body on underwear and bedding so after taking the medication, clean "risk areas" thoroughly to prevent reinfection:
● Clean beds and bedrooms thoroughly. Wash all bedlinen, sleepwear, towels, cuddly toys, and vacuum mattresses. Don't allow eating in the bedroom.
● Make sure the whole family washes their hands thoroughly after going to the lavatory and before eating. Use a nail brush to clean the nails properly.
● Don't share towels or flannels.

6 Ask your pharmacist for a medicine that the whole family can take, even those with no symptoms but who may still be infected. You can also get this on prescription.

Epilepsy

Epilepsy, which causes recurrent convulsions, affects about one in 200 people. Many people with epilepsy experience their first seizure before the age of 20. A seizure is caused by excessive electrical discharges by brain cells. The most common cause of convulsion in children is a high fever (see page 194), but this is not normally a form of epilepsy. A single seizure does not mean your child has epilepsy, but do seek medical advice to rule out any serious underlying condition.

What is it?

Epilepsy is currently defined as a tendency to have recurrent seizures, caused by an abnormal electrical discharge in the brain. In many cases the cause of epilepsy is unknown (see page 194), but only a quarter of children who have suffered a seizure will go on to develop epilepsy. With treatment, many children grow out of it. There are several different types of epilepsy; two common forms in childhood are absence attacks and generalized seizures (see symptoms box).

What can I do?

1 During a generalized seizure, stay with your child and protect her from injury by removing any harmful objects nearby. Don't try to restrain her.

2 After the seizure, turn her on her side in the recovery position (see page 241). Don't wake her if she falls asleep, but make sure that she is breathing properly (see page 238).

3 Try to avoid letting your child get into situations that could be dangerous if she has a seizure – for example, put a guard at the top of the stairs, and don't leave her alone in the bath. But don't be over-protective – she shouldn't feel that her epilepsy makes her abnormal.

Symptoms

Absence attacks (petit mal convulsions)
- Sudden cessation of movement
- dazed expression
- complete recovery in a few seconds.

Generalized seizures (grand mal convulsions)
- Sudden unconsciousness, so your child falls down
- stiff arms and legs
- twitching or jerky movements
- sometimes urination
- sleeping, or gradual return to consciousness, after the twitching movements have stopped.

☎ Call an ambulance

Call an ambulance now if your child has:
- a major seizure for the first time
- a major seizure lasting more than three minutes
- a series of seizures in rapid succession.

Consult your doctor if you think your child has absence attacks.

What might the doctor do?

The doctor may send your child to hospital for tests. He may also prescribe a drug to help control the seizures; if so, tell the doctor if your child's behaviour changes in any way, but don't stop giving her the drug.

The recovery position
If your child has a seizure, place her in the recovery position, and tilt her chin to keep her airway open, and ensure that she is breathing properly. Leave her in this position until she regains consciousness. If she falls asleep, let her wake naturally.

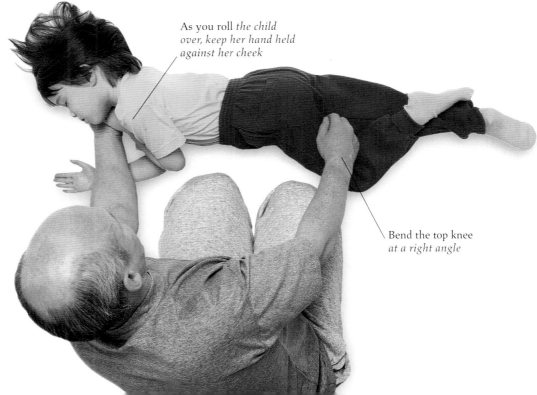

As you roll *the child over, keep her hand held against her cheek*

Bend the top knee *at a right angle*

Your child's safety

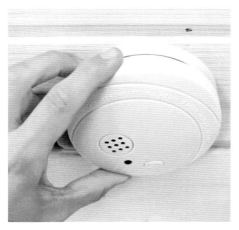

Small children are accident prone, especially when they are tired or hungry, or you are preoccupied. The best way to keep your child safe is to keep him under your watchful eye, particularly in an unfamiliar environment. Make sure that the safety equipment you buy for the house conforms to European safety standards, and use it only for the age of child it is designed for. Buy new if possible. Second-hand items may not comply with safety regulations.

Safety in your home

Children are vulnerable to accidents because their desire to explore and experiment far outstrips their common sense and forethought. Many accidents can easily be prevented, and it is your responsibility to make sure that your child can't injure himself and his world is safe for him to play in and explore.

Kitchen

Your kitchen is full of potential hazards for a child, and these dangers are increased if you are busy. Keep him away from the cooking area when you are cooking – a bouncing cradle or a playpen is ideal. Don't forget that cooker rings, kettles, and irons stay hot long after you have switched them off. At mealtimes, keep hot dishes near the centre of the table so that your child can't grab them. Don't use a table cloth because he can pull it, and spill hot things over himself.

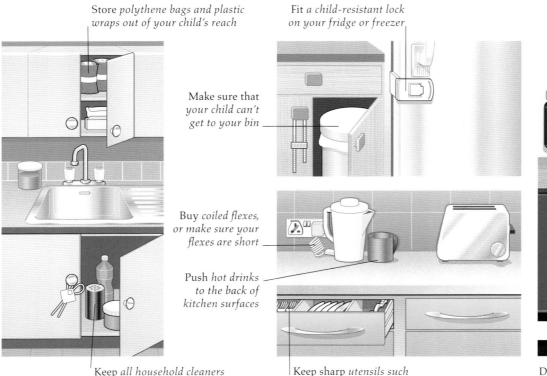

Store *polythene bags and plastic wraps out of your child's reach*

Fit *a child-resistant lock on your fridge or freezer*

Make sure that *your child can't get to your bin*

Buy *coiled flexes, or make sure your flexes are short*

Push *hot drinks to the back of kitchen surfaces*

Keep *all household cleaners and bleaches in a cupboard with a child-resistant catch*

Keep sharp *utensils such as kitchen knives in a drawer with a child-resistant catch*

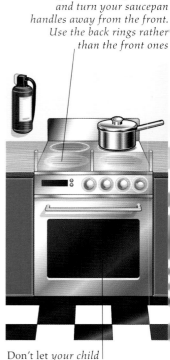

Fit a guard *around your hob, and turn your saucepan handles away from the front. Use the back rings rather than the front ones*

Don't let *your child touch the oven door while it is hot*

Keeping your baby safe

With each new skill he develops, your baby will find ways of running into danger, so you must think ahead to avoid hazards. He will learn to roll over when he is very young, so if you need to lay him down for even a moment, put him on the floor.

He will soon grab things, so make sure that anything he can reach is safe to handle, and too large to swallow or choke on. Don't eat, drink, carry anything hot, or smoke while you are holding your baby. Never leave him alone with a bottle – he could choke. Always use

safety straps on his pram and high-chair. Don't put him in a bouncing cradle on a high surface – it could easily fall off. Don't leave a young child alone with your baby: he might pick him up and drop him, or give him dangerous objects to play with.

Bedroom

Your child will spend a lot of time in his bedroom, so make sure it is safe. Don't put a pillow in his cot until he is at least two, and don't use loose plastic sheeting as a waterproof mattress cover. Never attach his toys to the cot with cords – they might wind around his neck. Keep large toys out of the cot – your child could use them as stepping stones to climb out – and don't string toys across the cot once he can stand. His toys should be non-toxic and non-flammable, and must have no sharp edges or pieces small enough to swallow.

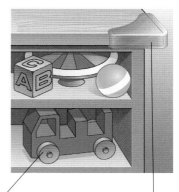

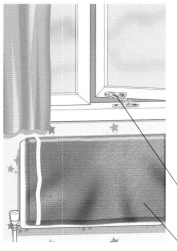

Fix *catches on the windows, so that they can be opened only a little way. Open sash windows from the top*

Cover *hot radiators with a towel*

Store *toys in a low cupboard or shelf, so your child can reach them without climbing*

Make *sure that your furniture is sturdy and has rounded edges. You can buy corner pieces to fix on to sharp edges*

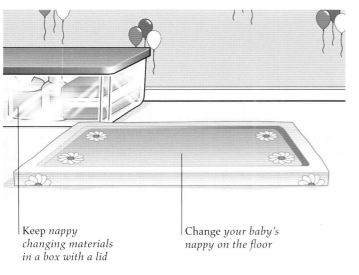

Keep *nappy changing materials in a box with a lid*

Change *your baby's nappy on the floor*

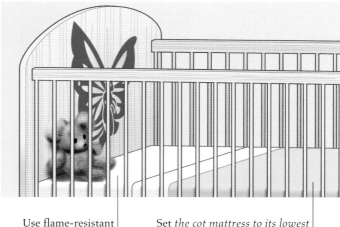

Use flame-resistant *bedding and sleepwear*

Set *the cot mattress to its lowest position before your baby can pull himself to standing*

Bathroom

Never leave a child under four alone in the bath, or in the bathroom if the bathtub is full, even for a few seconds. Use a non-slip bath mat. Set your water heater lower than 55°C (130°F), and run the cold water into your child's bath first. Test the temperature before putting your child in. Other accidents that may occur

in the bathroom can easily be prevented:
● Keep all medicines out of your child's reach in a cabinet with a lock or a child-resistant catch.
● Cover any heated towel rails with towels.
● If you have an electric heater, it should be wall-mounted, and have a pull-string switch that your child can't reach.

● Keep cleaning fluids and the toilet brush in a cupboard with a child-resistant catch.
● Put razors and cosmetics out of your child's reach.
● If you have a shower with a glass screen, replace the screen with a curtain, or install safety glass.

Garden

Keep an eye on your child when he is playing in the garden. Never let your child play in or near a paddling pool without supervision, and empty the pool after use. If you have a pond, cover or fence it securely. Make sure that the plants in your garden aren't poisonous. Teach your child not to eat any berries. Fix child-resistant locks on all gates. Don't let your child play in an area where you have recently used pesticide, weed-killer, or fertilizer.

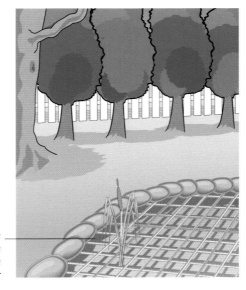

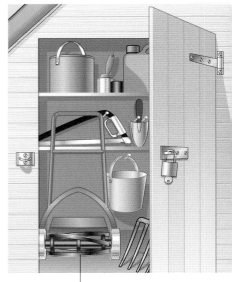

Keep the whole pond covered with wire netting or surround it with a sturdy fence. Children can drown in a few centimetres of water

Lock away all your gardening and DIY tools, and any weed-killer, fertilizer, and pesticide

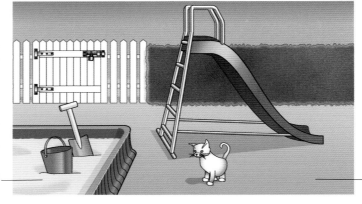

The sand in your child's sandbox should be too shallow for him to bury himself. Teach him not to throw sand. Cover the sandpit when not in use, as dogs and cats could foul the sand, which is a hygiene risk

Put your child's play equipment on grass or sand, not on a hard surface

Living room

When you buy upholstered furniture, make sure that it will not give off toxic fumes if you have a fire. Fix a guard round all fires. Keep the television out of your child's reach.

Don't leave cigarettes, matches, alcohol, sewing equipment, or coins lying around. Keep indoor plants out of his reach, as some are poisonous.

If you have low glass panels in doors or windows, use toughened, laminated, or wire-net glass, or apply a transparent safety film, or put coloured stickers on them, so that your child can see where the glass is. Avoid glass-topped tables.

Hall and stairs

Fix safety gates at the top and bottom of the stairs before your child can crawl or climb. Make sure that the hall, stairs, and landings are well lit, and that the banisters aren't so wide apart that your child could fall through. Make sure that the front door latch is out of his reach. Install a smoke detector. Repair loose tiles or tears in rugs. On polished wooden floors don't let your child wear socks without shoes.

Cars

Your child should always travel in a car seat that is officially approved for his age and weight. Check your vehicle manufacturer's handbook to see if it will take a "Universal" child seat, or conforms to ISOFIX standards (see page 158). Children should never travel in the front seat of a car with air bags. Use child-proof locks on the doors, and don't let your child lean out of the window or put his hand out while you are travelling.

Don't leave your child by himself in the car for more than a few moments, and when he is alone, make sure the handbrake is on, take the keys out of the ignition, and leave the car in gear. Check where he is before closing the door or reversing.

Electricity

Electric shocks from the mains can be very serious, so minimize the chances of your child getting a shock:
● Switch off electrical appliances when you are not using them.
● Never leave a socket switched on with nothing plugged into it.
● Cover unused sockets with dummy socket covers, or mask them with heavy insulating tape.
● Check all flexes regularly, and renew those with exposed wires.
● Don't let your child play with toys powered from the mains until he is at least four years old.

First aid

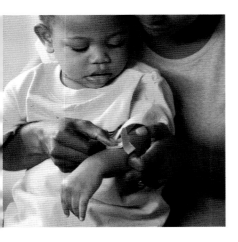

This chapter will help you deal with various injuries yourself and indicate when medical help is necessary. Always treat the most serious injury first. Sometimes it may be faster to take your child to hospital rather than call an ambulance, but see below for occasions when you must call an ambulance. If your child is badly injured, she will need urgent medical treatment, but you should give first aid while waiting for emergency help to arrive.

Getting your child to a hospital

Call for an ambulance, or better still ask someone else to phone, if:
- your child is unconscious
- you think your child might have a head or spinal injury
- you think she needs special treatment while travelling.

If you take your child to the hospital yourself, there should be one person to drive, while the other sits in the back with your child and continues to give first aid.

If your child is unconscious, don't leave her alone even to call an ambulance. If she is not breathing and you are on your own, give her cardiopulmonary resuscitation (CPR) (see page 239) for one minute before calling for help.

Warning

If there is a chance that your child has injured her neck or spine – for example, after a fall from a height – don't move her unless her life is in danger. Leave her in the position you found her while you check whether or not she is breathing. If you need to perform cardiopulmonary resuscitation (CPR), turn your child on her back very gently, keeping her head, neck, and back aligned. Ideally, get help so that one person supports her head and neck while you turn her body.

First aid kit

Keep a supply of first aid equipment in a clean, dry container, and replace anything you use as soon as possible. Take some antiseptic wipes with you on outings, to clean cuts and scrapes.

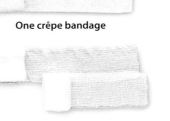

One crêpe bandage

Two gauze bandages

Hypoallergenic tape
This is useful for sticking on dressings, and drawing together the edges of large cuts.

Calamine lotion
This will soothe sunburn and insect bites and stings.

Non-adherent, absorbent, sterile wound dressings
These peel off a wound easily.

Triangular bandage
This can be used to make a sling or secure a dressing.

Resuscitation mask
This plastic pocket mask protects you and the casualty from cross infection during CPR.

Alcohol-free antiseptic wipes

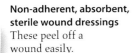

Tweezers

Scissors

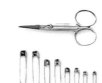

Safety pins

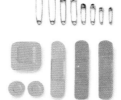

Assorted adhesive plasters
Use these for dressing minor cuts and grazes.

Prepared wound dressings
These consist of a pad attached to a bandage, and are easy to use.

Non-latex disposable gloves

Life-saving techniques

Every second counts. If your child appears to be unconscious, follow the steps on these pages before you attend to any other injury as it's a life-threatening condition. If she is not breathing normally, her heart could also stop beating, so it's vital to begin cardiopulmonary resuscitation (CPR) immediately. CPR is a combination of rescue breaths and chest compressions. By breathing into her lungs with rescue breaths, you can maintain her oxygen levels, and by giving chest compressions you can artificially "circulate", or pump, the oxygenated blood around her body. If you need to give CPR, keep going until emergency help arrives or you become too exhausted to continue.

> The CPR procedures described in the first aid section of this book conform to the guidelines as set by the International Liaison Committee on Resuscitation at the time of the book's publication. For the latest information please go to www.ilcor.org

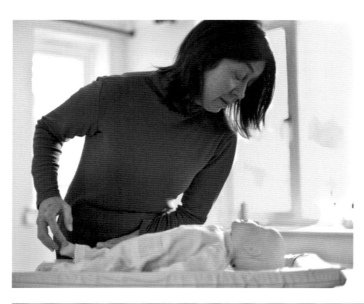

Checking for consciousness

Unconsciousness is a potentially life-threatening condition that requires immediate medical assistance. To assess whether your baby is unconscious, tap the soles of her feet, for a child, tap her shoulder and call out her name loudly. If there is no response, it is likely that she is unconscious. **Never** shake a baby.

If she responds, she's conscious. Assess and treat any other injuries. Don't move her unless it's absolutely essential, and attend to life-threatening injuries, such as breathing difficulties, severe bleeding, or burns first.

If she doesn't respond, she is unconscious, check to see if she is breathing (see below).

Emergency

Call for emergency help immediately if your baby or child becomes unconscious, even if this is only for a few seconds.

Opening the airway and checking breathing

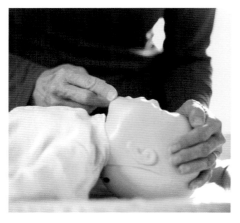

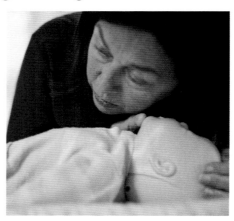

If she is breathing normally, cradle her in your arms with her head lower than her body (see page 241), and call for emergency help.

If she is not breathing normally, ask someone to call an ambulance while you begin CPR immediately. If you are on your own, continue CPR for one minute before stopping to call for help.

1 Place your baby on a firm surface. Put one hand on her forehead, and tilt her head back slightly. Place the forefinger of your other hand on the point of her chin and lift it. For a child, put two fingers on the chin. Keep your fingers away from her neck.

2 Put your ear near to your baby's mouth and nose, and look along her chest to see if it is moving. Listen for breathing sounds, and feel for breaths against your cheek. Check for no more than 10 seconds to see if she is breathing.

Cardiopulmonary resuscitation (CPR) for a baby up to 12 months

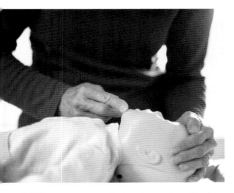

1 Make sure your baby is on her back on a firm surface, such as a table. Check that her airway is still open by keeping her head tilted, and lift her chin.

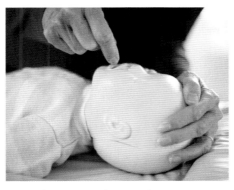

2 Pick out any obvious obstructions you see in her mouth. Be very careful not to push anything down her throat, and don't sweep your finger around her mouth to search for obstructions.

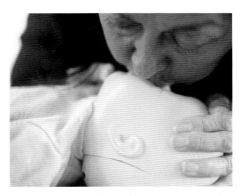

3 Begin rescue breaths. Take a normal breath, then seal your lips around her mouth and nose, and blow gently into the mouth for about one second until you see the chest rise.

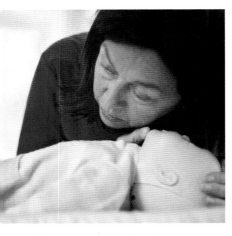

4 Still supporting her head, remove your lips and watch the chest fall back. Repeat to give **five** rescue breaths.

If the chest does not rise, the airway may not be open correctly, adjust the head position and try again.

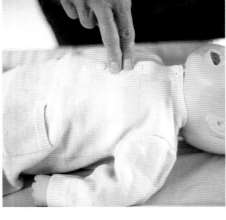

5 Begin chest compressions. Support your baby's head with one hand, and place two fingers of your other hand on the centre of her chest (on the breastbone). Press straight down sharply to compress the chest by one-third of its depth.

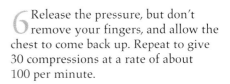

6 Release the pressure, but don't remove your fingers, and allow the chest to come back up. Repeat to give 30 compressions at a rate of about 100 per minute.

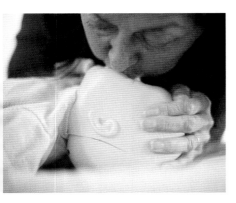

7 Go back to the head and give **two** rescue breaths this time, followed by another 30 chest compressions. Continue to give chest compressions and rescue breaths at a rate of 30:2 until the baby begins to breathe again, the emergency help arrives, or you are too exhausted to keep going.

If you are on your own, give CPR for one minute before stopping to call an ambulance.

If she starts breathing normally, hold her in the recovery position (see page 241).

Life-saving techniques *continued*

Cardiopulmonary resuscitation (CPR) for a child over one year

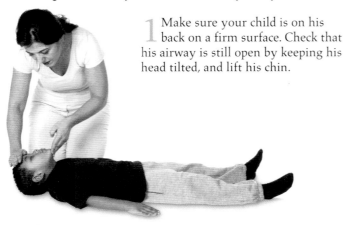

1 Make sure your child is on his back on a firm surface. Check that his airway is still open by keeping his head tilted, and lift his chin.

2 Pick out any obvious obstructions you see in his mouth. Be very careful not to push anything down his throat, and don't sweep your finger around his mouth to search for obstructions.

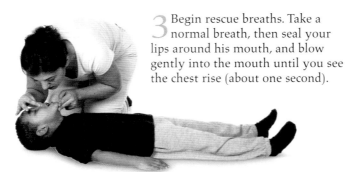

3 Begin rescue breaths. Take a normal breath, then seal your lips around his mouth, and blow gently into the mouth until you see the chest rise (about one second).

4 Still supporting his head, remove your lips and watch his chest fall back. Repeat to give **five** rescue breaths.

If the chest does not rise, the airway may not be open correctly; adjust the head position, and try again.

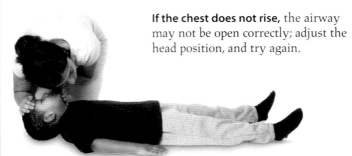

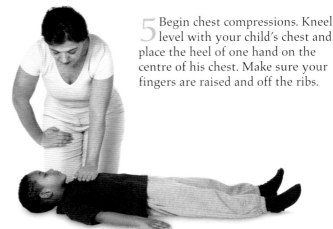

5 Begin chest compressions. Kneel level with your child's chest and place the heel of one hand on the centre of his chest. Make sure your fingers are raised and off the ribs.

6 Press straight down sharply to compress the chest by about one third of its depth. Release the pressure, and allow the chest to come back up. Repeat to give 30 compressions at a rate of about 100 per minute.

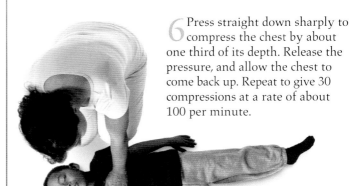

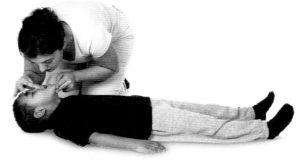

7 Go back to the head and give **two** rescue breaths this time, followed by another 30 chest compressions. Continue to give chest compressions and rescue breaths at a rate of 30:2 until your child begins to breathe again, the emergency help arrives, or you become too exhausted to keep going.

If you are on your own, give CPR for one minute before stopping to call an ambulance.

If he starts breathing normally, place him in the recovery position (see opposite).

The recovery position

Put your child into this position if she is unconscious but breathing normally. This keeps the airway open as the tongue cannot fall back and block the airway, and it allows any fluid to drain from her mouth. For a baby, see right.

For a child over one year

1 Kneel beside your child. Tilt her head back and lift her chin forwards. This keeps her air passages open while you put her in the recovery position.

Her head must be tilted well back with the chin jutting forward

2 If necessary, straighten her legs. Bend the arm nearest to you so that it makes a right angle and lay it on the ground, with the palm of the hand upwards.

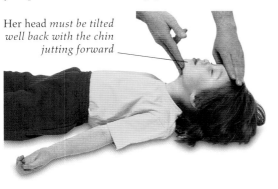

3 Bring her other arm across her chest. Hold the back of her hand against her opposite cheek.

Move her furthest arm across her chest and bend it

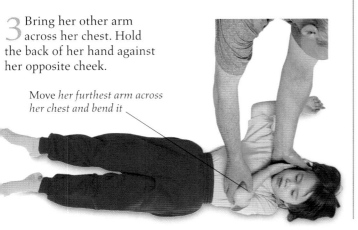

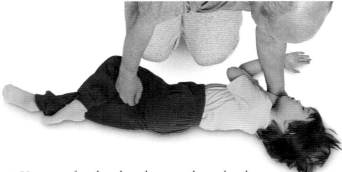

4 Use your free hand to clasp gently under the thigh furthest from you. Leaving the foot flat on the ground, pull the knee up to bend the leg. Keeping your child's hand against her cheek to support her head, pull on the thigh of the bent leg to roll her towards you and onto her side.

5 Adjust her arm and leg so she cannot fall forwards, and tilt her head. Call an ambulance.

Bend her top leg into a right angle at the hip and knee to prevent her from rolling forwards

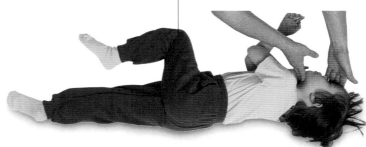

Recovery position for a baby

A baby under the age of one should be cradled in your arms with her head tilted down to avoid obstruction of her airway and prevent her from choking on her tongue.

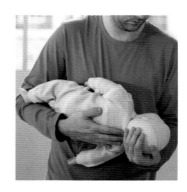

Choking

This happens when a small object or piece of food blocks the windpipe, causing coughing and breathing difficulty. It is important to dislodge the object quickly, so that the child can breathe normally. Choking is common in young children who tend to put everything they get hold of into their mouths.

Helping a baby under 12 months

1 Hold your baby face down with his head low along your forearm. Support his head and shoulders on your hand. Give five sharp blows to the upper part of his back.

Keep his head low and give five sharp blows on the back

2 Turn him face up along your other arm. Look in his mouth and remove any obvious obstruction with one finger. **Do not** feel blindly down the baby's throat.

Turn him on to his back along your other arm

3 If back blows fail, give chest thrusts. Place two fingers on the lower half of his breastbone, and give five sharp downwards thrusts at a rate of one every three seconds. These act as artificial coughs. Check the mouth again.

4 If the blockage hasn't cleared, repeat steps 1–3 until help arrives. Take your baby with you to call an ambulance.

Helping a child over one year

1 Your child may be able to cough up the object on his own. Encourage him to do this, but do not waste time. If this fails, make him bend forwards. Give him five sharp blows between the shoulder blades.

Give five sharp blows on the back

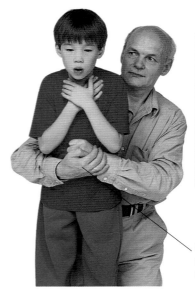

Give him abdominal thrusts

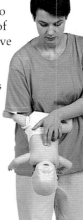
Warning
- If the baby or child loses consciousness at any point, begin CPR (see pages 239–40).
- Any baby or child who has been given thrusts must be checked by a doctor afterwards.

2 Check his mouth. Remove any object you can see. Do not put your finger into his mouth trying to find something.

3 If back blows fail, give abdominal thrusts. Place a fist in the middle of the upper abdomen below his rib cage. Hold your other hand over it. Give five inward and upward thrusts. Check his mouth.

4 If the abdominal thrusts fail, repeat steps 1–3 three times. If still unsuccessful, call an ambulance. Repeat the cycle until help arrives, the child recovers, or he becomes unconscious.

Suffocation

Anything that is lying across your child's face may block his mouth and nose, and prevent him from breathing.

What can I do?

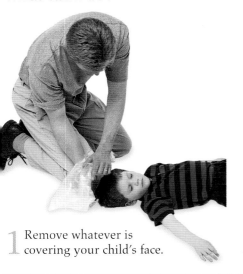

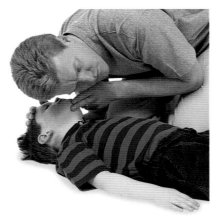

1 Remove whatever is covering your child's face.

2 Check to see if your child is conscious and breathing (see page 238).

If he is not breathing, start CPR immediately (see pages 239–40), and ask someone to call for emergency help.

If he is unconscious but breathing, place him in the recovery position (see page 241), then call for emergency help.

If he is conscious, simply comfort and reassure him while you wait for emergency service to arrive.

Drowning

Babies and children can drown even in very shallow water. When a young child's face is submerged, her automatic reaction is to take a deep breath to scream, rather than to lift her face up out of the water.

What can I do?

Get the child out of the water if it is safe to do so. Lift her very gently, and make sure you do not twist her back. Carry her with her head lower than her body, so that water can drain from her mouth. Once she is out of the water, lay her down and check for consciousness and breathing (see page 238).

If she is conscious, take off her wet clothes, replace them with dry clothes, and wrap her up to keep her warm.

If she is breathing normally but is unconscious, place her in the recovery position so that water can drain from her airways. Call for emergency help. If possible lay her on a coat or blanket, and replace any wet clothing with dry clothes. Wrap her in a blanket to keep her warm.

If she is not breathing, ask someone to call for emergency help. Clear any obvious debris, such as seaweed, from her mouth, and begin CPR. If you are on your own shout for help, but give CPR for one minute before stopping to call the emergency services.

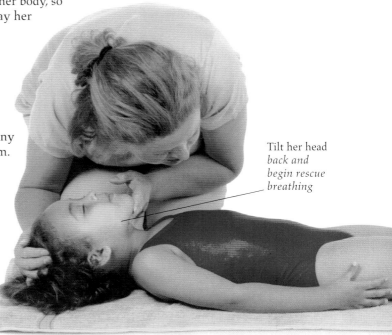

Tilt her head *back and begin rescue breathing*

Warning

It is vital to keep your child warm as children can develop hypothermia after even a short period in cold water.

Shock

Shock is a condition in which blood pressure suddenly drops, depriving the body's vital organs of oxygen. It can occur as a reaction to any severe injury, especially heavy bleeding or severe burns.

Symptoms

- Pale, cold, sweaty skin
- blue or greyish tinge inside the lips or under the fingernails
- rapid and shallow breathing
- restlessness
- drowsiness or confusion
- unconsciousness.

Emergency

Call for emergency help immediately if your child is in shock.

What can I do?

1 Lay your child down, ideally on a blanket to protect him from the cold ground. Raise and support his legs high on a pile of cushions or a chair. If you suspect a broken leg, or a poisonous bite on his leg, do not raise the affected area.

2 Cover him with a blanket or coat, or cuddle him, to keep him warm. **Do not** try to warm him up with a hot water bottle or an electric blanket – this only draws blood away from the vital body organs to the skin.

3 If he complains of thirst, moisten his lips with a damp cloth. **Do not** give him anything to eat or drink, unless he has burns in his mouth. In this case, give him sips of water.

4 If he becomes unconscious, check his breathing (see page 238).

If the child is not breathing, start CPR immediately (see pages 239–40).

If the child is breathing normally, put him into the recovery position (see page 241).

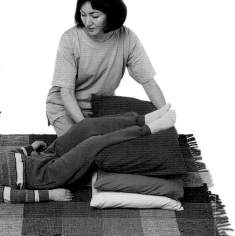

Poisoning

Children tend to be curious so it is vital to keep poisonous substances out of their reach. It is one of the most common emergencies in young children.

What can I do?

1 Find out what your child has taken; if she is conscious, ask her. Look for clues nearby. There may be a medicine bottle or poisonous plants near her.

2 Call the emergency services and give them as much information as you can. It helps them to know what was taken, how much, and when.

3 If you see signs of burning around the child's mouth and she is fully conscious, give her sips of water or milk to drink. Wipe her face and mouth. Do not try to make her vomit – a substance that burned on the way down will burn again on the way back up.

4 If the child vomits, keep a sample, as this can help the emergency services identify what she took, and so give the appropriate treatment.

If she loses consciousness, check breathing, and be prepared to begin CPR if she is not breathing.

If she is unconscious but breathing, place her in the recovery position.

Symptoms

Your child's symptoms will depend on the type of poison she has swallowed. You may notice any of these signs:

- stomach pain
- vomiting
- symptoms of shock (see above)
- seizures
- drowsiness
- unconsciousness
- burns or discolouration around the mouth if your child has swallowed a corrosive poison
- poison or empty container nearby.

Warning

If a child needs CPR and there is poison around her mouth, place a pocket mask over her mouth first.

Burns and scalds

All burns and scalds carry a serious risk of infection. A burn that causes only superficial reddening of the skin and is less than 2–3cm (1in) is a minor burn, and can be treated at home first before you seek medical advice. Any deeper burn or burns that affect a larger area need immediate medical attention as there is also a risk of shock if a lot of fluid is lost from the burn.

Emergency

Get your child emergency medical help immediately if:

- the burn covers an area of more than about 2–3cm (1in)
- the burn was caused by an electric shock (see page 251)
- the casualty is a baby
- the burn has affected all the layers of skin (deep), however small it is.

Minor burns

What can I do?

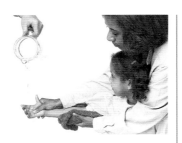

1 Cool the burn immediately by holding it under cold running water for 10 minutes or until the pain eases.

2 Cover the injury with cling film or a plastic bag. If neither is available, then cover with a clean non-fluffy dressing. Don't use a plaster as the burned area may be more extensive than you think. Seek medical advice.

Do not burst any blisters – they protect the damaged area underneath while the new skin is growing.

Do not put any cream, lotion, or adhesive dressing on the burn.

Burning clothes

What can I do?

1 Stop the child moving as movement will fan the flames. Drop him to the floor to stop flames rising to his face.

2 Wrap the child in a non-flammable coat or blanket to help smother the flames.

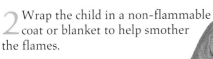

3 Roll the child on the ground. This will help to put out the fire.

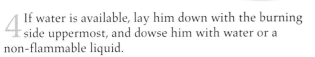

4 If water is available, lay him down with the burning side uppermost, and dowse him with water or a non-flammable liquid.

Do not let the child run about in panic; movement will fan the flames.

Major burns

What can I do?

1 To stop the burning and relieve the pain, cool the burn with cold running water for 10 minutes or until pain eases.

Do not immerse a young child in cold water as there is a risk of hypothermia.

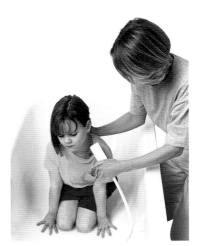

2 While cooling the burn, remove clothing from around the burned area before it swells. Cut clothing away if required.

Do not remove anything sticking to the burn. Never touch or burst any blisters.

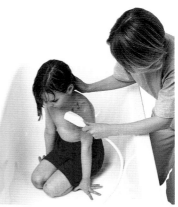

3 Cover the burn with cling film laid along the injury (don't wrap it around the limb as the injured area will swell), or place a hand or foot in a plastic bag. If neither is available use a clean, non-fluffy material (such as a pillow case) to protect it from infection. The dressing does not need to be secured. Ensure that the child remains warm to prevent the onset of hypothermia. Seek emergency medical help.

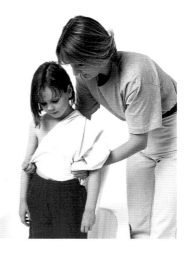

Do not give her anything to eat or drink, and watch for signs of shock (see p244).

Serious bleeding

If blood spurts from a wound or if bleeding continues, try to stem the flow so that the blood has a chance to clot. Use disposable gloves; alternatively wash your hands before and after treatment.

> ## Emergency
> **Take your child to hospital as soon as you have given first aid** if he has been bleeding heavily.

What can I do?

1 Press a sterile dressing or pad of clean non-fluffy material over the wound. If there is a foreign object embedded in the wound, treat as below.

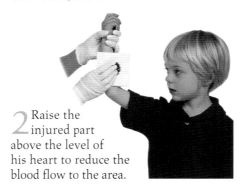

2 Raise the injured part above the level of his heart to reduce the blood flow to the area.

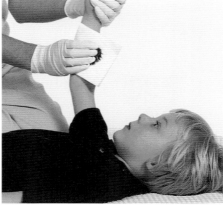

3 Lay your child down, keeping his injury raised and supported. Keep pressing on the injury for at least 10 minutes.

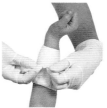

4 Secure the original pad with a bandage. If blood seeps through the first dressing, place another one on top and secure it.

5 If blood seeps through the second dressing, too, then the pressure is probably not on the right point. Take both dressings off, and press a clean one on the wound directly over the point of bleeding.

6 Check for symptoms of shock (see page 244), and treat your child for this if necessary.

Embedded objects

Small pieces of dirt in a cut will be washed out by bleeding. However, if your child has a foreign object stuck in a wound do not attempt to remove it as you may cause more damage. Try to stop the bleeding (see above), bandage, and take your child to the hospital.

> ## Emergency
> ● **Take your child to hospital as soon as you have given first aid** if he has something embedded in a wound.
> ● Treat for shock if necessary (see page 244).

What can I do?

1 Help your child rest. Apply pressure on either side of the object and raise the injured part above the level of your child's heart. **Do not** try to remove any objects that are embedded in a wound as you may cause further damage and bleeding.

Apply pressure *on either side of the wound*

2 Loosely place a piece of clean gauze over the wound and object to minimize the risk of infection.

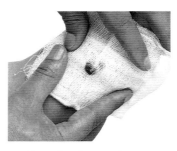

3 Use spare bandage rolls to build up padding to the same height as the embedded object.

Bandage *over padding*

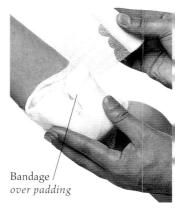

4 Secure the padding by bandaging over it, being careful not to press on the embedded object. Take your child to hospital.

Cuts and scrapes

Cuts and scrapes are common throughout childhood, and you can treat most of them yourself. Make sure that you keep your child's tetanus injections up to date. Treat an animal bite as a cut, but if your child receives a poisonous bite or sting, see page 252.

Emergency
Take your child to hospital as soon as you have given first aid if:
- the cut is large or deep
- the cut is jagged or gapes open
- your child has cut his face badly
- the cut or scrape is very dirty
- your child has a puncture wound (a deep cut with a small opening in the skin) caused by something dirty

☎ Seek medical help
Seek medical help as soon as possible if the area around the wound later becomes tender and red – it may be infected.

What can I do?

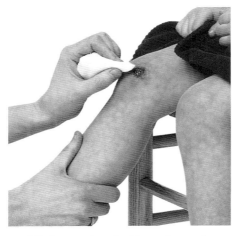

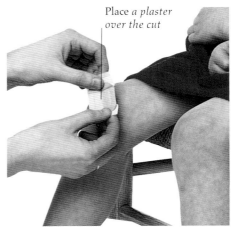

Place a plaster over the cut

1 Wash your hands. Clean the cut by holding it under running water for some time, or wiping gently around it with an antiseptic wipe or cotton wool soaked in warm water. Use a clean piece of cotton wool for each stroke. **Do not** remove anything that is embedded in the cut (see opposite).

If your child has been bitten by an animal, wash the wound thoroughly with soap and water.

2 If the cut continues to bleed, press a pad such as a clean handkerchief or a non-fluffy cloth firmly on it for a few minutes.

3 Put a plaster or dressing over the cut to help protect the wound and keep it clean. **Do not** put any antiseptic ointment on your child's cut.

4 Keep the cut covered with a sticking plaster or a dressing until it has completely healed. This ensures that the area remains moist, and helps the cut heal more quickly. Change the plaster or dressing every day – soak sticking plaster in water to remove it easily.

Nose bleeds

Nose bleeds are very common in young children and can result from a bump on the nose, nose-picking, or excessive nose-blowing. A few children seem prone to nose bleeds, which can be because they have fragile blood vessels in their noses.

What can I do?

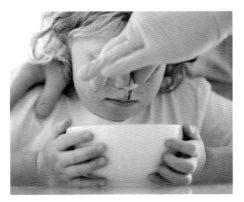

1 If your child experiences a nose bleed, you will need to apply direct pressure on her nose. To do this, help your child to lean forwards over a bowl or washbasin, and pinch the soft part of her nostrils.

2 If her nose is still bleeding, pinch her nose for another 10 minutes. Try holding a cloth wrung out in very cold water over her nose for a few minutes.

3 Don't let your child blow her nose for about four hours after the bleeding has stopped.

☎ Seek medical help
Seek medical help if your child's nose is still bleeding just as badly after half an hour. Consult your doctor if your child has frequent, severe nose bleeds.

Head and face injury

Bumps on the head are common in young children. A cut on the forehead or scalp, even a small one, is likely to bleed profusely. If your child has had a severe blow to her head, she may have concussion, which results when the brain is shaken within the skull, or compression caused by bleeding inside the skull – this may not be apparent for some hours.

What can I do?

1 If your child's head is bruised, hold a cloth that has been wrung out in very cold water, or an ice pack wrapped in a damp cloth, over the bruise. This may stop it from swelling. Check the skin underneath the pack

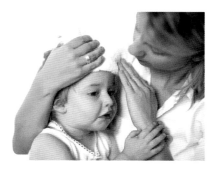

every minute, and remove the pack if a red patch with a white waxy centre develops.

2 If there is a wound, place a clean cloth over the cut and press against the wound, just as you would for bleeding anywhere else on the body (see page 246).

Emergency

Call for emergency help immediately if your child has injured her head and shows any unusual behaviour or has any of these symptoms up to 24 hours later:
- unconsciousness, however brief
- vomiting more than twice
- noisy breathing or snoring if your child doesn't normally snore
- difficulty in waking, or abnormal drowsiness
- discharge of clear or blood-stained fluid from her nose or ear
- unusual crying
- severe headache
- dislike of bright light.

3 Watch your child carefully for the next 24 hours in case she develops any of the emergency signs listed above. If she bumped her head badly, wake her every three hours – **if she won't wake up, call for emergency help immediately.**

If a discharge of clear or blood-stained fluid trickles from your child's nose or ear, lay her down with a pad of clean material placed under her nose or ear. If she deteriorates or loses consciousness, assess her condition (see page 238). Be prepared to begin CPR (see page 239–40). If breathing, place her in the recovery position (see page 241). **Call an ambulance.**

Broken teeth

If your child has broken a tooth, or one has become dislodged, put the broken piece in some milk, and take your child and her tooth to your dentist or to hospital immediately.

Put *your child in the recovery position*

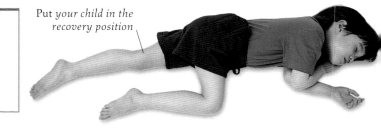

Bruises and swelling

A bruise appears when a fall or blow causes bleeding into the tissues beneath the skin, causing swelling and discolouring.

Crushed fingers and toes

If your child has crushed his fingers in a door or window, or dropped something heavy on his foot, hold the injured area under cold running water for a few minutes. If it is very swollen, or still painful after about half an hour, take your child to the hospital.

What can I do?

1 Hold a pad that has been wrung out in very cold water, or an ice pack wrapped in a damp cloth, over the bruise for about 10 minutes, repeat if necessary. This should help to reduce pain and swelling.

Apply *a cold compress*

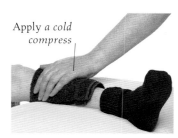

2 If your child seems to be in great pain or if it hurts him to use a bruised limb, especially if the swelling is severe, check for any signs of a sprained joint or a broken bone (see opposite).

Sprained joints

If the ligaments that support a joint are damaged, it is said to be sprained. This can cause symptoms very similar to those of a broken bone: if you are not sure which it is, treat as a broken bone (see below).

What can I do?

1 Taking care not to pull or twist the injured joint, gently take off your child's shoe and sock, or any other items that might constrict swelling around the injury.

2 Raise and support the injured joint in the most comfortable position for your child, then hold a cloth wrung out in ice-cold water, or an ice pack wrapped in a cloth, on the joint for 10 minutes, to reduce swelling and pain.

3 Wrap a thick layer of cotton wool round the joint, then bandage it firmly, but not too tightly from the joint below the injury up to the joint above it (from the toes to the knee for a sprained ankle).

Emergency
Get medical help as soon as you have given first aid.

Symptoms
- Pain in the injured area
- swelling and, later, bruising
- difficulty moving the joint.

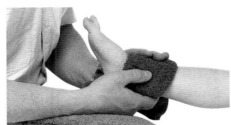

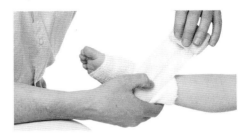

Fractures and dislocated joints

Broken bones are unusual in young children – their bones have not hardened, so they are flexible and tend to bend rather than break. Sometimes there may be a partial break, which mends easily. A joint is dislocated if one or more bones slip out of place.

Symptoms
- Severe pain in the injured area
- swelling and, later, bruising
- difficulty moving the injured part
- misshapen appearance to the injured part – a limb may be bent in an odd way, or may look shorter than the uninjured limb.

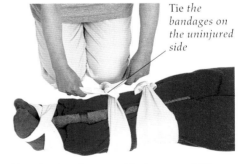

Tie the bandages on the uninjured side

For a broken leg or ankle, lay your child down and put padding round the injured area and between his knees and ankles. Bandage the injured leg to the uninjured one, securing it above and below the injury. Put some padding under the knots.

What can I do?

1 Gently take off your child's shoe and sock, or anything that might constrict swelling around the injured area. Do not move him unless it is absolutely essential.

2 Support an injured part in the most comfortable position for your child. For a broken wrist, arm, or collar-bone, put padding round the injured area and, if your child will let you, gently fold his arm across his chest, then support it in an arm sling, fastening the bandage with a reef knot tied just below the shoulder. Don't try to force his arm into this position. If he can't bend it, surround it with padding, and put a folded triangular bandage right

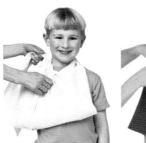

Arm sling   **Elevation sling**

around the arm and body. If there is bleeding that needs to be reduced, the arm should be raised in an elevation sling. The fingertips are brought up to the level of the opposite shoulder, the sling is wrapped around the arm, passed from the elbow across the back, and tied at the shoulder.

3 Check for symptoms of shock and treat him for this if necessary (see page 244). If you think he has a broken leg, don't raise his legs.

Emergency
Call for emergency help as soon as you have given first aid.

Foreign object in the eye

Eyelashes or particles of dust can easily get into the eye. If your child's eye seems irritated but you can't see anything in it, it may be an eye infection (see page 209).

Symptoms
- Pain in the eye
- red, watering eye
- your child may rub her eye.

Chemicals in the eye
If your child has splashed any chemicals or corrosive fluids in her eyes, wash her eyes out immediately under cold running water, keeping her eyelids apart with your fingers. If only one eye is affected, tilt her head so that the injured eye is lower, and the chemical cannot wash over into the uninjured one. Then cover the eye with a pad, and take your child to a hospital. If possible, take the chemical bottle with you.

What can I do?

1 Wait a few minutes to see if the natural watering of the eye washes the foreign object away. Try to stop your child from rubbing her eye.

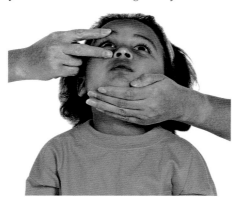

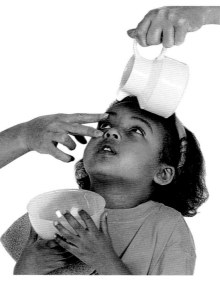

2 Sit your child down, facing the light. Separate the eyelids. Ask her to look right, left, up, and down. Make sure that you examine all of the eye.

3 If you can see the foreign object, wash it out using a jug of clean water. Aim for the inner corner, so that water will wash over the eye. Or, use a damp swab or handkerchief to lift it off.

4 If an object is under the eyelid, you can ask an older child to clear it by lifting the upper eyelid over the lower. You will need to do this for a younger child; wrap her in a towel first to stop her grabbing your arms. If the eye is still red or sore once the object has been removed, take her to the hospital.

A foreign object that cannot be removed
Cover the eye with a sterile dressing. Reassure the child and take her to the hospital.

Foreign object in the ear

Insects may crawl into your child's ear, and children may push small objects into their ears. Don't let your child play with beads or similar small objects until she is old enough to understand that they should not be put into her ears.

Symptoms
- Tickling in the ear
- partial deafness
- your child may rub or tug at her ear.

What can I do?

1 If your child has an insect in her ear, she may be very alarmed. Sit her down and support her head with the affected ear uppermost. Gently flood the ear with tepid water so that the insect floats out. If you can't remove the insect, take your child to hospital.

2 Children often push things into their ears. A hard object may become stuck. This may result in pain and temporary deafness; it may damage the ear drum. Do not attempt to remove the object, even if you can see it. Reassure your child and ask her what she put into her ear. Take your child to the hospital.

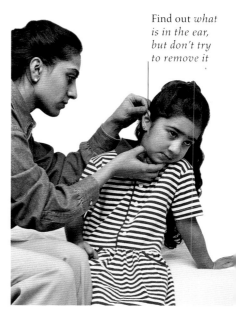

Find out what is in the ear, but don't try to remove it

Foreign object in the nose

Children sometimes stuff small pieces of food or other objects, such as beads or marbles, up their noses.

Symptoms
- Smelly, blood-stained discharge from the nose.

What can I do?
If your child can blow her nose, help her to do so, one nostril at a time. If this does not dislodge the object, take her to the hospital straightaway.

Electric shock

A mild electrical shock gives only a brief pins-and-needles sensation. A severe one can knock your child down, render her unconscious, and stop both breathing and heartbeat. Electric current can also burn. Factors that affect the severity of the injury are: the voltage, the type of current, and the path of the current. Be aware that a high-voltage jolt may cause the child to fall resulting in spinal injuries and fractures.

Electrical burns
Electricity can burn where the current enters the body and where it leaves, so your child may have burns where she touched the electrical source and anywhere that was in contact with the ground. Although these burns may look small, they are often very deep.

What can I do?

1 Switch off the current, at the mains if possible.

If you can't do this, stand on an insulating material – such as a rubber mat, a pile of dry newspapers, or a phone directory. Separate your child from the electrical source by pushing the cable away, using a dry, non-conducting object, such as a wooden chair or broom handle.

If nothing is available, drag your child away, insulating your hand as much as you can by wrapping it in a dry cloth or newspaper. Grasp your child's clothes, and avoid touching her skin.

2 Check to see if your child is conscious (see page 238).

If she is unconscious, check her breathing. If she is not breathing, start CPR (see page 239–40) immediately. If your child is breathing, put her in the recovery position (see page 241).

If she is conscious, comfort and reassure her. Look for symptoms of shock (see page 244).

3 Examine her for any burns: check areas that were in contact with the electrical source or the ground (burns will look red or scorched, and may swell). If you find any, treat them as severe burns (see page 245).

Emergency
Call for emergency help as soon as you have given first aid if:
- your child was unconscious, even if only for a few seconds
- she has any electrical burns.

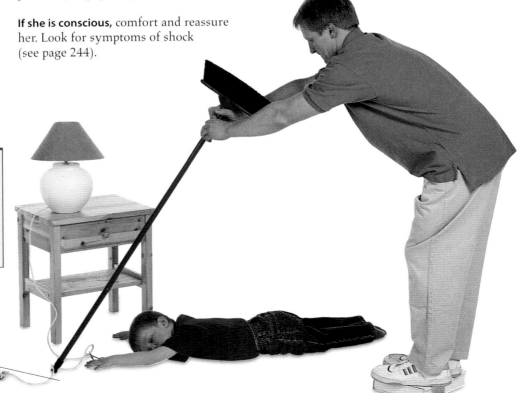

Move *the cable rather than your child's arm*

Minor bites and stings

While they may be painful and uncomfortable, most bites or stings from plants, insects, and jellyfish are not usually life-threatening for your child. However, a few people develop a serious allergic reaction to stings that can lead to shock, and therefore need urgent medical treatment.

Symptoms
- Sharp pain
- redness
- slight swelling
- itching.

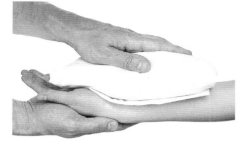

What can I do?

1 If your child has been stung by a bee, check whether the sting has been left in the skin. Brush or scrape it off with a flat object, such as a bank card. Do not use tweezers as you will inject more poison into your child.

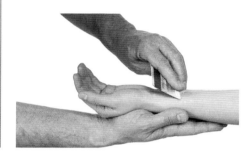

2 Hold a cloth that has been wrung out in ice cold water over the sting.

3 Soothe the area around the sting, which will quickly become red, swollen, and itchy, by dabbing it gently with cotton wool dipped in calamine lotion, or by applying antihistamine ointment around the sting.

If your child has been stung in his mouth, the swelling of tissues in the mouth may cause the airway to become blocked. Give him a cold drink or, if your child is over two, let him suck an ice cube. This will help to reduce the swelling.

Emergency
Take your child to accident and emergency department as soon as you have given first aid if he:
- has difficulty breathing
- develops a widespread rash with weals
- feels dizzy, or faints
- develops symptoms of shock (see page 244)
- has a sting inside his mouth.

Snake and spider bites, and scorpion stings

Bites from snakes and poisonous spiders and scorpion stings are always serious for young children. Snake bites carry a risk of tetanus, but your child can be vaccinated against this. The only poisonous snake in Britain is the adder.

Symptoms
Your child's symptoms will depend on what has bitten or stung him; some symptoms may not appear for a few hours:
- severe pain
- one or two puncture marks
- swelling
- nausea or vomiting
- difficulty breathing
- shock (see page 244)
- seizures
- drowsiness
- unconsciousness.

Emergency
Call an ambulance immediately. Give first aid while waiting for help, if your child has been bitten by a snake, spider, or a scorpion.

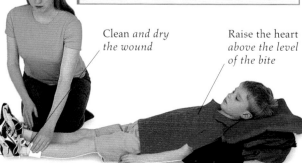

Clean *and dry the wound*

Raise the heart *above the level of the bite*

What can I do?

1 Calm your child, and help him lie down. Keep the bitten part still, and position it below the level of his heart.

2 Call for emergency help. Meanwhile, wash thoroughly around the area, but do not suck out any poison.

3 Carefully place a clean, sterile dressing over the affected area.

4 Place a conforming bandage around the affected limb.

5 Immobilize the limb with padding. If the hand or foot feels numb or cold, loosen the bandages.

6 Reassure your child. Keep him still to stop the venom from spreading through the body.

Jellyfish stings

In Europe, the only jellyfish that gives a severe sting is the Portuguese Man-of-War. Found throughout Europe, it looks like a pale blue translucent sac floating in the water. The venom is contained in stinging cells that stick to the skin. A child stung by one will need medical attention.

Symptoms
- Burning pain
- redness
- shortness of breath
- fainting.

What can I do?

1 Pour vinegar over the affected area to incapacitate the stinging cells.

2 Help the child to lie down with head and shoulders raised, and treat as for a snake bite (see opposite page).

☎ Seek medical help
Ask someone to call for emergency help as you give first aid.

Thorns and splinters

Thorns or tiny splinters of wood, glass, or metal will often become embedded in a child's hands or feet. They carry a risk of infection because they are rarely clean.

What can I do?

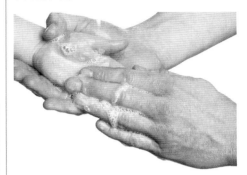

1 Clean the area around the splinter with soap and water, and gently pat it dry.

Grasp the end of the splinter with tweezers

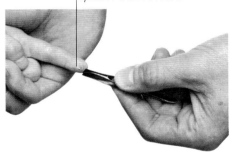

2 Using a pair of tweezers, grasp the end of the splinter as close to the skin as you can. Carefully draw it out at the same angle that it entered the skin.

☎ Seek medical help
Get medical advice if:
- a splinter is embedded
- the embedded splinter is glass or metal
- the area around a splinter becomes red, swollen, or tender 48 hours later.

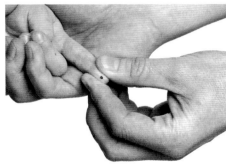

3 Squeeze the wound to encourage it to bleed, as this will "wash" the dirt out of the wound.

4 If a small thorn or splinter has gone straight down into the skin, and is not painful, it is best to leave it alone. It will probably work its own way out.

Blisters

Blisters form when burns, scalds, or repeated friction damage the skin. The fluid-filled blister forms on the top layer of the skin to protect the new skin that is forming underneath.

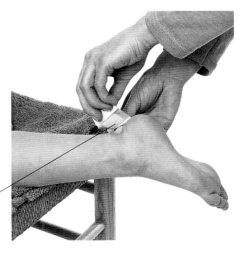

Cover the blister with a special blister plaster to prevent your child's shoe from rubbing it

What can I do?

1 Don't burst or prick the blister or try to remove the top layer of skin. This will leave the raw skin below open to infection. Protect it with a dressing. Dress your child in clothes that will not rub against it.

2 If the blister bursts, cover with a plaster with a large enough pad to cover the whole blister, or a special blister plaster.

Growth charts: girls

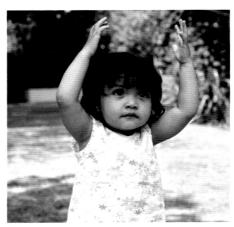

Growth charts are an important way to monitor your child's growth. They provide you with the information to interpret how well your child is growing. The charts below show average growth (the solid line), and the range of normal measurements. You can check your baby's progress by weighing and measuring her regularly and marking her own growth curve on a similar chart. The shape of her curve should run parallel to the "average" curve: this shows a healthy rate of growth.

Head circumference

Your health visitor or doctor will pass a tape measure around your baby's head (see page 81). During the first year, head circumference is an easy-to-measure yardstick of healthy growth.

Key to graphs

— — Average and normal range

○ Age in months

□ Age in years

Data sources:
UK 1990 reference data, reanalysed 2009 and WHO Child Growth Standards (WHO Multicentre Growth Reference Study Group).

Your child's height

Once your child is able to stand unaided, measure her against a wall every six months. She should stand close to it, without shoes and with feet together. Use a ruler at right angles to the wall to mark her height, then measure the distance to the floor. Don't worry if your child has periods of slow growth interspersed with spurts; but if two consecutive measurements seem very low, consult your doctor.

Data sources:
UK 1990 reference data, reanalysed 2009 and WHO Child Growth Standards (WHO Multicentre Growth Reference Study Group).

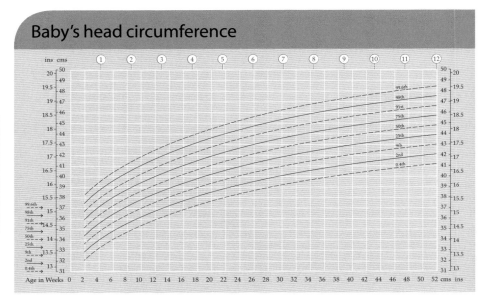

Baby's head circumference

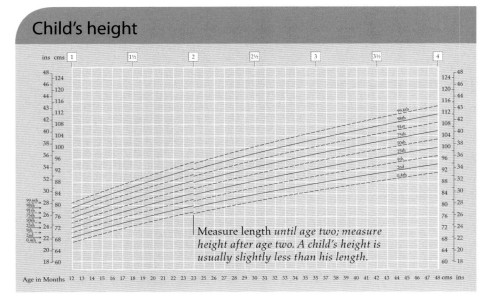

Child's height

Measure length until age two; measure height after age two. A child's height is usually slightly less than his length.

Your baby's weight

Your baby's weight gain is a vital indicator of her general health and well-being throughout the first year. Do remember that the range of "normal" weights at a given age is very wide. Ask your health visitor or doctor to weigh your baby once a month, and more often if you are at all worried that she might not be gaining normally.

Data sources:
UK 1990 reference data, reanalysed 2009 and WHO Child Growth Standards (WHO Multicentre Growth Reference Study Group).

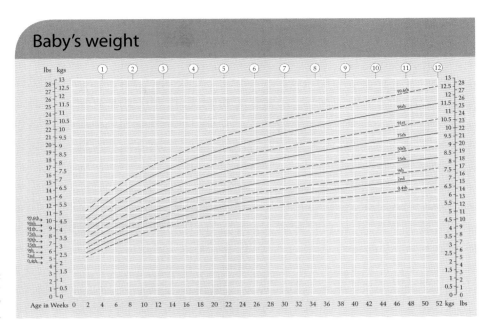

Your child's weight

After her first birthday, weigh your child naked about every six months. She won't put on weight steadily, but the periods of slow and rapid growth should balance out. She shouldn't lose weight. If she seems overweight, she probably only needs to mark time until her height catches up. Ask your doctor's advice if her weight drops, or if two consecutive measurements are less than you would expect. Although it's normal, try to resist comparing her weight to others of her age.

Data sources:
UK 1990 reference data, reanalysed 2009 and WHO Child Growth Standards (WHO Multicentre Growth Reference Study Group).

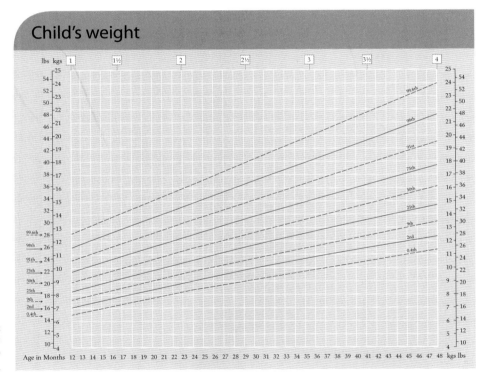

Your child's clothes sizes

Finding the right size of clothes for your child can be a daunting task. In this chart you will find an approximation of general sizes for baby girls based on their age. Since these are all approximations, it's best to measure your child and simply refer to her height measurement when inquiring about sizes.

Rough guide to clothes sizes

Age	Size	Age	Size
0–3 months	45–65cm	2–2½ years	80–95cm
3–6 months	60–70cm	2½–3 years	85–100cm
6–12 months	65–80cm	3–3½ years	90–105cm
12–18 months	70–90cm	3½–4 years	95–110cm
18–24 months	75–95cm		

Growth charts: boys

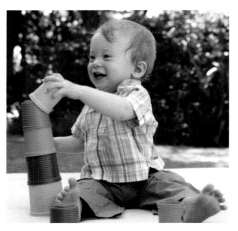

The charts below show average growth (the solid line), and the range of normal measurements. You can check your baby's progress by weighing and measuring him regularly and marking his own growth curve on a similar chart. The shape of his curve should run parallel to the "average" curve: this shows a healthy rate of growth. However, the growth charts are not diagnostic instruments, but just tools that contribute to forming an overall clinical impression for the child being measured.

Head circumference

Your health visitor or doctor will pass a tape measure around your baby's head (see page 81). During the first year, head circumference is an easy-to-measure yardstick of healthy growth.

Key to graphs

— Average and normal range

♀ Age in months

♀ Age in years

Data sources:
UK 1990 reference data, reanalysed 2009 and WHO Child Growth Standards (WHO Multicentre Growth Reference Study Group).

Your child's height

Once you child is able to stand unaided, measure him against a wall every six months. He should stand close to it, without shoes and with feet together. Use a ruler at right angles to the wall to mark his height, then measure the distance to the floor. Don't worry if your child has periods of slow growth interspersed with spurts; but if two consecutive measurements seem low, consult your doctor.

Data sources:
UK 1990 reference data, reanalysed 2009 and WHO Child Growth Standards (WHO Multicentre Growth Reference Study Group).

Baby's head circumference

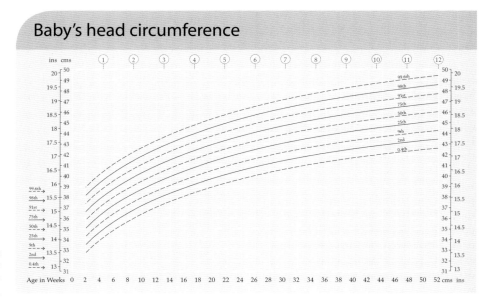

Child's height

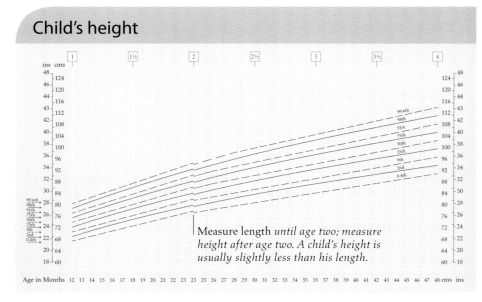

Measure length until age two; measure height after age two. A child's height is usually slightly less than his length.

Your baby's weight

Your baby's weight gain is a vital indicator of his general health and well-being throughout the first year. Ask your health visitor or doctor to weigh him once a month, and more often if you are at all worried that he might not be gaining normally.

Data sources:
UK 1990 reference data, reanalysed 2009 and WHO Child Growth Standards (WHO Multicentre Growth Reference Study Group).

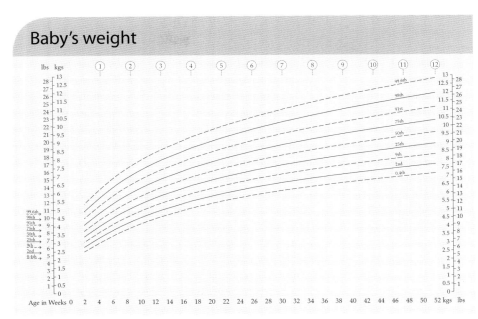

Your child's weight

After his first birthday, weigh your child naked about every six months. He won't put weight on steadily, but the periods of slow and rapid growth should balance out. He shouldn't lose weight: if he seems overweight, he probably only needs to mark time until his height catches up. Ask your doctor for advice if his weight drops, or if two consecutive measurements are less than you would expect. Your doctor will help evaluate your child's weight using tools such as body mass index (BMI) and growth charts.

Data sources:
UK 1990 reference data, reanalysed 2009 and WHO Child Growth Standards (WHO Multicentre Growth Reference Study Group).

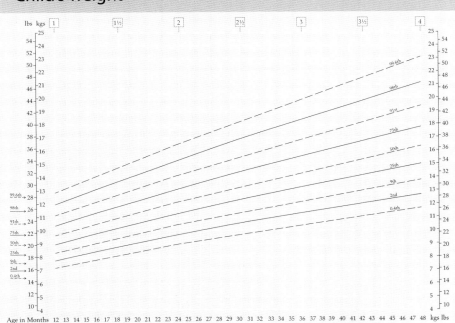

Your child's clothes sizes

Refer to this chart for an approximation of general sizes for baby boys based on their age. Since these are all approximations, it's best to measure your child and simply refer to his height measurement when inquiring about sizes.

Rough guide to clothes sizes

Age	Size	Age	Size
0–3 months	45–65cm	2–2½ years	80–100cm
3–6 months	60–70cm	2½–3 years	85–105cm
6–12 months	65–80cm	3–3½ years	90–110cm
12–18 months	70–90cm	3½–4 years	95–115cm
18–24 months	80–95cm		

Useful addresses

Antenatal support

AIMS (Association for Improvements in the Maternity Services)
Tel: 0300 365 0663
www.aims.org.uk

APEC (Action on Pre-eclampsia)
2c The Halfcroft
Syston
LE7 1CD
Tel: 0116 2608088
www.apec.org.uk

ARC (Antenatal Results and Choices)
73 Charlotte Street
London
Wl T 4PN
Tel: 020 7631 0285
www.arc-uk.org

The Independent Midwives Association
PO Box 539
Abingdon
OX14 9DF
Tel: 0845 4600 105
www.independentmidwives.org.uk

Postnatal Support

Association of Breastfeeding Mothers
PO Box 207
Bridgwater
TA67YT
Tel: 0 8444 122 949
www.abm.me.uk

Association for Postnatal Illness
145 Dawes Road
Fulham
London
SW6 7EB
Tel: 020 7386 0868
http://apni.org

Caesarean Support
55 Cooil Drive
Douglas
Isle of Man
Tel: 01624661269 (after 6pm)
www.caesarean.org.uk

Community Practitioners and Health Visitors Association
Unite the Union
Unite House
128 Theobald's Road
Holborn
London
WC1X 8TN
www.unitetheunion.com/cphva

Family Planning Association
50 Featherstone Street
London
EC1Y 8QU
Tel: 0845 122 8690
www.fpa.org.uk

MAMA (Meet-a-Mum Association)
54 Lillington Road
Radstock
BA3 3NR
Helpline: 0845 120 3746
www.mama.co.uk
Support for postnatal depression

National Childbirth Trust
Alexandra House
Oldham Terrace
Acton
London
W3 6NH
Tel: 0844 243 6000
www.nct.org.uk

Parents' groups

BLISS (Baby Life Support Systems)
9 Holyrood Street
London Bridge
London
SE1 2EL
Tel: 020 7378 1122
www.bliss.org.uk

CRY-SIS Support Group
BM Cry-Sis
London
WC1N 3XX
Tel: 0845 122 8669
www.cry-sis.org.uk
Advice on babies who cry excessively

Foundation for the Study of Infant Death
11 Belgrave Road
London
SW1V 1RB
General enquiries: 020 7802 3200
Helpline: 080 8802 6868
http://fsid.org.uk

Gingerbread
255 Kentish Town Road
London
NW5 2LX
General enquiries: 020 7428 5400
Helpline: 0800 802 0925
www.gingerbread.org.uk
For one-parent families

La Leche League
PO Box 29
West Bridgford
Nottingham
NG2 7NP
Tel: 0845 456 1855
www.laleche.org.uk
Breastfeeding support and advice

The Miscarriage Association
c/o Clayton Hospital
Northgate
Wakefield
West Yorkshire
WFl 3JS
Tel: 01924 200799
www.miscarriageassociation.org.uk
For advice, information, and support

Multiple Births Foundation
Level 4
Hammersmith House
Queen Charlotte's and Chelsea Hospital
Du Cane Road
London
W12 OHS
Tel: 020 8383 3519
www.multiplebirths.org.uk

Parentline Plus
520 Highgate Studios
53–79 Highgate Road
London
NW5 1TL
Tel: 020 7284 5500
Helpline: 0808 800 2222
www.parentlineplus.org.uk

SANDS (Stillbirth and Neonatal Death Society)
28 Portland Place
London
W1B 1LY
Tel: 020 7436 5881
www.uk-sands.org
Helpline for bereaved parents

TAMBA (Twins and Multiple Birth Association)
2 The Willows
Gardner Road
Guildford
Surrey
GU1 4PG
Tel: 01483 304442
Helpline: 0800 138 0509
www.tamba.org.uk
Support for families with twins or higher multiples, also local clubs

Vegetarian Society
Parkdale
Dunham Road
Altrincham
Cheshire
WA144QG
Tel: 0161 9252000
www.vegsoc.org

Care and Education

British Association for Early Childhood Education
136 Cavell Street
London
El 2JA
Tel: 020 7539 5400
www.early-education.org.uk

National Childminding Association
Royal Court
81 Tweedy Road
Bromley
BR1 1TG
Tel: 0845 880 0044
www.ncma.org.uk

Preschool Learning Alliance
The Fitzpatrick Building
188 York Way
London
N7 9AD
Tel: 020 7697 2500
www.pre-school.org.uk

First Aid and Safety

British Red Cross
44 Moorfields London
EC2Y 9AL
Tel: 0844 871 11 11
www.redcross.org.uk

British Standards Institute
389 Chiswick High Road
London
W4 4AL
Tel: 020 8996 90010
www.bsi-global.com

Child Accident Prevention Trust
Canterbury Court
1–3 Brixton Road
London
SW9 6DE
Tel: 020 7608 3828
www.capt.org.uk

Royal Society for the Prevention of Accidents (RoSPA)
Edgbaston Park
353 Bristol Road
Edgbaston
Birmingham
B5 7ST
Tel: 0121 248 2000
www.rospa.com

Special Needs

Association for Spina Bifida and Hydrocephalus (ASBAH)
Asbah House
42 Park Road
Peterborough
PEl 2UQ
Tel: 0845 450 7755
www.asbah.org

Contact-a-Family
209–211 City Road
London
EC1V 1JN
Tel: 020 7608 8700
www.cafamily.org.uk

Down's Syndrome Association
The Langdon Down Centre
2A Langdon Park
Teddington
Middlesex
TW11 9PS
Tel: 0845 230 0372
www.downs-syndrome.org.uk

Hyperactive Children's Support Group
71 Whyke Lane
Chichester
West Sussex
PO19 7PD
Tel: 01243 539966
www.hacsg.org.uk

MENCAP
Mencap National Centre
123 Golden Lane
London
EC1Y ORT
Tel: 020 7454 0454
www.mencap.org.uk
For people with learning disabilities

Index

Acknowledgments

Dorling Kindersley would like to thank **Elizabeth Fenwick**, the author.

This revised edition
Our thanks to:
Medical consultants: **Dr Elizabeth Owen** and **Dr Su Laurent**
Healthcare consultant: **Ann Peters R.N H.V**
First-aid consultants: **Jemima Dunne** and **Dr Viv Armstrong**

Child Growth Charts provided and approved by **WHO Multicentre Growth Reference Study Group**

Editorial assistance: **David Isaacs** and **Kate Meeker**
Design styling: **Sara Kimmins**
Artworks: **Debbie Maizels** and **Philip Wilson**

Picture credits
Picture Researcher **Jenny Baskaya**
Picture Librarian **Romaine Werblow**

The publisher would like to thank the following for their kind permission to reproduce their photographs:
(Abbreviations key: t=top, b=bottom, r=right, l=left, c=center)
Alamy: Janine Wiedel Photolibrary 64bl;

INSADCO Photography 117tl; Oredia 21tl; Peter Griffin 140bc; vario images GmbH & Co. KG 119tr; imagebroker 234tl ; **Corbis:** Andrew Brookes 195tl; Aurelie and Morgan David de Lossy/ cultura 159tc; Centers for Disease Control 203br; Corbis Yellow 117cc; Fabrice Lerouge/Onoky 158tr; Image Source 97br; JGI/Jamie Grill/Blend Images 188; Kevin Dodge 156tl; Laura Dwight 146b; Left Lane Productions 159br; Marina Dempster/First Light 68tl; Nico Hermann/Westend61 54tl; Tammy Hanratty 174tl; JGI/Jamie Grill/Blend Images 188tl; Jupiterimages 175t; **Genesis Film Productions Limited:** Neil Bromhall 23crb; **Getty Images:** American Images Inc 117cl; Andersen Ross 12tl; Ariel Skelley 237tl; ColorBlind Images 168cl; Dennis O'Clair 1c; Elyse Lewin 125bl, 204bc; Jamie Grill 32tl, 104br, 192tl; Jose Luis Pelaez Inc 17tr; Jupiterimages 175tr; Keith Brofsky 43tl; LWA 70cr; Michael Krasowitz 87tl; PNC 158cl; Steve Wisbauer 148tr; Stockbyte 237cc; Studio Tec/ailead 173bl; Thinkstock 159cc; Vanessa Gavalya 71br; VCL/Justin Pumfrey 166-7c; Victoria Blackie 134tl; **iStockphoto.com:** Steve Debenport 141cr; **Meningitis Research Foundation:** 208br; **Mother & Baby Picture Library:** Eddie Lawrence 67cr; Ian Hooton 17bl, 32, 33tr,

35tl, 36br, 59tr, 74-75, 80cc, 83r, 89, 162-163, 178-179, 181c, 198cr, 199cr, 200tl, 202, 224cr, 244cr, 248tc; Moose Azim 96bl; Paul Mitchell 2-3, 8-9, 57tr, 160tl; Ruth Jenkinson, 81br; ©**Mothercare:** 156, 157b; **Science Photo Library:** AJ Photo 70bl; Dr H.C.Robinson 206br; Laurent BSIP 65br; **St John's Institute of Dermatology:** 228cl, 231tr; **St Mary's Hospital:** 183tl; **Sue Ford, Western Ophthalmic Hospital:** 183bl, 209r; **The Wellcome Institute Library, London:** 209cl, 213bl, 226l, 227cla, 232l; **Dr Ian Williams/ msl:** 182tl, 203r, 210l 214cr, 227bl, 229br, 230tr;

Original edition
Senior Art Editor **Carole Ash**
Project Editors **Sarah Pearce**
Pregnancy and Birth **Tanya Hines**
Health Care **Claire Le Bas**

Art Editors
Pregnancy and Birth **Rowena Alsey**
Health Care **Tina Hill**
Production Manager **Michel Blake**
Editorial Direction **Daphne Razazan**

Picture credits
Picture Researcher **Anna Grapes**
Picture Librarians **Melanie Simmonds, Marcus Scott**

Illustrators
Coral Mula: all line artwork except 14t;
Nick Hall: 14t; **Kevin Jones Associates:** 234, 235, 236; **Richard Tibbitts:** 14, 16, 18, 20, 22, 24, 28, 30

Photography
Andy Crawford assisted by Gary Ombler, **Antonia Deutsch** assisted by Pamela Cowan, **Trish Gant, Steve Gorton, Dave King, Ray Moller, Stephen Oliver, Susannah Price, Steve Shott**

Loan or supply of props
Avent (baby feeding equipment); Mothercare; Baby B's, Fulham, London, England; Diana Dolls Fashions Inc., Stoney Creek, Ontario; The Nursery Collection, Watford, England; Porter Nash Medical, London, England; Seward Ltd., London, England. **Special thanks to:** Mary Snyder at Snugli, Inc.; Gerry Baby Products Company, Denver, Colorado; Judi's Originals, Scottsdale, Arizona.

Consultants
Dorling Kindersley acknowledges the contribution of the following consultants to the original edition:
Professor R. W. Taylor MD, FRCOG, Head of Department of Gynaecology, The United Medical Schools of Guy's and St. Thomas's Hospitals, London; **Professor Jon Scopes** MB, PhD, FRCP, Department of Paediatrics, St. Thomas's Hospital, London; **Christine Williams** RGN, HV, FWT, Health Visitor and Family Planning Nurse; **Janice Leighton** RGN, RM, Community Midwife; **Alan McLaughlin** RGN, Department of Clinical Neurology, St Thomas's Hospital, London.